Introduction to the Science of Medical Imaging

Introduction to the Science of Medical Imaging

Edited by

R. Nick Bryan

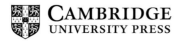

CAMBRIDGE
UNIVERSITY PRESS

CAMBRIDGE UNIVERSITY PRESS
Cambridge, New York, Melbourne, Madrid, Cape Town, Singapore,
São Paulo, Delhi

Cambridge University Press
The Edinburgh Building, Cambridge CB2 8RU, UK

Published in the United States of America by
Cambridge University Press, New York

www.cambridge.org
Information on this title: www.cambridge.org/9780521747622

© Cambridge University Press 2010

First published 2010

Printed in the United Kingdom at the University Press, Cambridge

A catalogue record for this publication is available from the British Library

ISBN 978-0-521-74762-2 Paperback

Contents

List of contributors   *page* vi

Introduction
R. Nick Bryan   1

Section 1:   Image essentials   13

1. **What is an image?**
   R. Nick Bryan   13

2. **How to make an image**
   R. Nick Bryan and Christopher R. B. Merritt   38

3. **How to analyze an image**
   R. Nick Bryan and Christopher R. B. Merritt   82

Section 2:   Biomedical images: signals to pictures   117

Ionizing radiation   117

4. **Nuclear medicine**
   Suleman Surti and Joel S. Karp   117

5. **X-rays**
   Andrew D. A. Maidment   133

Non-ionizing radiation   147

6. **Ultrasound imaging**
   Peter H. Arger and Chandra M. Sehgal   147

7. **Magnetic resonance imaging**
   Felix W. Wehrli   160

8. **Optical imaging**
   Nathan G. Dolloff and Wafik S. El-Deiry   172

Exogenous contrast agents   183

9. **Contrast agents for x-ray and MR imaging**
   Peter M. Joseph   183

10. **Nuclear molecular labeling**
    Datta Ponde and Chaitanya Divgi   196

Section 3:   Image analysis   207

11. **Human observers**
    Harold L. Kundel   207

12. **Digital image processing: an overview**
    Jayarama K. Udupa   214

13. **Registration and atlas building**
    James C. Gee   230

14. **Statistical atlases**
    Christos Davatzikos and Ragini Verma   240

Section 4:   Biomedical applications   251

15. **Morphological imaging**
    R. Nick Bryan   251

16. **Physiological imaging**
    Mitchell D. Schnall   265

17. **Molecular imaging**
    Jerry S. Glickson   275

Appendices
1. *Linear systems*
   Paul A. Yushkevich   292
2. *Fourier transform and* k-*space*
   Jeremy Magland   302
3. *Probability, Bayesian statistics, and information theory*
   Edward H. Herskovits   308
Index   316

Contributors

Peter H. Arger
Emeritus Professor of Radiology
Department of Radiology
University of Pennsylvania
Philadelphia, PA, USA

R. Nick Bryan
Eugene P. Pendergrass Professor of Radiology and
Chairman
Department of Radiology
University of Pennsylvania
Philadelphia, PA, USA

Christos Davatzikos
Professor of Radiology
Chief Section of Biomedical Image Analysis
Department of Radiology
University of Pennsylvania
Philadelphia, PA, USA

Chaitanya Divgi
Professor of Radiology
Chief Nuclear Medicine and Clinical Molecular
Imaging
Department of Radiology
University of Pennsylvania
Philadelphia, PA, USA

Nathan G. Dolloff
Post-doctoral Scientist (Drexel)
University of Pennsylvania
Philadelphia, PA, USA

Wafik S. El-Deiry
Professor of Medicine
Chief Optical Imaging Laboratory
University of Pennsylvania
Philadelphia, PA, USA

James C. Gee
Associate Professor
Chief of Biomedical Informatics
Department of Radiology
University of Pennsylvania
Philadelphia, PA, USA

Jerry S. Glickson
Research Professor of Radiology
Chief Laboratory of Molecular Imaging
University of Pennsylvania
Philadelphia, PA, USA

Edward H. Herskovits
Associate Professor of Radiology
Department of Radiology
University of Pennsylvania
Philadelphia, PA, USA

Peter M. Joseph
Professor of Radiology
Department of Radiology
University of Pennsylvania
Philadelphia, PA, USA

Joel S. Karp
Professor of Radiology
Chief PET Center
University of Pennsylvania
Philadelphia, PA, USA

Harold L. Kundel
Emeritus Professor of Radiology
Department of Radiology
University of Pennsylvania
Philadelphia, PA, USA

Jeremy Magland
Assistant Professor
Laboratory for Structural NMR Imaging
Department of Radiology
University of Pennsylvania
Philadelphia, PA, USA

Andrew D. A. Maidment
Associate Professor of Radiology
Chief Medical Physics
Department of Radiology
University of Pennsylvania
Philadelphia, PA, USA

Christopher R. B. Merritt
Professor of Radiology
Department of Radiology
Thomas Jefferson University Medical College
Philadelphia, PA, USA

Datta Ponde
Research Assistant Professor
Department of Radiology
University of Pennsylvania
Philadelphia, PA, USA

Mitchell D. Schnall
Matthew J. Wilson Professor of Radiology
Department of Radiology
University of Pennsylvania
Philadelphia, PA, USA

Chandra M. Sehgal
Professor of Radiology
Chief Ultrasound Laboratory
University of Pennsylvania
Philadelphia, PA, USA

Suleman Surti
Research Assistant Professor
Department of Radiology
University of Pennsylvania
Philadelphia, PA, USA

Jayarama K. Udupa
Professor of Radiology
Chief Medical Image Processing Group
Department of Radiology
University of Pennsylvania
Philadelphia, PA, USA

Ragini Verma
Assistant Professor of Radiology
University of Pennsylvania
Philadelphia, PA, USA

Felix W. Wehrli
Professor of Radiology
Director Laboratory for Structural NMR Imaging
Department of Radiology
University of Pennsylvania
Philadelphia, PA, USA

Paul A. Yushkevich
Research Assistant Professor
Penn Image Computing and Science Laboratory
Department of Radiology
University of Pennsylvania
Philadelphia, PA, USA

Introduction

R. Nick Bryan

The title of this book refers to two components – *science* and *imaging*. Science, by usual definitions, has two aspects: a body of knowledge and a methodology. The former is the organized body of information that we have gained about ourselves and our environment by rigorous application of the latter. The scope of the scientific body of knowledge is vast; indeed, it is the total knowledge we have of our universe and everything in it. However, there is a restriction on this knowledge: it must have been derived through the scientific method. This carefully circumscribed method uses observation and experimentation in a logical and rational order to describe and explain natural phenomena. Scientific imaging, which is the specific topic of this presentation, likewise has two aspects: it is a body of knowledge – knowledge gained from the application of imaging – and a scientific methodology to answer scientific questions. While both of these elements, knowledge and methodology, are equally important, this book will focus on the methodological aspects of scientific imaging. However, this methodology will be extensively illustrated by examples from the commensurate body of knowledge. Hopefully the reader will be able to appreciate not only how to make and analyze a scientific image, but also what might be learned by doing so.

In a very broad sense, science is the study of the universe and all aspects of its components. It is the goal of science to understand and be able to explain everything about us. This goal is perhaps unachievable, but that does not diminish its importance or its validity. Science has greatly expanded our knowledge of the world, and it continues to do so. However, there are great voids in our knowledge about our world that provide the rationale and stimulus for future scientific activity – activity in which imaging will be a central element. Imaging has played, plays, and will continue to play a critical role in scientific investigation for two main reasons: the nature of the universe and human nature.

Though it may appear presumptuous, this presentation of the science of imaging will begin by addressing the general question of the universe: the whole space–time continuum in which we exist along with all the energy and matter within it. While vastly more complex than we can currently comprehend, this universe (U) can be grossly simplified, in the macroscopic sense, as the collection of all mass (m) and energy (E) distributed over three-dimensional space (x,y,z) evolving with time (t). This conceptualization of the universe can be formally expressed as:

$$U = (m, E)(x, y, z)(t) \qquad (1)$$

Science is the study of this spatial and temporal distribution of mass and energy. What makes imaging so critical to this enterprise is that mass and energy are not spread uniformly across space. This fact is readily appreciated by observing almost any aspect of nature, and it is beautifully illustrated by *The Powers of 10*, a film by Charles and Ray Eames illustrating the universe from its largest to its smallest elements, in 42 logarithmic steps (Figure 1). What is perhaps even more striking than the spatial magnitude, i.e., size, of the universe is its spatial complexity, reflected by extraordinary spatial variation at all levels. Mass and energy tend to be aggregated in local collections, albeit collections which vary greatly in their mass/energy make-up, spatial distribution, and temporal characteristics. Some collections are small, discrete masses that are relatively stable over time, like a diamond, while others are enormous, diffuse, rapidly evolving energy fields, like the electromagnetic radiation of a pulsar. Broadly defined, a coherent collection of mass/energy may be considered as a pattern or object: the former

Introduction to the Science of Medical Imaging, ed. R. Nick Bryan. Published by Cambridge University Press. © Cambridge University Press 2010.

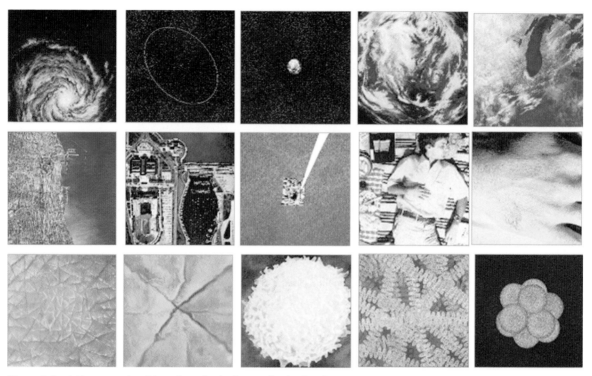

Figure 1. Spatial heterogeneity of the universe by the Powers of 10 by C. and R. Eames (www.powersof10.com). © 1977 Eames Office, LLC. Used with permission.

more diffuse and obtuse, the latter more discrete and well-defined. The critical point is that the universe is spatially and temporally heterogeneous. What is *here* is different than what is *there*! What is *here* today may be *there* tomorrow! Furthermore, this concept of spatial heterogeneity applies to most objects within the universe. From afar, the earth might be viewed as a simple, discrete object; however, on closer inspection its geographic heterogeneity is striking. There is a hierarchy of patterns and objects characterized by spatial heterogeneity at all levels. Biological systems, particularly a complex organism such as a human body, are incredibly heterogeneous objects, macroscopically and microscopically. Within the abdomen, the liver may be near to, but is distinctly separate from, the right kidney (Figure 2). Furthermore, this spatial heterogeneity is not just physical or anatomic, but also functional. The liver uses energy to make bile (among many other things), while the kidney makes urine. At the microscopic level organs are spatially segregated, with renal glomerular cells that filter urine distinct from nearby blood vessels. It is this intrinsic, spatially heterogeneous nature of the universe and objects within it that makes imaging so important to science.

In order to understand why imaging is so important to science, it is necessary to understand what an image is. In general, an image is defined as a representation of something, usually an object or local collection of objects (a scene). There are many different kinds of images: mental, auditory, abstract, direct, etc. Some images are permanent, others fleeting; some precise, others vague; some imaginary, others real. For purposes of this presentation, an image is defined as a representation or reproduction of a scene containing patterns or objects that explicitly retains and conveys the spatial aspects of the original. Specifically, we shall be dealing with what I call "scientific" images. A scientific image is an attempt to produce an accurate or high-fidelity reproduction of pattern(s) or object(s) based on spatially dependent measurements of their mass and/or energy contents. An image is a spatially coherent display of mass/energy measurements. This definition of an image can be formalized as:

$$I = f(m, E)(x, y, z)(t) \qquad (2)$$

Note that this is virtually the same as Equation 1, except that it is formally presented as a mathematical function, and the elements do not represent actual

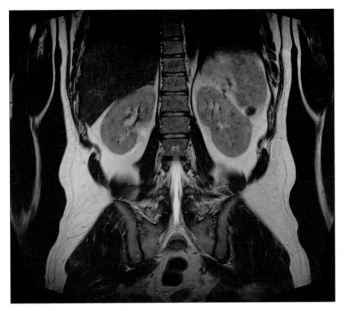
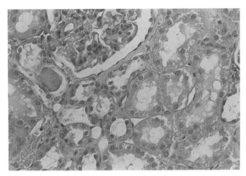

Figure 2. Macroscopic and microscopic spatial heterogeneity of the abdomen (magnetic resonance imaging) and kidney (light microscopy), respectively.

mass, energy, space, or time, but *measurements* of these physical features of the universe or of an object. Measurements of mass and energy are often modeled as signals, particularly in the engineering environment. There are many ways that these measurements can be made and subsequently displayed; this incredible smorgasbord of phenomena will be a large part of our story.

The original painting of a white pelican by Audubon is an image that is based on "measurements" of the amplitude and wavelength of visible light by the observer's (Mr. Audubon's) eye (Figure 3). The light signal measurements are spatially dependent. The light signal from the bird's left wing is more intense and of broader frequency (whiter) than the signal from the bird's left leg. Mr. Audubon's visual system integrated this signal and spatial information into an internal or mental image that he then rendered via his psychomotor system, a brush, paint, and canvas into a reproduction or representation of the original object, a pelican.

In this example, the imaging "system" was Mr. Audubon, his gun and his painting tools. The image is scientific because it is an attempt at a faithful, high-fidelity reproduction of the natural object under investigation, a pelican. Essentially all scientific images are variants of this theme: some kind of imaging device makes spatially dependent signal measurements and then renders a reproduction based on these measurements. An image such as this explicitly preserves and conveys spatial information as well as that relative to mass/energy.

Images such as these are robust forms of data. Such data are the descriptive heart of natural science. They reflect a rigorous interrogation of an object. The more faithfully, i.e., accurately, the image reflects the object, the higher the potential scientific quality of the image. Of obvious but special note is the fact that an image is the only way to fully investigate a spatially heterogeneous object. Non-spatially dependent scientific measurements may be, and often are, made, but they can never fully describe a spatially heterogeneous object. Measuring the amplitude and wavelength of light reflected from a pelican without explicit spatial information tells us something about the object, perhaps enough to distinguish a white pelican from a flamingo, although perhaps not enough to distinguish a white pelican from a swan. On the other hand, the barest of spatial information can convey a wealth of information. An image is necessary to fully describe and distinguish spatially heterogeneous objects.

This presentation on scientific imaging will proceed in a series of steps, beginning with a brief but more refined definition of a pattern, object, or sample – the thing to be imaged. Then the general principles of measurement will be reviewed. It should be emphasized that science is greatly, if not completely, dependent on

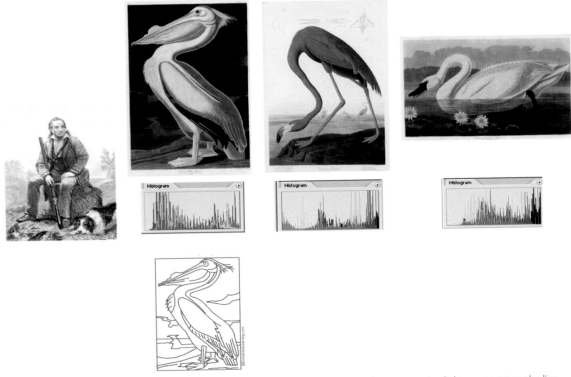

Figure 3. John James Audubon and his watercolors of a pelican, flamingo, and swan, with accompanying light spectrograms plus line drawing of pelican. Paintings used with permission: Audubon, John James, by J. Woodhouse Audubon (1974.46); others by John J. Audubon: American White Pelican (1863.17.311), Greater Flamingo (1863.17.431), Tundra swan (1863.17.411), all from the collection of The New-York Historical Society http://emuseum.nyhistory.org/code/emuseum.asp; drawing used with permission of EnchantedLearning.com.

measurements. This applies to descriptive as well as experimental science. Oddly, measurements, especially accurate, quantitative measurements, have been a major challenge and weakness of scientific imaging. There are no explicit measurements, much less numbers, associated with Audubon's paintings. Roentgen made the first x-ray image (of his wife's hand) with a mechanical apparatus that performed no explicit mathematical operation and produced no numbers (Figure 4). Today a radiologist typically interprets a CT scan of the brain in an empirical, qualitative, non-quantitative fashion. However, this aspect of scientific imaging is rapidly changing, and this is one of the major stimuli for this book. Today's CT scan may be interpreted qualitatively by the human eye, but the actual image is numeric, digital, and was created by a very sophisticated machine using advanced mathematics (Figure 5). Furthermore, the interpretation or analysis of scientific images will increasingly be performed with the aid of a computer in a quantitative fashion. Robust scientific images demand a strong quantitative component. Therefore this text will introduce the basic mathematics of scientific

imaging, which includes the superset of measurement as well as the related topics of probability and statistics.

The unique aspect of imaging is the inclusion of spatial information. *Space* is the central element of imaging. This is evident in the formulae of the universe and of an image. Scientific imaging requires the explicit measurement of space, in addition to the measurements of mass or energy. The nature and importance of space seems intuitively obvious to humans. However, space is a very complex ideation that has multiple definitions and related applications that will require significant exposition and illustration. This will be important for understanding how human observers deal with images and their content. Psychologically it turns out that space is not as innate a concept as one might think: people actually have to learn what space is. As a result of this learning process, there is significant variability among different individuals' conceptions and perception of space, which can influence how they view and interpret images.

Furthermore, space is a key concept of the mathematics of imaging, and mathematicians define, think

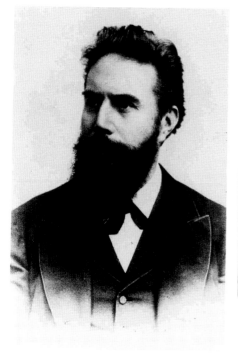

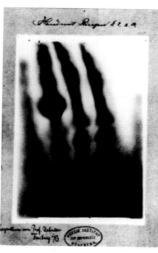

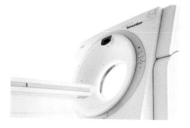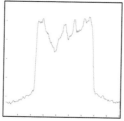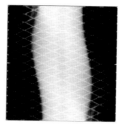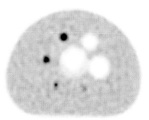

Figure 5. Contemporary CT scanner, CT data projection, reconstructed sinogram, and conventional Cartesian images of physical phantom containing seven rods of different sizes and radiodensities. Scanner photo courtesy of Siemens Healthcare. Others courtesy of J. S. Karp.

about, and use space very differently than many of the rest of us. Mathematical space is not only important conceptually, but also practically, as it is essential for scientific application.

Early cartographers might be considered the founders of scientific imaging, in that they first dealt with the explicit measurement and representation of real, physical space, in contrast to mathematicians, who dealt in abstract, metric space. Cartography is the science of spatially defined measurements of the earth (and other planets); maps form a subclass of scientific images. Early cartography focused on the new methodologies of space measurement in order to address the "where" (spatial) question. The very earliest maps were essentially one-dimensional, initially showing the

order and then the distances between locations in one direction (Figure 6). Early spatial metrics were very crude, often in rough physical units such as spans (of a hand) or even more imprecise units of time equivalents (days of travel). This limited spatial view was expanded by the twelfth century to include refined two-dimensional flat maps, and by the fifteenth century three-dimensional globes of the world based on well-defined spatial units such as rods and sophisticated geometric concepts appeared. Early "mappers" paid less attention to the "what" question, the other essential component of an image. Usually there was only a rudimentary, qualitative description of "what" (post, village, river), located at a quantitatively defined location. However, the "what" of a cartographic map is

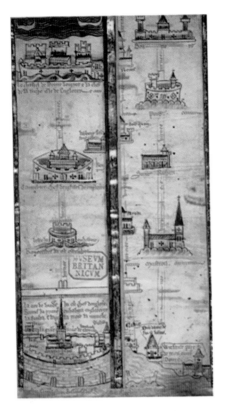

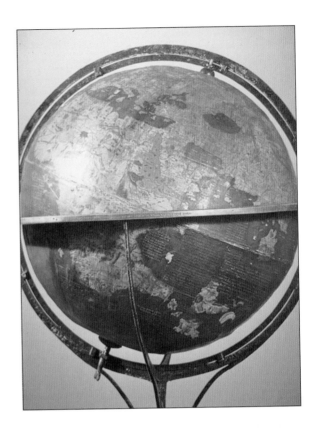

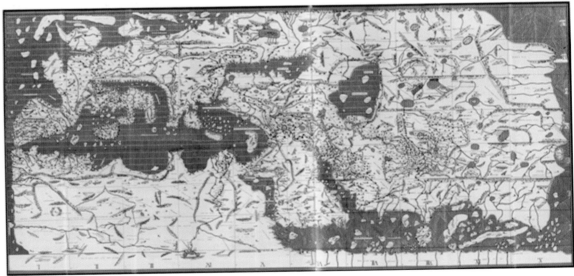

Figure 6. One-dimensional map of route from London, England to Beauvais, France by Dover ca 1250; two-dimensional map of Eurasia by al-Idrisi in 1154; three-dimensonal world globe by Martin Behaim in 1492, which still does not include America. London route owned by the British Library; image appeared in Akerman JR and Karrow RW, *Maps*, University of Chicago Press, 2007. Muhammad al-Idrisi's map appears on http://en.wikipedia.org/wiki/Tabula_Rogeriana. Globe photo courtesy of Alexander Franke, http://en.wikipedia.org/wiki/Erdapfel.

equivalent to the m,E measurement in a generic scientific image. Beginning in the seventeenth and eighteenth centuries, the introduction of more precise physical measurements of the "what" (number of people, temperature, wind direction) that was located at specific geographical locations resulted in rich *functional* maps that are not only exquisite, but classical examples of scientific images.

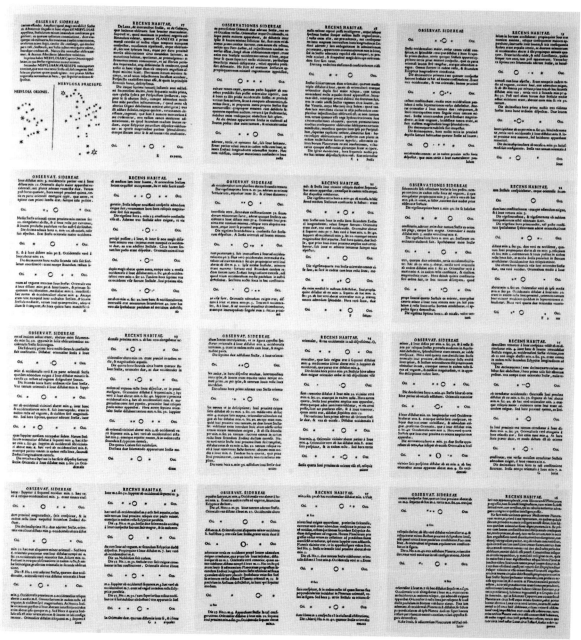

Figure 7. Notes from Galileo's notebook depicting a series of nightly observations of Jupiter and its four previously unknown moons. As appeared in Edward R. Tufte, *Beautiful Evidence*, Graphics Press LLC, Cheshire, Connecticut, 2006. Used with permission.

If there were to be challengers to cartographers as the first scientific imagers, it would have to be the astronomers (unless, that is, astronomy is deemed to be cartography of the skies, and astronomers thus the first cartographers). Certainly the two disciplines evolved very closely, as both are dependent on the same mathematical principles and related instrumentation for their spatial measurements. As with cartography, early astronomers focused on the spatial measurements of an image, with only crude measurements of the mass/energy of the objects they were observing. I would propose Galileo's astronomical observations of Jupiter's moons as perhaps the first modern scientific images (Figure 7). His work included not only careful

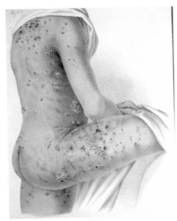 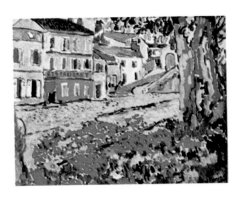 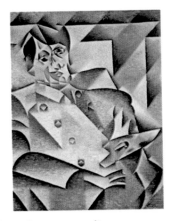

Figure 8. High-fidelity artist's rendering of dermatologic disease accurately depicts signal (color) and spatial components of image. Deliberate color distortion of the village of Marley by the Fauvist Vlaminck, and spatial distortion of Picasso in his portrait by the cubist Juan Gris. *Depiction of Infected Atopic Dermatitis*, by Dr. Louis Duhring, University of Pennsylvania. *Restaurant de la Machine at Bougival* by Maurice de Vlaminck, 1905, is at the Musée d'Orsay in Paris. Used with permission of Erich Lessing/Art Resource, NY and © 2009 Artists Rights Society (ARS), New York/ADAGP, Paris. Juan Gris' *Portrait of Picasso*, 1912, is at The Art Institute of Chicago. http://en.wikipedia.org/wiki/Juan_Gris.

measurements of mass/energy, space, and time, but also a mathematically tested and proven hypothesis. Contemporary scientific imaging now reflects very refined spatially dependent measurements of almost any imaginable body, object, view, or scene of our universe.

Mass/energy and spatial measurements are of two different physical domains and are relatively independent; however, a "complete picture" is dependent on the accurate amalgamation of the two. This combination of spatial and physical measurements is the methodological core of imaging and the source of its power. An artist may inadvertently or deliberately misrepresent or distort spatial or m,E information, but a scientist must not (Figure 8). Science requires that significant attention be given to the accuracy of spatially dependent measurements and their subsequent display and analysis.

In this book the basic concepts of a scientific image will be presented in Section 1 (Chapters 1–3), followed by a survey of contemporary biomedical imaging techniques in Section 2 (Chapters 4–10). Technology – in this context, instrumentation – is intimately related to scientific imaging. Imaging instruments generally include devices that improve on the human visual system to observe or measure objects within a scene, specifically including their spatial aspects. The Whipple Museum of the History of Science at the University of Cambridge is filled with fascinating scientific contraptions; notably, over 60% of these are imaging devices (Figure 9). While the human visual system alone may have been an adequate imaging device for a natural scientist in Audubon's time, or

perhaps for a contemporary dermatologist, it is severely limited in terms of what types of objects or samples it can interrogate. Specifically, the unaided human visual system cannot image very small objects; it cannot image signals other than those within the wavelength of visible light; it cannot image below the surface of most objects; and it cannot image remote objects. The ongoing revolution in scientific imaging is defined by and dependent upon the discovery and development of new imaging devices that improve our ability to image not only with light signals (microscope, fundiscope), but also with different types of signals: x-rays for computed tomography (CT) scans, radio signals for magnetic resonance imaging (MRI), and sound waves for ultrasonography (US) (Figure 10). An important aspect of many newer imaging techniques is their non-destructive nature. While this feature greatly complicates the imaging process, it is obviously of great practical value for many applications. Prior to the late nineteenth century, imaging of the inside of the body required cutting into it, an event that took place after or immediately prior to death (Figure 11). Today, modern medical ultrasound provides universally compelling 3D images of a living, moving fetus with neither pain nor harm to baby or mother.

Once an image has been created, it must then be interpreted or analyzed, as elaborated on in Section 3 (Chapters 11–14). Traditionally this function has been performed by the human "eye" using empirical, qualitative methods dependent on visual psychophysics. This very human process is highly individualized, and thus it can be rather mundane or highly creative

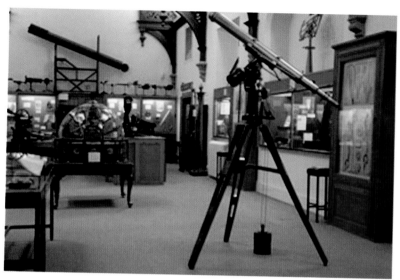

Figure 9. Scientific imaging devices at the Whipple Museum, the University of Cambridge. Photo courtesy of the museum. www.hps.cam.ac.uk/whipple/index.html.

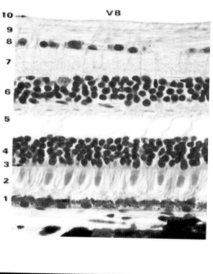

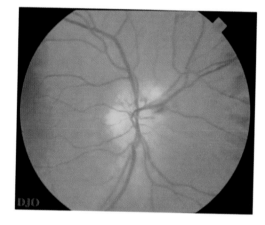

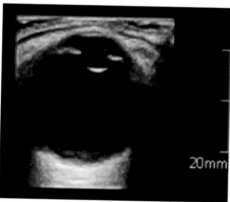

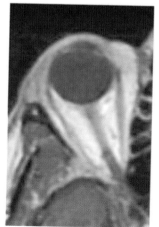

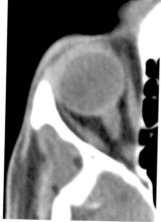

Figure 10. Multimodality images of the human eye: histological, fundiscopic, ultrasound, MRI, and x-ray CT. Histological image appeared in Young B and Heath JW, *Wheater's Functional Histology: A Text and Colour Atlas*, Churchill Livingstone, Edinburgh and New York, 2000. © Elsevier. Used with permission. Fundoscopic image appeared online in Neuro-ophthalmology Quiz 1 of *Digital Journal of Ophthalmology* by Shiuey Y, MD. www.djo.harvard.edu/site.php?url=/physicians/kr/468. Used with permission from *Digital Journal of Ophthalmology*.

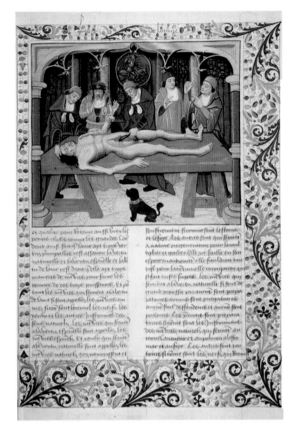

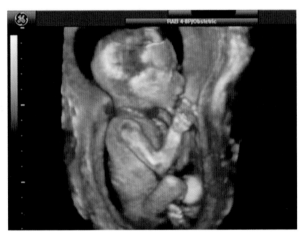

Figure 11. Medieval invasive morphological imaging; contemporary non-invasive ultrasound imaging of fetus. *Dissection Scene,* from De Proprietatibus Rerum, by Bartolomeus Anglicus, late fifteenth century. Owned by Bibliothèque Nationale de France.

and "artistic." There may be "art" not only in the creation of an image, but also great creativity in the interpretation of images. The artistic part of imaging is a function of the human observer and is probably inextricable as long as a human is involved in the creative and interpretive process. For aesthetics and the quality and variety of life, art is integral, important, and greatly desired. However, art can be a problem for scientific imaging. Art is intrinsically individualistic and therefore highly variable. Art is not restricted to "facts," does not require accuracy, and allows for the deliberate distortion of reality. Art is not science. Therefore scientific imaging must strive to control carefully the artistic aspects of imaging. This is a major challenge as long as humans participate in the imaging process. Images are made to be seen, looked at, and observed by people. This does not mean that machines, computers, mathematical algorithms cannot play a role in creating or even analyzing images, but at some stage a human has to look at a picture or image.

Human involvement is an integral part of imaging because imaging is, at its most basic level, a communication tool. Imaging is a language in the broadest sense. Imaging is the language of space. Imaging is how we most efficiently depict and convey spatial information from one person to another. Imaging's role as a communicating device is what keeps humans central to our discussion. The requisite involvement of humans in scientific imaging results in a persistent artistic component. While art is indeed an important element of scientific imaging, it is one that must be carefully coordinated with and, if necessary, subjugated to the methodological rules of science. The discussion of image analysis will include components related to the human visual system, psychophysics, and observer performance. Central to this discussion are information and communication theory relative to how effectively images convey information from one person to another. The incredible power of images to communicate should never be forgotten. "Seeing is believing" is deeply rooted in human psychology; indeed, it is human nature.

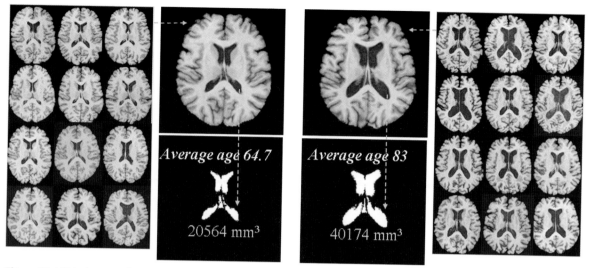

Figure 12. MRI brain scans of 12 younger (left) and older (right) subjects along with respective "average" brain slices and calculated ventricular volumes. Courtesy of C. Davatzikos.

Until recently these humanistic topics would have dominated the discussion of image analysis, but the incorporation of computers into scientific imaging now demands the inclusion of extensive sections on digital images and computer image analysis. In fact, essentially all contemporary scientific images are digital. Digital image analysis is revolutionizing imaging in many ways. Digital graphical displays immediately catch our attention, but more important is the computer's ability to quantitate, particularly in the spatial domain. The quantitative advantages of the computer over the human visual system are enormous. Digital image analysis allows remarkable operations that a human simply cannot perform, such as the statistical averaging and quantitative comparison of groups of human brains with detail and rigor (Figure 12).

The final section of this book (Section 4, Chapters 15–17) expands on specific biomedical applications of imaging. Many, if not most, medical images are used in a "descriptive" fashion. Though often used inappropriately as a pejorative term, descriptive applications of images are critical in research for describing the imaging characteristics of normal or diseased tissue and in clinical practice to find and diagnose a disease through imaging. However, after predominantly descriptive *natural science*, contemporary science quickly moves on to *experimental science*, which generally involves hypothesis testing. At this stage of science, images are just a form of data that may be used to test hypothesis. Images comprise the data for tests. We shall briefly review the principles of tests and testing and then expand on how image data in particular may be used to generate and test hypotheses related to biomedical questions. Specifically, principles of imaging as applied to morphological, physiological, and molecular questions will be presented. In the end, the reader should have a good understanding of what a scientific image is, how such images are made, and how imaging is incorporated into the rigorous analytical methodology of science.

Image essentials
What is an image?

R. Nick Bryan

What is to be imaged?

By definition an *image* is a representation or reproduction of something. Hence an image is dependent on what it represents. Therefore it is important to understand what an image might represent before tackling the derivative image itself. For purposes of scientific imaging, the "something" that images represent is the universe or, far more likely, portions thereof. The universe has been previously defined as

$$U = (m, E)(x, y, z)(t) \qquad (1.1)$$

An image is a representation or depiction of this distribution of mass/energy over three-dimensional physical space, varying with time. Let us now consider each of these fundamental aspects of the universe and nature. As explicitly defined in the above equation, the universe has three separate domains: mass and energy, space, and time. In classical physics, as in our everyday life, each domain is related to, but distinct from, the other.

Mass (*m*) and energy (*E*) can be conveniently thought of as the things and stuff of the universe. While this gross oversimplification may intuitively suffice, a slightly more detailed exposition is required in order to understand the relationship between these two entities and their role in imaging. For most of our purposes, the concepts of classical physics will suffice. Thus, mass and energy will generally be dealt with as distinct entities, as with time and space. *Mass* suggests a relatively discrete, particle-like object that, more importantly and by definition, resists displacement and specifically *acceleration* (Figure 1.1). The unit of mass is the kilogram (kg). Mass is not equivalent to weight, which is mass acted upon by the force of gravity. Amongst the smallest masses are subatomic particles such as electrons (9.109×10^{-31} kg) and protons, the latter having approximately 1800 times greater

mass than the former. Larger masses are just agglomerations of smaller masses – electrons, protons, and neutrons form carbon atoms that, in turn, form diamonds. Our sun has a mass of approximately 10^{30} kg, 60 orders of magnitude greater than an electron.

A stationary mass object, left alone, does not change its position; it remains at rest at a given spatial location. When acted upon by a force, a mass may change its position in space. The rate of change of position, *x*, over time, *t*, is defined as *velocity, v*:

$$v = \Delta x / \Delta t \qquad (1.2)$$

Velocity is a vector quantity with direction and magnitude; the magnitude being *speed*. *Acceleration, a*, is the rate of change of velocity over time and is also a vector quantity:

$$a = \Delta v / \Delta t \qquad (1.3)$$

A mass moving at constant velocity has *momentum, p*, in the direction of its velocity:

$$p = mv \qquad (1.4)$$

If no external force acts on an object, its momentum does not change. Masses are often described in terms of their actual mass, number, size (spatial extent), motion (velocity, acceleration), and, as we shall soon see, energy.

Force, F, is a vector quantity that reflects the push or pull on an object. Gravity acts as a force on objects that have mass. An electromagnetic field exerts a force on electrons. A mass in the absence of a force is either stationary or moving at a constant velocity, i.e., has constant momentum. Force acting on a mass produces acceleration (or deceleration) in the direction of the applied force:

$$F = ma \qquad (1.5)$$

Introduction to the Science of Medical Imaging, ed. R. Nick Bryan. Published by Cambridge University Press. © Cambridge University Press 2010.

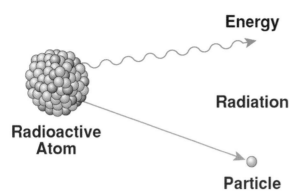

Figure 1.1. Mass and energy: particles and waves. C. R. B. Merritt.

A moving object has *kinetic energy*, E_k, a scalar quantity as defined by:

$$E_k = 1/2mv^2 \qquad (1.6)$$

Potential energy, E_p, is a property of an object in a force field and is a function of the strength of the field and the position of the object within the field. The *total energy* of a mass is the sum of its kinetic and potential energy, and this sum never changes (conservation of energy):

$$E_{total} = E_k + E_p \qquad (1.7)$$

In summary, a stationary object with mass has no associated energy in the absence of a force field, but has potential energy if in the presence of a force field. If the object is moving, it has kinetic energy. Energy moving through space (or matter) is called *radiant energy*. Radiant energy is energy on the move. A collection of neutrons (that have mass near that of protons) traveling through space is radiant energy. Radiant energy is of particular importance in our specific interest in non-destructive or *non-invasive* imaging.

There is another form of energy that has no mass – *electromagnetic* (EM) *energy*. EM energy might be contrasted to a stationary mass. The latter has mass, but no energy (absent a force field) while the former has no mass but energy. However, EM energy is always moving and, hence, is a type of radiant energy. EM radiation propagates as a pair of perpendicular forces – electric and magnetic (Figure 1.2). EM energy can be thought of or modeled in two non-exclusive fashions – wave-like (transverse) and particle-like. EM energy is very important in imaging and includes radiowaves, visible light, ultraviolet light, and x and gamma rays.

Waves, including EM waves, are characterized by six features: *amplitude, wavelength* (λ), *frequency* (f), *phase, speed,* and *direction* (Figure 1.3). Amplitude is the maximum height of a wave and is a measure of the wave's intensity. Wavelength is the distance between identical points (i.e., peaks) on adjacent wave cycles. Wavelength has two close correlates, frequency and phase. Frequency is the number of cycles per second. Phase is the temporal shift in a wave cycle relative to that of another wave. Waves move, *propagate*, in a specific direction and at a defined speed (c):

$$c = \lambda f \qquad (1.8)$$

In a classical sense, EM waves propagate at a constant speed, the speed of light, 3×10^8 meters/second. From this fact it follows that for EM energy, wavelength and frequency are inversely proportional:

$$f = c/\lambda \qquad (1.9)$$

Importantly, EM energy propagates in a *rectilinear* fashion, i.e., in a straight line.

Waves are frequently illustrated in the so-called *time domain* as amplitude versus time. The same information can be presented in the *frequency domain* as amplitude versus frequency. The mathematical tool that links these two presentations of the same information is the *Fourier Transform* (*FT*). The *FT* expresses a mathematical function as a series of sine and cosine terms. The *FT* is an important mathematical tool for imaging, and we shall see more of it later (Appendix 2).

While EM energy can be modeled as orthogonally propagating waves (electric and magnetic), it can also be modeled in a particulate fashion as non-mass packets of energy called *photons*. As a form of EM energy, a photon travels through space rectilinearly at the speed of light. The energy of a photon, where h is Planck's constant, is:

$$E = h\nu = hc/\lambda \qquad (1.10)$$

When E is expressed in kiloelectronvolts (keV) and λ in nanometers (nm):

$$E = 1.25/\lambda \qquad (1.11)$$

EM energy may be defined in units of wavelength, frequency, or energy. E increases with ν and decreases with λ.

Classical physics treats mass and energy separately, with separate conservation laws for each. This turns out to be true for "slowly" moving masses, but Einstein's theory of relativity states that these two states become interchangeable at the speed of light:

$$E = mc^2 \qquad (1.12)$$

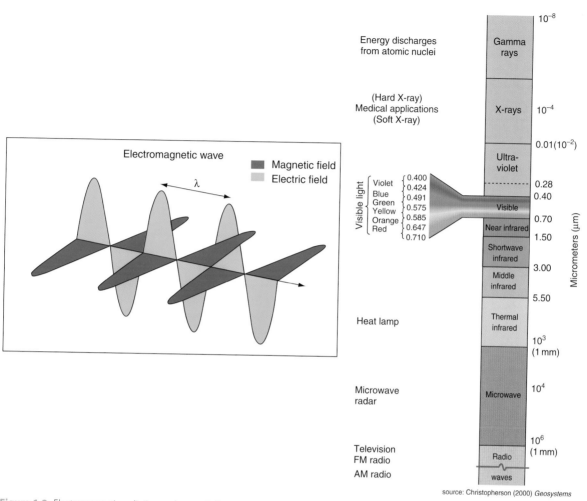

Figure 1.2. Electromagnetic radiation: orthogonal electric and magnetic force fields of varying wavelength. Wave diagram by C. R. B. Merritt, after an animated graphic by Nick Strobel for www.astronomynotes.com, used with permission. Frequency chart from Christopherson R, *Geosystems*, Prentice-Hall, 2000. Used with permission.

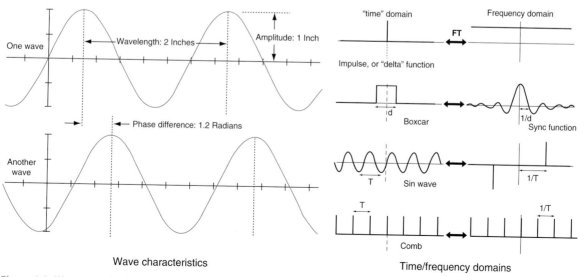

Figure 1.3. Wave properties in time and frequency domains, linked by the Fourier transform. C. R. B. Merritt.

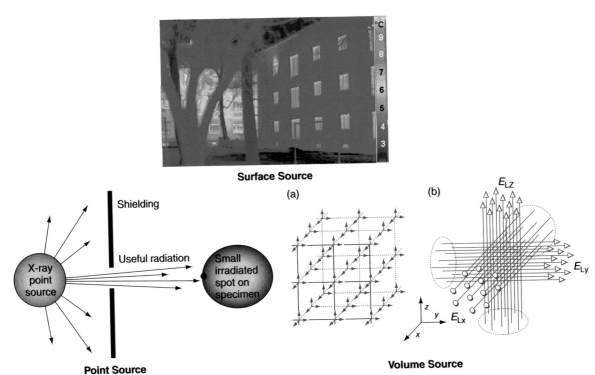

Figure 1.4. Geometry of energy sources. Surface image courtesy of Passivhaus Institut, Germany, available at http://en.wikipedia.org/wiki/Thermography. Point image from NIST GCR 05-879 by T. Pelsoci. Used with permission of the author and the Technology Innovation Program of the National Institute of Standards and Technology. Volume diagram from Malmivuo J, Plonsey R, *Bioelectromagnetism: Principles and Applications of Bioelectric and Biomagnetic Fields*, Oxford University Press, 1995. Used with permission.

From simple multiplication it follows that the electron, with a mass of 9.109×10^{-31} kg, has an associated energy of 511 keV. As previously noted, most of our discussion need only involve classical physics, using either the wave or photon model of EM energy when appropriate.

The bouncing balls and sinuous waves of mass and energy are the fundamental constituents of nature and as such are often the quest of scientific inquiry, including scientific imaging that attempts to represent these entities in relationship to space and time. Jumping forward a bit, in order to make an image, mass and energy are measured as a function of location and time. It turns out that imaging measurements are seldom of mass but almost universally of energy. Imaging measurements may reflect mass, but are nearly always based on measurements of radiant energy, energy emanating from the object of interest or *sample*. Radiant energy as energy traveling through space or matter is easy to intuit, but relatively difficult to mathematically describe. An abbreviated introduction to this topic follows.

Radiant energy may be viewed as direct emission of energy from an object or energy derived from an external source that may be transmitted, reflected, or scattered by an intervening object. Radiant energy may be modeled as originating from one-, two-, or three-dimensional sources – point, surface, or volume radiators, respectively (Figure 1.4). From an imaging perspective, volume sources are most important, and they can be defined by the very intimidating *phase–space distribution function* (or *distribution function* for short). This function is denoted as $w(\tau, s, \varepsilon, t)$ and defined by:

$$w = \frac{1}{\varepsilon} \frac{\Delta^3 Q}{\Delta V \Delta \Omega \Delta \varepsilon} \tag{1.13}$$

In photon terms, this function can be interpreted loosely as the number of photons contained in volume ΔV centered on point τ, traveling in solid angle $\Delta \Omega$ about direction s, and having energies between ε and $\varepsilon + \Delta \varepsilon$ at time t. We shall not belabor this complex description of radiant energy at this time, but will further elaborate in Chapter 2 when we discuss in more detail how an image is made. For now, just remember that imaging involves taking measurements of radiant energy emanating from a sample.

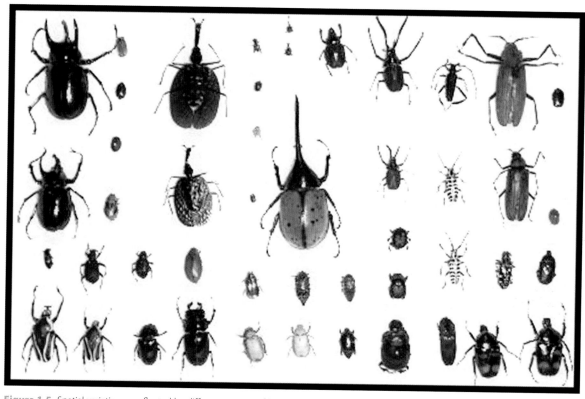

Figure 1.5. Spatial variation as reflected by different species of beetles (Coleoptera). Courtesy of J. Culin, Clemson University.

Imaging is particularly concerned with space, which has many aspects and definitions. For this immediate discussion, space is defined as *"real" space*, that is, the physical space of the universe represented by the three naturally perceived orthogonal spatial dimensions we observe in our daily environment, as symbolized by x, y, z in Equation 1.1. As previously noted, the distribution of m,E is not uniform throughout this "real" space. In fact, the contents of the universe are very non-uniform, and distinctly heterogeneous. Mass/energy tends to clump together and form "things" or create patterns of "stuff." It is this spatial heterogeneity that makes the universe interesting and imaging so very important.

While imaging the whole universe is perhaps a goal or fantasy of some scientists, most are interested in a piece of the universe, some particular aspect of nature – perhaps a large piece like the Milky Way, a small piece like a carbon atom, or a medium-sized piece like the magnetic field of a superconducting MRI magnet. Most scientific investigators are therefore interested in imaging their special part of the universe. Biological organisms, such as the human body, are special parts of the universe that interest biomedical researchers and medical practitioners. A local piece of

the universe can be defined as a *scene*, which by refining Equation 1.1 can be expressed as:

$$S = (m, E)(x, y, z)(t) \qquad x, y, z < \infty \qquad (1.14)$$

A scene is spatially bound, but otherwise has no limitations on its m,E content, properties, or distribution. Generally a scene is also temporally bound, but discussion of this condition will be deferred. The definition of a scene will be very important when we address an image, and it is one of the key aspects of imaging that differentiates it from other types of scientific measurements. A spatially restricted portion of the universe is a scene. An *image* is a representation of a *scene*.

Pieces of the universe are not only spatially heterogeneous, but are also relatively unique. The m,E that collects at one site is nearly always different from the m,E that collects at another site. If the universe were spatially heterogeneous but repetitive, it would be boring and imaging would be much less exciting. Just take beetles! What if there were only one kind of beetle (a local collection of m,E), instead of over 300 000? Instead of the visually rich and captivating *Atlas of Tropical Beetles*, there would be either one picture or 46 pictures of the same beetle (Figure 1.5). By the way,

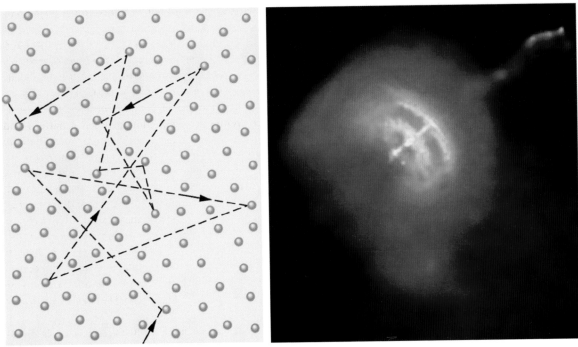

Figure 1.6. Spatial patterns: random (Brownian motion of gas molecules) versus non-random (x-ray emissions from a pulsar). Diagram of C. R. B. Merritt. Photo courtesy of NASA.

the highly repetitive genotype of beetles provides few clues to the rich spatial variety of the species. Given that essentially every piece of the universe is different than another, and given the vastness of the universe, it is not surprising that some scenes are quite simple, while others are incredibly complex. Local complexity reflects the organized aspects of the universe. Scenes with greater local complexity and higher-order organization are often those of greatest scientific interest. In science one must be prepared to deal with complexity, and much of that complexity is spatial.

In the physical sense, a scene is a function of its contents. In the real world, a scene complete with water molecules acts as a liquid at room temperature. A scene complete with oxygen acts as a gas that is warmer if it has greater kinetic energy. This physical relationship has a mathematical correspondence:

$$S = f(m, E)(x, y, z)(t) \qquad x, y, z < \infty \qquad (1.15)$$

This mathematical expression of a scene is obviously applicable at the universe level. The universe is a *function* of the spatial distribution of mass and energy over time. *Function* is described here in the physical sense, but is also being introduced as its mathematical formalism.

As previously noted, the m,E contents of a scene vary in enormously different ways. There may be

different forms of m,E within a scene: a piece of "outer space" may contain no mass and little energy, while a piece of lead shielding of an x-ray room may contain much mass and relatively little energy (kinetic, at least). Different parts of the universe are very different from each other in a real physical sense. Furthermore, within a scene m,E may be spatially organized in two relatively distinct fashions; unpredictably, randomly, or in predictable, non-random patterns. There is one key word and one key concept in the previous sentence: *relatively* and *predictable/ unpredictable* – or synonymously *non-random/random*. Newton's classical description of nature, along with his novel mathematical concepts that were incorporated into the calculus, were predicated on a smooth, continuous, highly organized universe that followed the "Rules of Nature" and were completely predictable. This model, which has little room for unpredictable or random events, has great practical advantages that science still utilizes, but it has been found wanting. Contemporary models recognize that nature is only relatively predictable; it is replete with "random" events that limit but do not prohibit prediction. Energy in a relatively empty piece of "outer space" may be moving as a relatively predictable wave form in a particular direction, perhaps as x-rays away from a pulsar, while hydrogen molecules in a balloon may be bouncing about in a highly unpredictable, random fashion (Figure 1.6). The spatial distribution of m,E creates a *pattern* that helps characterize a scene and differentiates one scene from another. Scenes whose m,E contents are the same and similarly distributed are indistinguishable from one another. The spatial distribution of m,E, the pattern, of some scenes is highly predictable, while in others the spatial pattern is random. From the scientific viewpoint, non-random patterns are generally the more interesting aspects of the universe. From a communications perspective, only non-random patterns carry information. It is the spatial distribution of m,E that results in identifiable patterns and objects in nature, and this suggests a rationale for a mathematical definition of patterns:

$$S = f_{nr}(m, E)(x, y, z)(t)$$
$$+ f_r(m, E)(x, y, z)(t) \quad x, y, z < \infty \quad (1.16)$$

$$P_{nr} = f_{nr}(m, E)(x, y, z)(t)$$
$$P_r = f_{Nr}(m, E)(x, y, z)(t) \quad (1.17)$$

with $_{nr}$ being non-random functions and patterns, and $_r$ being defined as random functions and patterns. The problem with these definitions is that predictability or randomness is relative; patterns and objects are defined by probability. This non-deterministic view of nature creates conceptual, mathematical, and semantic difficulties. For the sake of practicality and simplicity, unless otherwise stated, I will use *random* and *unpredictable* (and their respective opposites) interchangeably and relatively. That is, a non-random pattern is one that is relatively predictable. It should be admitted that this very simple definition of a pattern is related to a difficult concept, one that is still evolving, and one that will be addressed in more detail in Chapter 3 and Section 3, *Image analysis*. While the universe may consist of much disorder and randomness, and even tends towards this state (Second Law of Thermodynamics), this is not the focus of most scientific investigation, which searches for predictable patterns reflecting more highly organized parts of the universe.

Sometimes m,E aggregates in very localized, adherent patterns or in collections somewhat arbitrarily called *objects*. While most people are intuitively comfortable with the concept of an object, the explicit definition of an object is not easy, either in the physical or in the mathematical sense. Solid structures such as a diamond are easily and usually appreciated as objects,

but what about the Gulf Stream (Figure 1.7)? Some would argue that the Gulf Stream is a *pattern*, not an *object*. There is a continuum from pattern to object, with the latter being more self-adherent or possibly having a less random structure than a pattern. "Real" physical patterns and objects exist in "real" space, which is often called "object" or rarely "pattern" space. While the distinction between a pattern and an object can be of considerable importance in many situations and applications, it is not so important in terms of an image *per se*. An image represents the contents of a scene regardless of whether the m,E distribution is random or a non-random pattern or object. However, image analysis will strive to identify patterns and/or objects within a scene. *The goal of scientific imaging is to identify patterns and objects within nature.* In essence, science, at least applied science, strives to identify and study the non-randomness of nature, and imaging is one of its critical tools, as only an image can reflect spatial non-randomness.

A scene is a defined, bounded area of space within which there are things that scientists want to investigate, ideally and generally by measurements. Science is dependent on measurements, and the more rigorous the measurements, the better. Measurement, as a specific topic, will be dealt with in the next chapter. Now, however, is an appropriate time to further consider the contents of a scene in preparation for measurement. In the classical Newtonian sense, the contents of a scene are not only non-random but continuous. That is, if one begins to break up the contents of a scene, including a pattern or an object, one will find that the piece can always be divided further. Patterns and objects have an infinite number of parts that are smoothly and continuously related to their neighbors. The universe is a continuum. All aspects of the universe or a scene within it are continuous. Mass and energy are continuums. A solid physical object such as a rubber ball can be divided into an infinite number of smaller and smaller masses; the spectrum of visible light can be divided into an infinite number of wavelengths of different energy. Space is also a continuum: a scene may have finite dimensions of its outer boundaries, but within that scene there is an infinite number of smaller spaces. Likewise, time is a continuum.

Such physical continuity should be reflected by any related mathematics. Therefore, measurements of a continuous universe should be based on *continuous numbers* and explicative mathematical functions as *continuous functions*. A basic mathematical tool of continuous numbers and functions is calculus, of

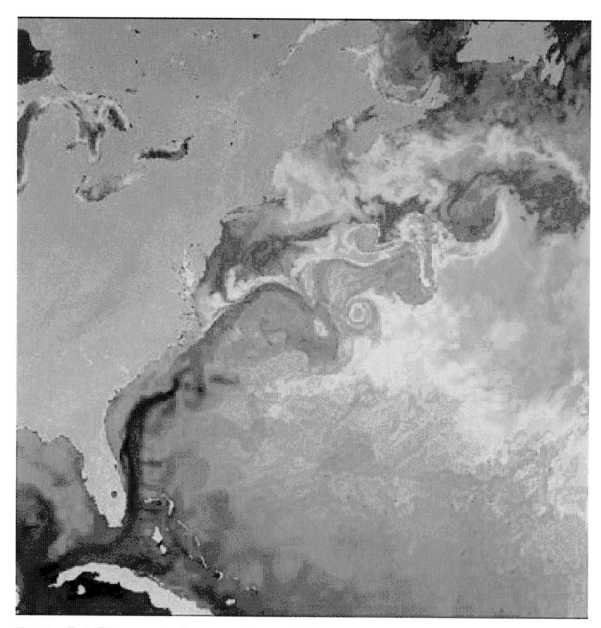

Figure 1.7. The Gulf Stream, a pattern of seawater flow. Courtesy of NASA.

which a basic (but only a very basic) understanding is needed to appreciate contemporary scientific imaging.

However, the Newtonian view of the world has been superseded by the modern view of a relatively predictable, discontinuous universe. This view is certainly true at the quantum level and is even evident macroscopically. Consider the seashore, which consists of the relatively infinite, continuous ocean water and the relatively finite, discrete sand (Figure 1.8). Is the pail of water more "Newtonian" than the pail of sand? Regardless,

measurement tools for random, discrete aspects of nature are needed for this non-Newtonian world, and the mathematics of *discrete numbers* and *probability* will be necessary. More importantly, not only must nature be considered in continuous as well as discrete fashions, but so also must images. To complicate matters, while nature viewed classically may be relatively continuous, contemporary images are usually discrete.

The universe and portions thereof, i.e., scenes, consist of spatially random and non-random distributions

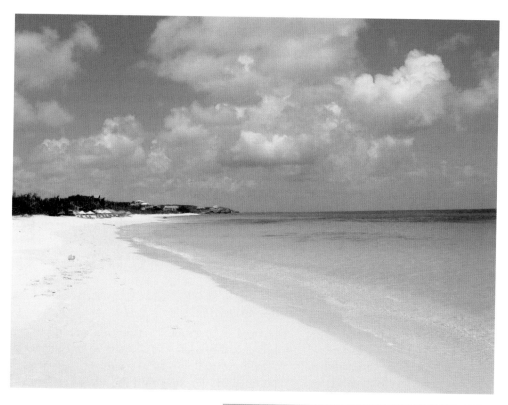

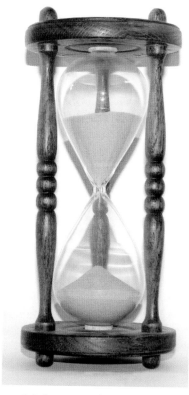
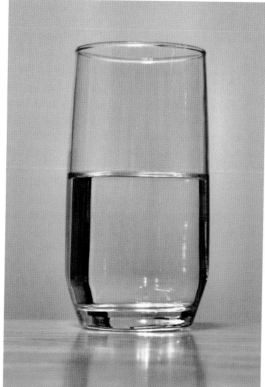

Figure 1.8. Nature, a combination of continuous (water) and discrete (sand) objects.

of m,E that are the potential contents of a scientific image – of a particular time. *Time*, the third domain of the universe, like m,E and space, is generally intuitive – but perhaps the most subtle. We intuitively recognize our lives, experience, nature as constantly changing. Time is the unit of measure of this sequence of change. Time marks change, only goes forward, and is necessary for describing any aspect of nature. All scientific measurements, including images, have at least an implicit expression of time (when the measurement was made) and sequential measurements have explicit expressions of time denoting the interval between measurements. Now our description of the universe, elements of which as scientists we will be investigating, is complete, as expressed in Equation 1.1.

What is an image?

Although there are many types of images, three aspects of images – nature, space, and accuracy – will be used to define our topic, scientific images, and to restrict the discussion. Scientific images represent the universe – nature is our subject. Spatial information distinguishes scientific images. A scientific image explicitly expresses the spatial attributes of a scene, pattern, or object. Furthermore, it attempts to do so accurately. Mental, verbal, auditory, gustatory, imaginary, hallucinatory images – these are all images in that they are representations of something, and usually something related to our environment and the universe. Moreover, they can include elements of m,E, space, and time. However, they are greatly different in what they attempt to represent, how it is represented, and how the representation is stored and disseminated. Most of these image types do attempt to reproduce some aspect of our universe, but not necessarily accurately. Imaginary images may or may not attempt to accurately reflect a scene, and hallucinatory images are almost by definition inaccurate and distorted reflections of reality. These are not scientific images, which strive to be accurate reproductions of nature. Tactile, auditory, and gustatory images may accurately reflect their respective aspects of the universe and may be very important imaging modalities for some species, and even humans under certain circumstances. However, in the usual setting, the very limited spatial extent and content of these image types results in their being inferior and usually secondary imaging modalities. Even the auditory system with the incorporation of language has major limitations in terms of recording and conveying spatial information. The common saying, "A picture is worth a thousand words," is certainly

true when it comes to representing spatial information (Figure 1.9) [1]. Hence, for general, practical, and the immediate purposes of this book, visual images are of prime interest, specifically images that attempt to accurately reflect our universe and are intended at some point to be viewed by the human visual system.

Accurate, visually observable representations of nature are what we generally consider as scientific images. Since the purpose of images is to communicate, they can be categorized according to *what* they communicate and *how* they communicate. The *what* categorization relates to the content of an image. What an image communicates depends on what it represents. The *how* categorization relates to the physical nature of the image and its relationship to an observer. How an image communicates is very much dependent on the observer.

Image content

The value of a scientific image to a researcher is a function of the nature and accuracy of its contents, as well as its perceptibility. For our purposes, an *image* is a representation or reproduction of a portion of the universe with explicit spatial content. A *scientific image* is an attempt at an accurate reproduction of a piece of the universe or scene. The contents of scientific images are measurements of m,E, space, and time. An image is created by making spatially defined measurements of m,E and subsequently rendering these measurements in a spatially (and temporally) coherent fashion for subsequent observation and analysis. An image therefore consists of the following: up to three spatial dimensions, each corresponding to one or more of the "real" physical, spatial dimensions, one time dimension, and as many "m,E" dimensions as were measured in the scene. Note here the expanded use of the word and concept – *dimension*. In the most abstract sense, dimension may refer to any measurable condition. Real, physical spatial dimensions, i.e., length, width, depth (x, y, z), can be individually measured, as can time, another dimension. In the m,E domain, mass, or its derivative weight, is a measurable condition, as is light intensity or wavelength, acoustic pressure, molecular concentration, strength of a magnetic field, etc. Each of these measurable conditions can be mathematically considered as another dimension. Hence, an image must have at least three dimensions: one m,E, one spatial, and one temporal. At the other extreme, an image may have an infinite number of dimensions. While there may be an infinite number of potential

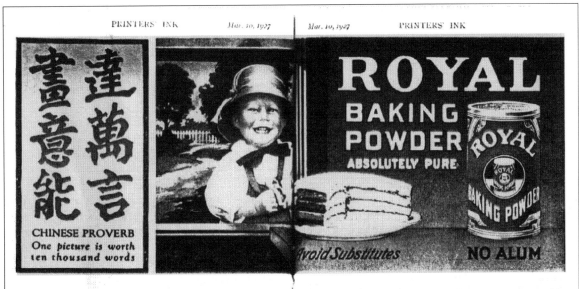

Figure 1.9. A picture is worth a thousand (or ten thousand) words. F. R. Barnard, in *Printer's Ink*, 8 December, 1921.

dimensions in an image, these dimensions are restricted to three distinct domains: m,E, space, and time. The space and time domains have a restricted number of dimensions (three and one, respectively); m,E does not. While in theory the m,E domain does not have a restricted number of dimensions, it does in practice.

Perhaps even more semantically confusing is the use of the word *space* as a set of any defined number of dimensions or measurable conditions. Earlier in this chapter "real" space was defined in the physical sense – the three orthogonal spatial dimensions we perceive as physical reality. However, in mathematical discussions and formulations, space is used in the broader sense of a set of quantifiable conditions. The x-ray CT "3D" video image of the beating heart can be said to

have five dimensions: three spatial, one temporal, and one m,E, the latter being the electron density of heart muscle (Figure 1.10).

The universe or a contained scene was previously noted to be a function of its "real" m,E, spatial, and temporal elements. Since an image consists of measurements of these elements, an image can be defined as a function of the measurements – m,E, space, and time – of its scene:

$$I = g(m, E)(x, y, z)(t) \quad x, y, z < \infty \quad (1.18)$$

This means nothing more than the fact that an image is a function of its contents' measurements. Function is now being used more in the mathematical sense rather than the physical sense.

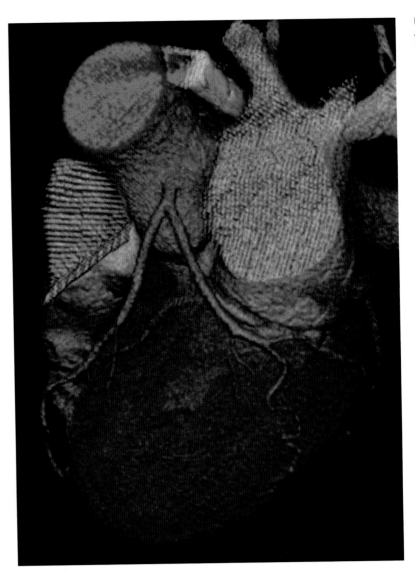

Figure 1.10. 3D x-ray CT of beating heart: a five-dimensional image. Courtesy of H. Litt.

As previously mentioned, the universe, in the classical sense, is a continuum, with most of its components being infinitely divisible and best described by continuous numbers. A faithful reproduction of such a system should also be of a continuous nature. An ideal image of a scene should therefore be continuous, accurately reflecting continuous measurements of its m,E, spatial, and temporal elements. The earliest scientific images were generally of a continuous nature. Human drawings are conceptually continuous, though not always as accurate as those of Audubon or Darwin. If quantitative measurements were made and incorporated into early scientific drawings, the measurements would have been performed in a continuous fashion based on human observations using rulers, protractors,

etc. Nearly all of the scientific instruments in the previously mentioned Whipple Museum at Cambridge are continuous measuring devices. After human drawings, photography was the earliest imaging format, and it also was a (relatively) continuous reflection of the photographed scene.

However, in the last quarter of the twentieth century, measurement and imaging devices became digital, measurements became discrete, and images became "pixelated." While the real world in many circumstances continues to be viewed as continuous, the scientific world has become digital and non-continuous. Most modern scientific images are not of a continuous nature in any sense. The m,E signals have been discretely sampled, space is divided into a discrete number of

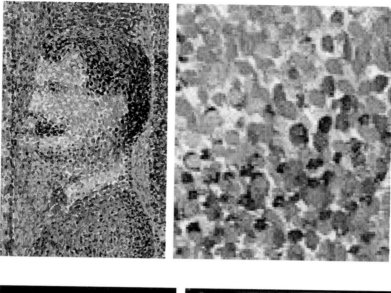

Figure 1.11. Artistic pixels: Seurat's points. Detail from *La Parade* (1889), Georges-Pierre Seurat. http://en.wikipedia.org/wiki/Georges-Pierre_Seurat. Pixel image from http://en.wikipedia.org/wiki/Pixel.

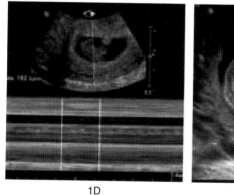
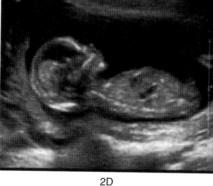
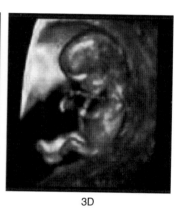

1D   2D   3D

Figure 1.12. Spatial dimensions in fetal ultrasounds. Courtesy of Women's Imaging Services, Perth, Australia.

pixels (picture elements) in a two-dimensional image, or *voxels* (volume elements) in a three-dimensional image, and even time is digitized (Figure 1.11). This transition is very important mathematically and will be discussed in more detail in Chapter 2 and subsequent sections when we discuss how images are made. For now it is important to remember that current scientific images are discrete samplings of a relatively continuous universe and hence only an approximation of the real world. As we shall see, there are other reasons that images and nearly all other measurement technologies are only approximations of reality.

Space is obviously crucial to imaging. An image exists in its own space, called *image space U*. This space is a reflection of "real" space, often called *object space V*, but distinct from it. Image space is a transformed version of "real" space. In practice, this transformation might be performed by the human visual system, an analog device such as a radiographic system, a digital device such as a CCD camera, or a combination as in a CT scanner. In engineering terms the transformation is performed by a *system*. Mathematically the transformation is performed by an *operator* **H** and expressed as:

$$I = HS \qquad (1.19)$$

or:

$$g(m, E)(x, y, z)(t) = Hf(m, E)(x, y, z)(t) \qquad (1.20)$$

This operation uniquely transforms scene *S* into image *I*, and it will be the main focus of Chapter 2. For now let us continue to focus on the image.

While real space always has three spatial dimensions, image space may have three or fewer (Figure 1.12). If an image has fewer than three spatial dimensions, then one

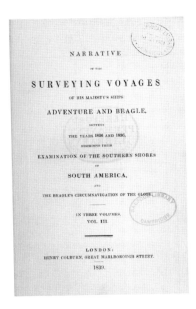

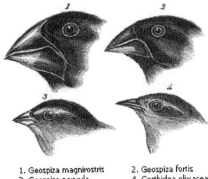

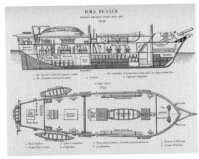

1. Geospiza magnirostris   2. Geospiza fortis
3. Geospiza parvula   4. Certhidea olivacea

Finches from Galapagos Archipelago

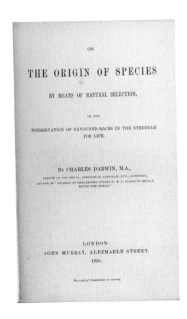

Figure 1.13. Darwin's finches: scientific images applied initially to "natural" science and then hypothesis development and testing. Used with permission from The Complete Work of Charles Darwin Online http://darwin-online.org.uk/.

or more of the three real spatial dimensions has been omitted or combined with another. If an imaging system can measure only two spatial dimensions, then it can only create a one- or two- (spatial) dimensional image. As a point of clarification, the common nomenclature of 1-D, 2-D and 3-D will be used in the book primarily in relationship to spatial dimensions. In general, image space for a particular scene is a result of the technical limitations of the imaging system and requirements of the *observer*.

The "real" space of a scientific image is almost always remote from the viewer, whereas image space is immediate. The imaging process involves moving a scene from remote "real" space to immediate "image" space. An image allows viewers to see what they otherwise could not see. A scientific image reproduces a scene of interest that is not immediately visible to the investigator. A scene may be invisible just because it is physically remote. This in and of itself can be of great importance and is the major asset of cartography. Darwin's drawings of Galápagos finches documented the distinguishing features of these previously geographically remote birds (Figure 1.13). Image remoteness is not just a function of physical distance. A scene may be remote because it is beyond the spatial

resolution of the naked eye. Leeuwenhoek's illustrations of microorganisms reproduced scenes that were invisible to human observers without a microscope (Figure 1.14). Galileo's telescopic images of Jupiter allowed him to see four moons that were not otherwise visible. Scientific images allow investigators to study places, as well as things, that they cannot get to or see with the naked eye. The rapid growth in scientific imaging is due to new imaging technologies that allow us to see new places, like the back side of the moon or gene expression in a living mouse (Figure 1.15). The nondestructive nature of newer imaging techniques is important both scientifically and practically: scientifically because it allows the observation of dynamic functions like glucose metabolism that are disrupted by destructive techniques; practically because it shows a tumor in a patient's brain that would otherwise be invisible unless a neurosurgeon performed a craniotomy (Figure 1.16). The ability to bring otherwise invisible real space to immediately visible image space is the practical rationale for scientific imaging.

Image space is not only in a different location than real space, but also is usually of a different physical scale. This is of great importance, both practically and

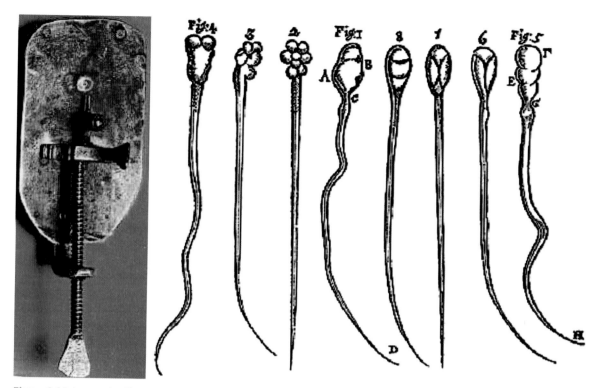

Figure 1.14. Leeuwenhoek's microscope and drawn images of ram sperm. A. van Leeuwenhoek, 1678. From www.euronet.nl/users/warnar/leeuwenhoek.html.

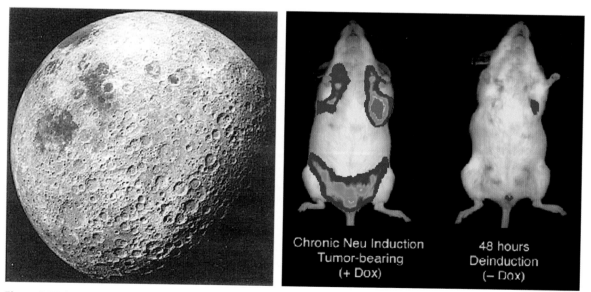

Chronic Neu Induction
Tumor-bearing
(+ Dox)

48 hours
Deinduction
(− Dox)

Figure 1.15. "Remote" images: far side of the moon and mouse gene expression. Photo courtesy of NASA. Optical images courtesy of W. El-Deiry.

symbolically. Cartography's challenge is not only to convey remote geographical information, but also to compress it into a more comprehensible and usable format. How much more practical for a traveler is a 1/60 000 scaled map of Texas than a physical model of the whole. In general, images of large objects are scaled down, while the images of small objects are scaled up (Figure 1.17). Though there is great latitude, scaling should be guided

27

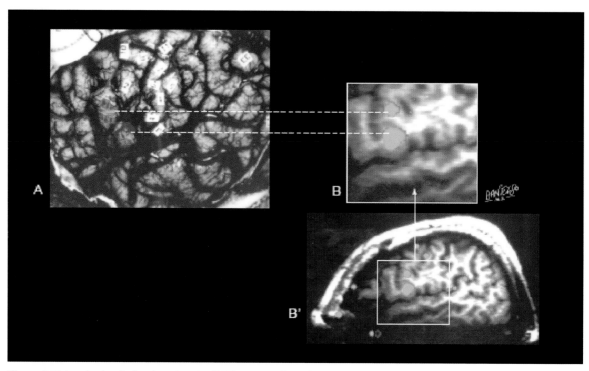

Figure 1.16. Invasive (surgical) and non-invasive (fMRI) imaging of brain function. From Yetkin FZ, *et al.*, Functional MR activation correlated with intraoperative cortical mapping. *AJNR Am J Neuroradiol* **18**: 1311–15, August 1997. Used with permission.

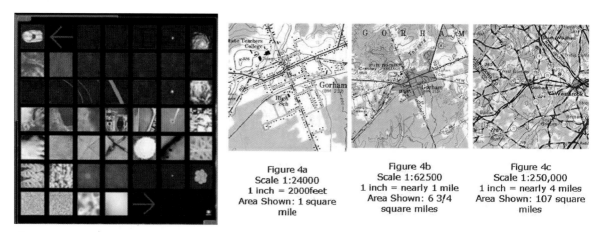

Figure 4a
Scale 1:24000
1 inch = 2000feet
Area Shown: 1 square
mile

Figure 4b
Scale 1:62500
1 inch = nearly 1 mile
Area Shown: 6 3/4
square miles

Figure 4c
Scale 1:250,000
1 inch = nearly 4 miles
Area Shown: 107 square
miles

Figure 1.17. Image scale: very small to very large scale images of universe. Map scale ratios. Scaled universe www.powersof10.com, © 1997 Eames Office, LLC, used with permission. Maps courtesy of U.S. Geological Survey.

by the needs of specific applications and the image scale should always be known, preferably by explicit and concise labeling on the image itself. In general, images are scaled to match the information density of an image and the viewing requirements of an observer.

Time is critical for scientific imaging, as nature is constantly changing. If it is not changing, a biological system is dead! However, the time frame of temporal changes varies enormously, from femtoseconds for radioactive decay to millennia for erosion of granite. All images incorporate time; even a single, static image is made at some specific time point. The more temporally dynamic an event, the more important is sequential imaging. Scientific images should attempt to match the time frame of the dynamics of their contents (Figure 1.18). There is a simple rule for how

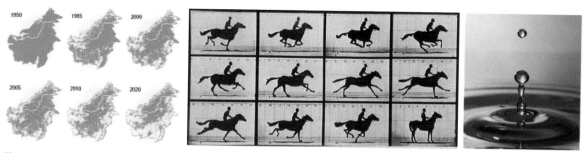

Figure 1.18. Application of the Nyquist sampling theorem to temporal changes: slow deforestation of Borneo, early cine of galloping horse, high-speed photography of drop of water. Map set used with permission from UNEP/GRID-Arendal, courtesy of WWF. *The Horse in Motion* by Eadweard Muybridge, 1878. Photo by Michael Melgar.

rapidly one should image a temporally dynamic process. One should collect images at twice the rate of any temporal change one wants to observe. To adequately image the motion of a heart beating at 60 beats/minute, or 1 Hz, an image should be made at least every 0.5 seconds – an imaging rate of 2 Hz. This is a temporal application of the sampling theorem of Nyquest:

$$U \geq \frac{1}{2\Delta x} \qquad (1.21)$$

U is the minimal sampling frequency needed to detect a change of Δx. The Nyquist sampling theorem actually applies to all types of measurements, as will be discussed in the next chapter.

An image should be an accurate, unbiased reflection of the physical contents of the scene it represents. From this perspective, the technical quality of an image should be judged only by the difference between it and reality. Unfortunately we rarely, if ever, know what reality is. The universe from the classical, Newtonian model could be fully described using accurate measuring tools and good scientific insight supported by rigorous mathematics. That world view or model was challenged not only by quantum physics, but also by advanced mathematical concepts of measurement, probability, and statistics. The earlier *deterministic* viewpoint has been supplemented by a *stochastic* perspective that we will pursue further in the next chapter. Suffice it to say that when we discuss image quality, we will have to deal not only with the image as an approximation of a scene, but also with the fact that the natural scene has intrinsic variability and a probabilistic component.

The universe and its component scenes are not continuous and fully predictable, but contain random and non-random distributions of m,E; the non-random aggregates define patterns and objects. Since

an image is a reflection of a scene, an image should also accurately reflect patterns and objects. However, an image is "of" a scene, not objects or patterns *per se*. This is a subtle point, but an image just contains m,E, spatial, and temporal information that may or may not contain or reflect a pattern or object. From a teleological perspective, the image does not care. The observer might, and it is the responsibility of the observer, not the image, to determine if a pattern or object exists within the scene. This subject will be reintroduced in Chapter 3 and extensively discussed in Section 3, *Image analysis*.

Image observer

Images are made to be "looked at" by someone or something. Usually an image is not only "looked at," but also analyzed to support a subsequent decision. It must always be remembered that images are tools of communication and hence are designed to convey information. The recipient of image information is often called an *observer*. An observer has two roles: one is the more passive role of perceiving the image; the other is the more active one of analyzing the image. Until recently observers were either humans or other organisms with imaging systems. This has rapidly changed since the introduction of digital images and computers, and the latter now play an increasingly active role as observers.

To serve its purpose – communication – an image has to be perceivable by the observer; visual images have to be seen. Hence, the physical nature of an image must be matched to the observer. At a minimum, an image must be in a physical form that can be detected by the observer. In the case of humans, an image must produce a physical signal that can be detected by either the olfactory, gustatory, auditory, tactile, or visual system – the human sensory systems. Given the requirement that images contain and convey spatial information, the dominant imaging system of humans

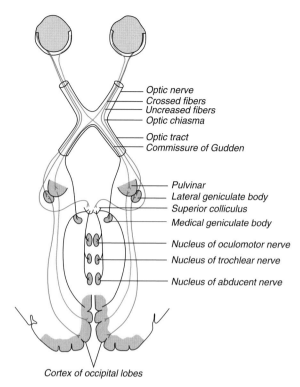

Optic nerve
Crossed fibers
Uncreased fibers
Optic chiasma

Optic tract
Commissure of Gudden

Pulvinar
Lateral geniculate body
Superior colliculus
Medical geniculate body

Nucleus of oculomotor nerve

Nucleus of trochlear nerve

Nucleus of abducent nerve

Cortex of occipital lobes

Figure 1.19. Human visual system. From *Gray's Anatomy*.

is the visual system, because of its superior spatial resolution and capacity to process abundant visible light that happens to reflect important environmental information. This capacity to process visible light reflects the evolutionary drive of the quite extraordinary human visual system. Such is not the case for a cave bat, which has only a crude visual system and lives in an environment lacking visible light. This creature uses its auditory system and ultrasound as its primary imaging system. In the case of a blind person, an effective image might consist of a tactile pattern, such as Braille. For the computer "observer," images have to be in electronic, digital format. However, visual images for human observation are of immediate interest, and are the subject to which the discussion will be limited unless otherwise noted.

The human visual system is an extraordinarily complex and sophisticated sensory system that is the "final" pathway to our appreciation and use of visual data (Figure 1.19). A basic understanding of this system is critical for creating and interpreting images, and Chapter 3 will provide a more detailed discussion of this topic. However, a few obvious but key points will be addressed now. This will also be our first exposure to an *imaging system*. The human visual system initially

detects visible light with chemical photoreceptors in the retina of the eyeball. These photoreceptors convert visible light energy into electrochemical energy that is subsequently processed by cells in the retina, midbrain, and multiple regions of the cerebral cortex. Different anatomic regions process different aspects of the visual image. For instance, motion and color information are processed by different sets of cells and anatomic structures. Different parts of the cerebral cortex appear to operate on different parts of an image. Human visual processing is "channelized." Distal to the retina, no part of the human brain actually receives a complete image of a scene, only components thereof.

A scientific image is a spatially dependent display of m,E measurements. Other than visible light, other forms of m,E, such as temperature, electron density, or MR spin density, are invisible to a human observer. An imaging device may detect and measure these signals, but the human eye cannot see them. Therefore, these measurements need to be converted into visible signals for human observation. The human visual system can only detect energy in the form of electromagnetic (EM) radiation in the range of what is commonly called "visible light." As previously noted, EM radiation is the most ubiquitous form of energy in the universe, and it plays many important roles in scientific imaging. Visible light has intermediate wavelengths of 400–700 nanometers that are of relatively low energy. Since the human visual system can only detect visible light, imaging device measurements are encoded into visible light using either a gray (shades of black/white) or color scale. In an optimal setting, the human visual system can distinguish up to 256 shades of gray and over a million different colors, the dynamic range of the visual system (Figure 1.20). Each shade of gray or color can be used to represent a single or range of measurement numbers.

However, if the eye only measured amplitude (brightness) and wavelength (color) of visible light, it would be a spectrometer, not an imaging device, and of little interest to our purpose. Fortunately, not only is the human eye extremely sensitive to light photons of different energy, but it is also very sensitive to the spatial origin of these photons. The unaided human visual system can spatially distinguish two extremely small, bright light sources separated from each other by only 0.5 mm at 40 cm.

The human visual system also has reasonably good temporal resolution. The retinal photoreceptors have "dead" times of approximately 10 milliseconds.

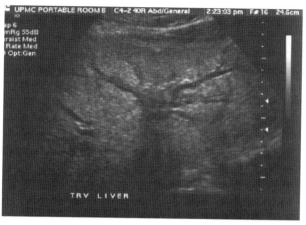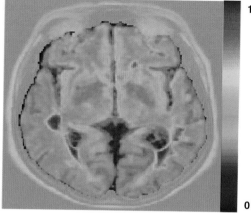

Figure 1.20. Gray-scale ultrasound image (16 shades of gray) and color-scale image of the probability of cerebrovascular disease (256 color hues). Courtesy of S. Horii and C. Davatzikos.

However, this front-end temporal resolution is not maintained through the visual system, and due to visual lag, individual images persist for 40–50 ms. Events that change faster than this rate cannot be detected by the unaided human visual system. Such rapidly changing events may be successfully recorded by some other imaging system with better temporal resolution and then played back in "slow motion" for human appreciation. Not only does the human visual system have the ability to temporally distinguish distinct images, but it also has the ability to integrate temporal image data. To take advantage of this temporal integrative ability, images should be presented with a frequency of at least 20 Hz. Hence most cine/video formats present individual images at 30–60 images per second, regardless of the temporal frequency of the initial image data.

This combination of spectral, spatial, and temporal sensitivity allows humans to see faint light from suns millions of light years away, count the legs of an ant, wonder at the colors of the rainbow, and track a baseball moving at 150 km per hour. The human visual system is the final observer for most scientific images. Hence, scientific images must be in an appropriate format to be effectively observed and analyzed by this system. The images must be in a visible light format, display the spatial distribution of the signal within the imaged scene, and convey appropriate temporal changes.

Simple physical aspects of an image may be mundane, yet very important. An ancient map rendered on stone was not easily reproduced, nor very portable, and was quickly superseded by more practical image recording formats, such as leather, papyrus, paper, and now electronic displays (Figure 1.21). How large, solid, permanent, and portable an image should be

depends on its purpose. In general, scientific images are designed to be appreciated with relative ease by multiple observers at multiple sites, so most are presented to the observer in either a standard printed format (hard copy) or electronic display (soft copy).

While earlier electronic displays could not match the spectral, spatial, or temporal resolution of the highest-resolution print formats, cathode ray (CR) monitors and liquid crystal displays (LCD) currently available can not only equal hard-copy image quality, but can also exceed the limits of the human visual system. However, with any form of physical presentation, lower-quality images can be produced that may compromise an observer's performance. A scientific imager should always be aware of the information density of the images of interest and ensure that the display device can accurately reproduce that information. For instance, a radiologist looking for a subtle bone fracture should be using a high-resolution 14-inch monitor with at least 2000 × 2000 pixel elements in order to see a fracture of 0.5 mm width; a cinematic presentation of the beating heart should be presented at 30–60 frames/second in order to detect irregularities in wall motion.

The rich literature of human psychophysics now provides abundant information on how human observers react to many aspects of images, and there exist numerous guidelines for effective image presentation. However, there are many poorly understood aspects of human image perception, and there remains an aesthetic component of image presentation that is psychologically important. The numerous publications of Edward Tufte nicely illustrate more versus less effective presentations of scientific data [2]. He

31

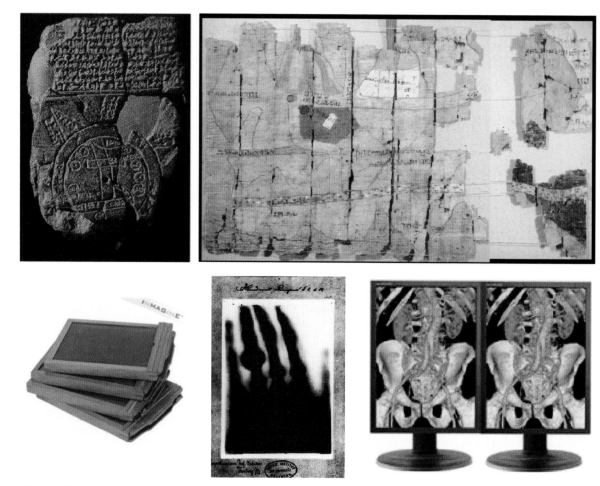

Figure 1.21. Image media: stone, papyrus, glass photographic plates, electronic monitor. Stone with permission from Henry Davis Co. Papyrus photo courtesy of J. Harrell. Monitor courtesy of Eizo Nanao Corporation.

particularly stresses the problem of "flatland," the challenge of displaying multidimensional data on flat, two-dimensional formats such as a sheet of paper or an LCD monitor (Figure 1.22). Effective images easily and fully communicate their content to observers; ineffective images confuse and mislead observers.

In the end, the quality of an image is determined by its ability to communicate, to convey information. Hence, the final evaluation of the quality of a scientific image depends on how well it performed its designated task, which implies that the purpose of a scientific image should be defined before the image is made. This is nothing more than good scientific forethought and methodology. A hypothesis is generated, methods are defined to test the hypothesis, data are collected, and the hypothesis is tested. Images are data, and the methods should explicitly define appropriate methodology to collect the data, i.e., create the images. The quality of the

image is then dependent on the ability of the image to provide the desired measurements and allow appropriate statistical testing of the hypothesis. This is the methodological aspect of the science of imaging.

Old and new scientific images

Before embarking in more detail in the technicalities of imaging, let us appreciate some examples of scientific imaging from its inception with cartography to a current medical application. Cartography is based on mapping, and it provides helpful illustrations of scientific multidimensional measurements, applied in this case to geography. The earliest cartographic maps were actually one-dimensional and consisted of nothing more than ordered representations of geographic points, such as villages, along a line. In this case the line represents one dimension of physical space defined by an ordinal

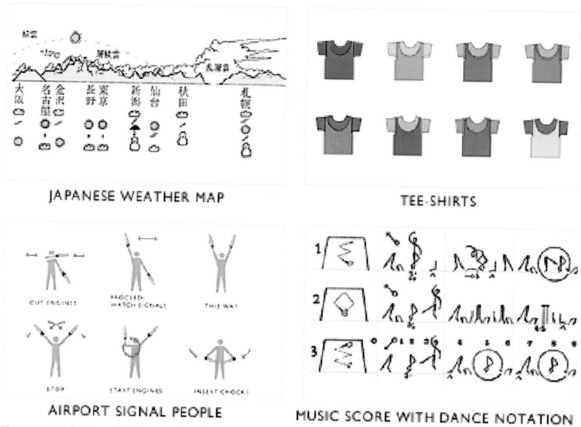

JAPANESE WEATHER MAP

TEE-SHIRTS

AIRPORT SIGNAL PEOPLE

MUSIC SCORE WITH DANCE NOTATION

Figure 1.22. Tufte's "flatland" challenge. Edward R. Tufte, *Envisioning Information*, Graphics Press LLC, Cheshire, Connecticut, 1990. Used with permission.

numeric system. Points along the line represent only order of occurrence; the points have no other numeric properties. This type of map is still in use for such applications as subway maps, but it was quickly followed by simple ratio maps upon which the points along a line represented not only the order, but the actual distance between geographic entities (Figure 1.23). This cartographic advance was dependent on the development of length-measuring technology such as measuring rods, one of the first scientific imaging devices.

The Greek development of Euclidean geometry, with its concept of angles as well as points, provided the means of simultaneously describing and analyzing multiple dimensions at the same time. A single number defines a point, two points define a line, two intersecting lines define a plane, and three intersecting planes describe a 3D space. Euclidean geometry provided the quantitative means to spatially describe many objects, including a sphere such as the earth. Simultaneously, early measuring devices such as rules, compasses, tridents, etc. that allowed distance and angle

measurements of the real world allowed cartography to expand from primitive one-dimensional displays to very sophisticated two- and three-dimensional displays of physical space. By the time of Ptolemy in 500 BC, accurate three-dimensional maps of the then-known world had been created using well-established geometrical techniques that also allowed remarkably accurate calculations, such as mountain heights or even the diameter of a round earth. Ptolemy calculated the diameter of a round earth at approximately 40 000 km, remarkably close to the present-day estimate of 40 075 km at the equator. Unfortunately, much of this knowledge was lost to most of the Western world for a thousand years. Fortunately, however, this was a temporary loss and Euclidean geometry, along with recent refinements, continues to be a key component of the mathematical basis for scientific investigation, particularly imaging.

Note a major difference between our previous discussions of scientific measurement and cartography. In the former, m,E is the measurement of interest, while for the latter, space is the measurement of

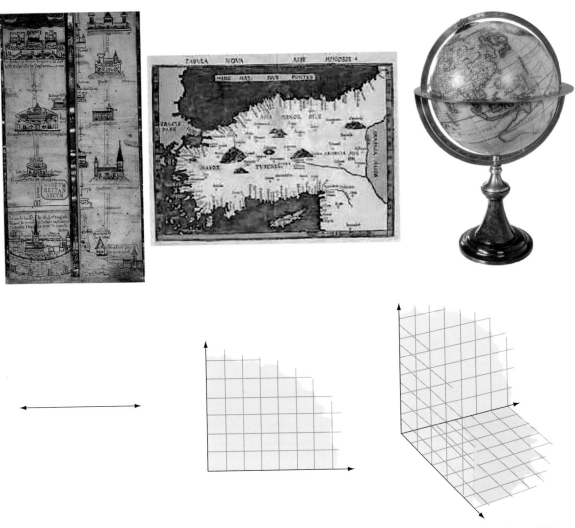

Figure 1.23. Cartesian geography: one, two, and three dimensions. London, England, to Beauvais, France, ca. 1250; Anatolia ca. 1531; world globe ca. 1745. London route owned by the British Library; image appeared in Akerman JR and Karrow RW, *Maps*, University of Chicago Press, 2007. Anatolia map, ca. 1531, from the *Atlas Ptolemeus Auctus Resitutus*, at http://turkeyinmaps.com/Sayfa4.html. Globe by Authentic Models. Graphs C. R. B. Merritt.

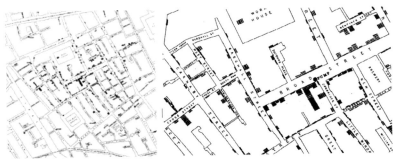

Figure 1.24. London cholera epidemic, 1855: the Broad Street pump. Map by Dr. John Snow, 1855. http://en.wikipedia.org/wiki/1854_Broad_Street_cholera_outbreak.

interest. While cartography developed very sophisticated quantitative techniques for handling physical spatial dimensions, only crude quantitation was applied to the other dimensions of nature – m,E and time. What was usually described at a particular spatial point was only a qualitative geographical name or structure, like a village or river. Mathematically, this is like saying $f(x) = Rome$, *Tiber River*, etc.

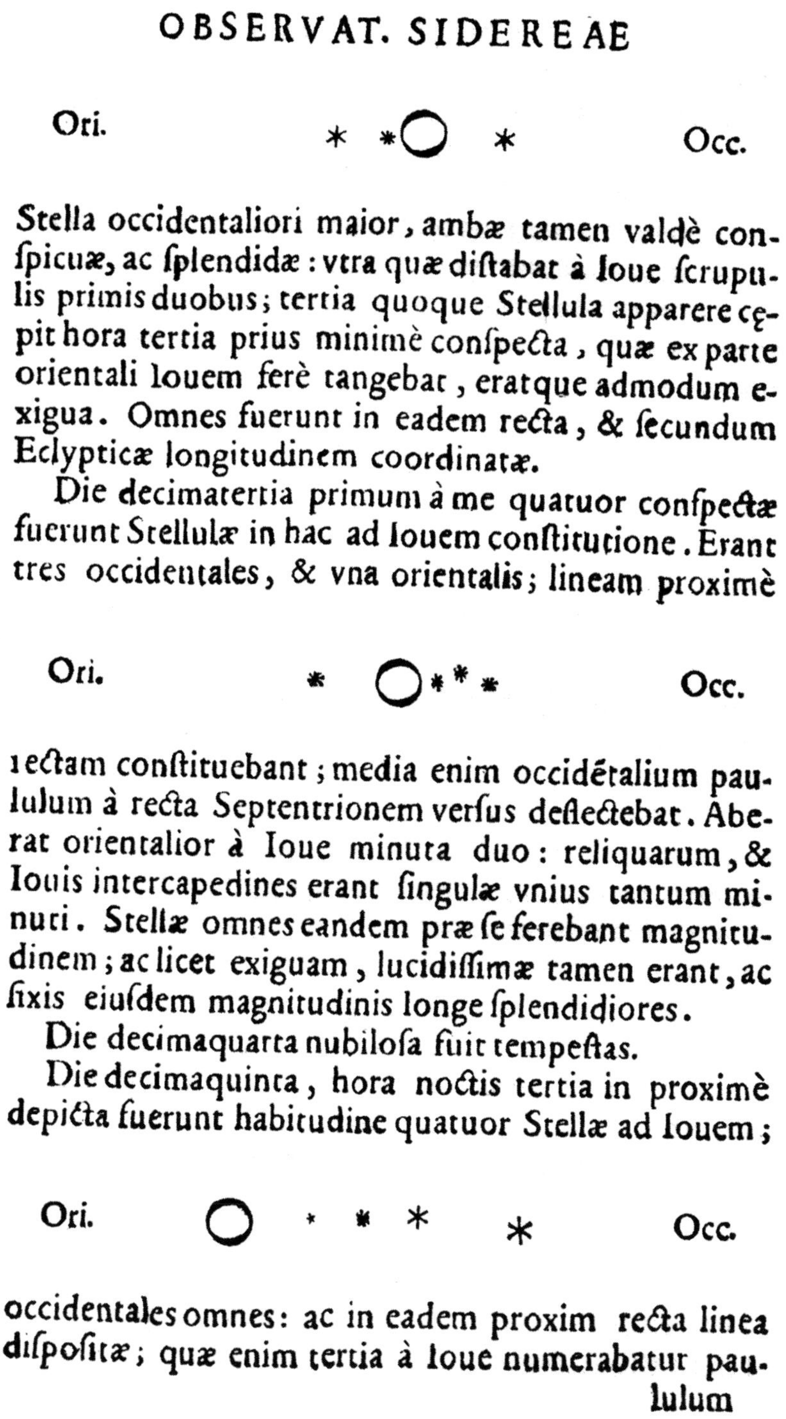

OBSERVAT. SIDEREAE

Ori.　　　　　✳ ✳○ ✳　　　　Occ.

Figure 1.25. Galileo's observations of the four moons of Jupiter, 1610. As appeared in Edward R. Tufte, *Beautiful Evidence*, Graphics Press LLC, Cheshire, Connecticut, 2006. Used with permission.

Stella occidentaliori maior, ambæ tamen valdè conſpicuæ, ac ſplendidæ: vtra quæ diſtabat à Ioue ſcrupulis primis duobus; tertia quoque Stellula apparere cępit hora tertia prius minimè conſpecta, quæ ex parte orientali Iouem ferè tangebat, eratque admodum exigua. Omnes fuerunt in eadem recta, & ſecundum Eclypticæ longitudinem coordinatæ.

　Die decimatertia primum à me quatuor conſpectæ fuerunt Stellulæ in hac ad Iouem conſtitutione. Erant tres occidentales, & vna orientalis; lineam proximè

Ori.　　　　✳　○✳✳✳　　　　Occ.

1ectam conſtituebant; media enim occidétalium paululum à recta Septentrionem verſus deflectebat. Aberat orientalior à Ioue minuta duo: reliquarum, & Iouis intercapedines erant ſingulæ vnius tantum minuti. Stellæ omnes eandem præ ſe ferebant magnitudinem; ac licet exiguam, lucidiſſimæ tamen erant, ac fixis eiuſdem magnitudinis longe ſplendidiores.

　Die decimaquarta nubiloſa fuit tempeſtas.

　Die decimaquinta, hora noctis tertia in proximè depicta fuerunt habitudine quatuor Stellæ ad Iouem;

Ori.　　○　·　✳　✳　　　✳　　　Occ.

occidentales omnes: ac in eadem proxim recta linea diſpoſitæ; quæ enim tertia à Ioue numerabatur paululum

lulum

Cartography remained spatially quantitative but non-spatially qualitative until the eighteenth and nineteenth centuries, when thematic maps were developed in conjunction with the development of social sciences and in response to political needs of governments.

Thematic maps report any variety of observations as a function of geographical location. An early example was John Snow's mapping of the locations of cholera victims in the London epidemic of 1854 (Figure 1.24) [3]. This simple thematic map emphatically demonstrated

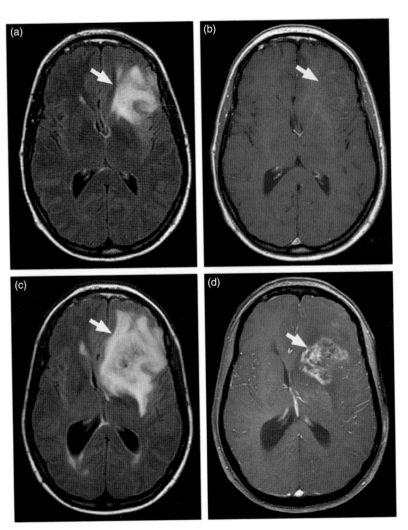

Figure 1.26. Growth of malignant brain tumor over 12 months (MRI). Reprinted by permission from Macmillan Publishers Ltd. Brat DJ, Van Meir EG. Vaso-occlusive and prothrombotic mechanisms associated with tumor hypoxia, necrosis, and accelerated growth in glioblastoma. *Laboratory Investigation* **84**(4); 2004.

the concentration of cholera-related deaths around the Broad Street water pump, which was thus established as the source of the deadly infection. Thematic maps are now routinely used to show local geology, temperature, population, per-capita income, death rates, etc. – anything that can be observed or measured at multiple geographic points. Thematic maps represent a subtle shift in the emphasis of cartography from determining and displaying the unknown location of a known entity (mountain) to defining and displaying an unknown entity (number of deaths) at a known location. The known and unknown, dependent and independent, variables are switched. Thematic maps are scientific images exactly as defined for this presentation, though the spatial domain is limited to geography.

Along with cartography, the basic principles of multidimensional measurements and images were utilized by astronomy. As mentioned previously,

perhaps the earliest example of modern scientific imaging was the astronomical study of Jupiter undertaken by Galileo in 1506 (Figure 1.25). For more than 30 evenings, Galileo focused his new scientific imaging device, the telescope, on Jupiter, whose astronomical location had long been known. He systematically measured the brightness and spatial location of previously unseen nearby objects, of which there were four. This was a scientific inquiry involving four dimensions – one m,E, two spatial, plus time. The m,E measurement was very crude, but included an important estimate of brightness, i.e., signal intensity. The locations of these new objects were carefully recorded as angular degrees from the planet in two spatial dimensions, x (horizontal) and y (vertical) (though most of the action was along the x-axis). The time dimension was discretely sampled at nightly (24-hour) intervals. From these primitive descriptive images, Galileo formed the hypothesis that these four objects could be modeled as moons orbiting about Jupiter. He subsequently proved his hypothesis by showing that his mathematical model not only explained his observations, but could also predict future behavior of these celestial objects. Galileo's observations involved four measurement dimensions that were displayed by a series of 3D images using a 2D format.

A contemporary example of a scientific image is an MR scan of a brain tumor (Figure 1.26). In this case a contemporary imaging device, an MR scanner, measured a form of m,E a radiosignal, at thousands of discrete locations in a patient's head. Scans were performed two months apart. The instrument defined the location of each measurement, a picture element or *pixel*, by a two-dimensional grid of spatial sampling points in a slice through the patient's head. The MR measurement unit in this case is T1 weighted. We could represent the signal measurement at each pixel as a vertical line perpendicular to the plane of the slice. For a single pixel this would look like a standard pseudo three-dimensional display. However, such a display of all pixels is confusing. This is a classical "flatland" problem: how to display three or more dimensions with a flat, two-dimensional format. A common solution is to use a *gray scale* in which greater signal measurements are assigned darker shades of gray within each pixel. This results in a typical 2D display of three-dimensional data. The fourth dimension, time, is reflected by the series of two-dimensional images made two months

apart. One can easily see the change, in this case growth, of the bright tumor. The most important information in these images is the increase in size, the change in the spatial characteristics of the tumor. When spatial information is important, imaging is mandatory.

References

1. Barnard FR. One look is worth a thousand words. *Printers' Ink* 1921 December 8.

2. Tufte ER. *Envisioning Information*. Cheshire, CT: Graphics Press, 1990.

3. Snow J. *On the Mode of Communication of Cholera*, 2nd edn. London: J. Churchill, 1855.

General reading

Akerman JR, Karrow RW, eds. *Maps: Finding our Place in the World*. Chicago, IL: University of Chicago Press, 2007.

Barrett HH, Myers KJ. *Foundations of Image Science*. Hoboken, NJ: Wiley-Interscience, 2004.

Epstein CL. *Introduction to the Mathematics of Medical Imaging*. Upper Saddle River, NJ: Pearson Education/ Prentice Hall, 2003.

Feynman RP, Leighton RB, Sands ML. *The Feynman Lectures on Physics*. Reading, MA: Addison-Wesley, 1963.

Robinson AH, Petchenik BB. *The Nature of Maps: Essays Toward Understanding Maps and Mapping*. Chicago, IL: University of Chicago Press, 1976.

Shah P, Miyake A. *The Cambridge Handbook of Visuospatial Thinking*. Cambridge: Cambridge University Press, 2005.

How to make an image

R. Nick Bryan and Christopher R. B. Merritt

Summarizing the previous chapter, a scientific image is a reproduction or representation of a portion of the universe, a scene. An image reflects the spatial distribution of matter and energy (m,E) in the scene at a particular point in time. A typical image is a graphical display of spatially and temporally dependent measurements of m,E. The reality of a natural scene is transformed by the imaging process into a representative image. Nature exists in its own physical space U while the image exists in its own, separate, image space V. The imaging process transforms the contents of U into V. Symbolized as $\mathbf{H}$, the imaging process is performed by a *system* that may be a physical machine, a computer algorithm, or a combination of the two. Mathematically the transformation may be termed an *operator* $\mathbf{H}$ and the imaging process expressed as:

$$I = \mathbf{H}S \qquad (2.1)$$

Or, considering I and S as their respective functions:

$$g(m, E)(x, y, z)(t) = \mathbf{H}f(m, E)(x, y, z)(t) \qquad (2.2)$$

The operator $\mathbf{H}$ uniquely transforms scene S of physical space U into image I in image space V.

The content of the scene is m,E, which is usually continuous in nature; the content of the image is measurement of m,E, of which the measurements may be continuous or discrete, often the latter. Importantly and specifically for images, the measurements of m,E are spatially defined or dependent. The m,E measurements are dependent on – and are a function of – their location. This dependence of m,E measurements on location is obviously what makes imaging so important as a scientific tool. It also creates major challenges. Not only is an m,E-measuring instrument required, but that instrument must also perform its measuring function in different locations. For many scientific images, the m,E measurements are made in thousands

of tiny, precisely defined parts of a scene, at perhaps hundreds of times a second. This is obviously much more difficult than making a measurement in one place at one point in time, e.g., like weighing an apple. This chapter will present the general process of imaging, and will illustrate the process with several examples of old and new scientific imaging systems.

Measurement

Because measuring some aspect of m,E is an integral component of imaging, let us briefly review the principles of measurement. Measurement is the association of numbers with observations, usually of physical quantities or phenomena. Therefore measurement begins with an observation; this implies an interaction between observed and observer. The "observed" is simply the object or *sample* that is to be measured. Though often under-appreciated, identification of the sample is not only the initial, but also the most critical step in measurement. If the sample is not appropriately defined, any subsequent measurement will be erroneous. If one sets out to measure the atomic mass characteristics of a protein by x-ray diffraction crystallography but starts with a contaminated protein, the resulting measurements may accurately reflect the characteristics of the contaminant rather than the protein of interest (Figure 2.1). Great care is necessary to ensure a *pure* sample, or in the case of a population, a *representative* sample. For many, if not most experiments, the sample is defined before any measurement is made. Interestingly, this is not usually the case with imaging measurements, as we shall later see.

Measurement involves work and therefore requires energy to drive it. Generally some type of exchange of energy is required for a measurement; a measuring device, the *detector*, must be energized. The force of gravity on a mouse provides the energy to the springs

Introduction to the Science of Medical Imaging, ed. R. Nick Bryan. Published by Cambridge University Press. © Cambridge University Press 2010.

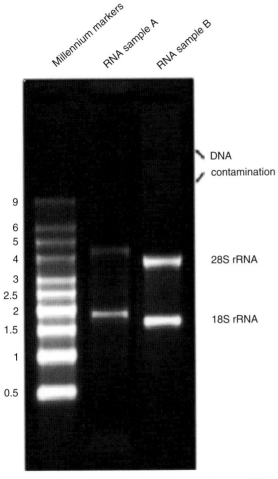

Millennium markers
RNA sample A
RNA sample B

DNA
contamination

9
6
5
4
3
2.5
2
1.5
1
0.5

28S rRNA

18S rRNA

Figure 2.1. Sample contamination: DNA contamination in RNA preparations. With permission from Applied Biosystems.

of a scale measuring the weight of a mouse. The energy required to determine the mass of a subatomic particle requires the force of a large beam of particles from a high-energy particle accelerator, such as the Collider Detector of Fermilab (Figure 2.2). Relative to the sample, the energy of detection may be relatively high and destructive, as in the case of the Collider Detector, or low and non-destructive, as in the case of weighing a mouse. If the sample is to be preserved, measurement energy is preferably negligible, minimally disturbing the sample. This is a requisite for non-destructive measurements, which are generally desired in imaging experiments.

In some situations energy from the object itself is sufficient to support the measurement. For instance, even a remote star creates enough light energy to expose photographic film or excite a solid-state detector. In this case, the detected energy is a direct reflection of the object being observed. In other experiments, energy must be applied to and interact with an object in order for a measurement to be made. In this case, the measurement is dependent on and may be derived from the added form of energy. The earth's sun adds visible light energy to surfaces in our environment that then reflect the energy of the incident light to our retinas for visual detection (Figure 2.3). The reflected light has been modified by the object. The light energy that our eyes detect originates from the sun, but after interaction with an intervening object it reflects the object's characteristics in addition to those of the sun. It is important to remember that such a measurement is

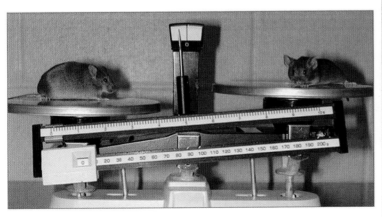

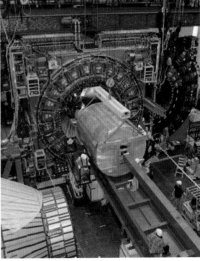

Figure 2.2. Measurement energy: non-destructive use of energy of gravity for measurement of mouse weight; destructive measurements of subatomic particles at Fermilab's Collider Detector using particle beams up to 1 TeV. Courtesy of Lexicon Genetics Incorporated and Fermi National Accelerator Laboratory, respectively.

dependent on both the external source of energy and the object of interest. Most scientific and nearly all biomedical measurements are of energy, not mass, and in most cases the energy detected is derived from an external source.

The detected energy is often called a *signal*, which is an engineering term for a mathematical function of one or more independent variables, such as measurement of light energy varying with time. Signals can be viewed as codified messages that contain information about their source, the sample. The whole measurement or sample/observer process can be thought of as the decoding of signals. Signals are commonly distinguished as either continuous or discrete. A continuous signal may involve any real or complex number, while a discrete signal involves only integers. As previously noted, the universe

Color	Wavelength interval	Frequency interval
Red	~ 625–740 nm	~ 480–405 nm
Orange	~ 590–625 nm	~ 510–480 nm
Yellow	~ 565–590 nm	~ 530–510 nm
Green	~ 520–565 nm	~ 580–530 nm
Cyan	~ 500–520 nm	~ 600–580 nm
Blue	~ 450–500 nm	~ 670–600 nm
Indigo	~ 430–450 nm	~ 700–670 nm
Violet	~ 380–430 nm	~ 790–700 nm

Continuous spectrum

~700 nm   ~550 nm   ~470 nm
Not drawn to scale

Figure 2.3. Visible light portion of EM spectrum. www.knowledgerush.com/kr/encyclopedia/Electromagnetic_spectrum.

and most of its components are continuous and would ideally be described by continuous signals. While some detectors are continuous in nature, such as a mercury thermometer or photographic film, more and more detectors operate in a discrete fashion, including solid-state detectors such as a charge capture device (CCD) camera. Even continuous signals from continuous detector systems often require subsampling of the signal for further transmission or processing. It might be necessary for a variety of reasons for a device to make or report measurements at specific, i.e., discrete, time points. A generic analog-to-digital (A/D) converter is a device that receives continuous input signal, which it intermittently samples and converts into a discrete output signal (Figure 2.4). The discrete output does not include all the information in the original signal and is therefore only an approximation of the original. Computers and other digital devices operate only with discrete signals. Hence, nearly all contemporary measuring systems are discrete. Therefore modern science usually involves discrete numerical approximations of continuous samples.

For measurement purposes, a detected signal must have a number assigned to it.

> When you can measure what you are speaking about, and express it in numbers, you know something about it, but when you cannot express it in numbers, your knowledge is of a meager and unsatisfactory kind; it may be the beginning of knowledge, but you have scarcely in your thoughts advanced to the state of science. Lord Kelvin [1].

A simple measurement M of a sample S by an operator H can be defined similarly to an image, without an explicit spatial component:

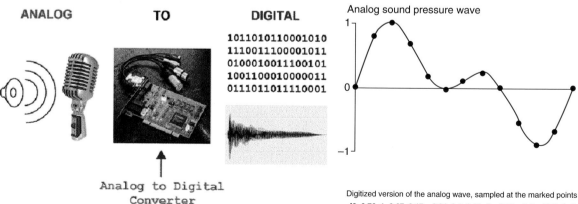

Figure 2.4. Analog-to-digital conversion: discrete temporal sampling of a continuous signal with digital or continuous signal measurements. From Gonzalez R, *The Musician's Guide to Home Recording*, http://home.earthlink.net/~rongonz/home_rec/. Graph C. R. B. Merritt (after M. Ballora, Penn State, with permission).

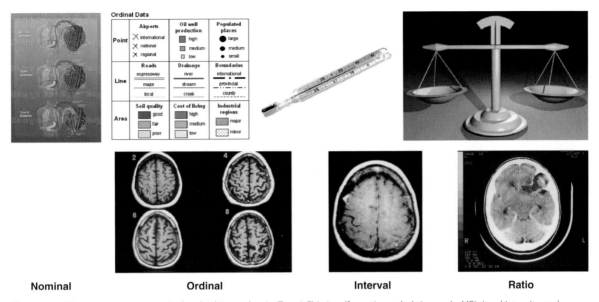

| Nominal | Ordinal | Interval | Ratio |

Figure 2.5. Measurement types: nominal, ordinal, interval, ratio. Type I Chiari malformation, sulcal size grade, MRI signal intensity, and SPECT cpm (counts per minute). Diabetes diagram courtesy of Novo Nordisk Inc. Ordinal table with permission from Natural Resources Canada 2009, courtesy of the Atlas of Canada. Scale courtesy of DOE. Chiari image from Secula RF, Dimensions of the posterior fossa in patients symptomatic for Chiari I malformation but without cerebellar tonsillar descent. *Cerebrospinal Fluid Research* 2005; **2**: 11, with permission.

$$M = \mathbf{H}S \qquad (2.3)$$

$$g(m, E)(t) = \mathbf{H}f(m, E)(t) \qquad (2.4)$$

The operator $\mathbf{H}$ uniquely transforms some observation of the sample in physical space U into a measurement M in some numeric space V.

According to Stevens, there are four types of numerical measurements [2]:

Nominal Discrete data assigning group membership; no order, numerical value, or zero

Ordinal Ordered without numerical value or zero

Interval Ordered with numerical value, arbitrary zero

Ratio Ordered with numerical value and non-arbitrary zero

Each type of measurement has its appropriate role, but for most scientific imaging applications *ratio* measurements are preferred (Figure 2.5). Ratio measurements involve comparison of a detected signal to a standard quantity of the same type. A length measurement, such as the height of a person, is reflected as the ratio of the actual physical measurement to a standard length, such as a standard meter. A two-meter person has a vertical physical measurement that is twice as long as the standard meter. Most scientific measurements are

SI base units		
Name	**Symbol**	**Quantity**
meter	m	length
kilogram	kg	mass
second	s	time
ampere	A	electric current
kelvin	K	thermodynamic temperature
mole	mol	amount of substance
candela	cd	luminous intensity

Figure 2.6. *Système International* (SI) base units for physical measurements. http://en.wikipedia.org/wiki/International_System_of_Units.

ratio measurements based on the scales of *Le système international d'unités* (SI) [3] (Figure 2.6).

Measurement can be considered or modeled as a *mapping*. Mapping is the establishment of *correspondence* among points, objects, or other entities. We shall use the mapping model extensively as it applies to many aspects of imaging. A most ancient application of mapping, *cartography*, involved correspondences between geographical sites and symbols, like dots, on some portable medium, like paper. Early

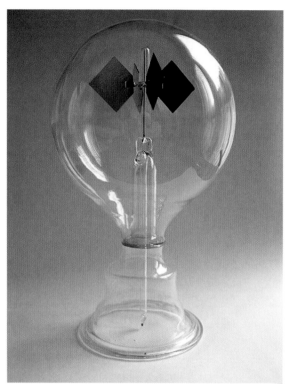

Figure 2.7. Continuous ratio measurement of light intensity. http://en.wikipedia.org/wiki/Radiometer.

geographical maps were amongst the first examples of scientific imaging. In the case of measurement, observations of states of nature are associated with or mapped to numbers of an appropriate numerical system. For instance, a photometer is calibrated to a standard light source of one lumen. It then detects incident light and compares its intensity to the standard. If the incident light is twice as bright as the standard, the instrument maps this ratio of detected signal/standard signal to the number 2 (lumen on the SI light intensity scale) (Figure 2.7). If the instrument next detects a light signal eight-and-a-half times greater than the standard 1 lumen signal, then the new signal will be mapped to the number 8.5 on the SI light scale. If the instrument were a spectrometer rather than a photometer, it would measure the intensity of the incident light as a function of wavelength, rather than overall intensity. However, the numerical mapping process would be the same. The wavelength of the detected signal would be compared to a set of standard visible light wavelengths and assigned to the appropriate number.

Geometrically the numbers to which an observation might be assigned can be thought of as a string of numbers that define a *line* (technically a curve). If the measurement is continuous, the line is a string of continuous numbers; for discrete measurements, the points (numbers) on the line are integers. One line of measurements defines one *dimension* or *metric space* of a sample object.

Measurement error and variability

Somewhat unexpectedly, at least from the eighteenth-century Newtonian perspective, measurements always have variability and therefore uncertainty. The Determinists thought that better measurement techniques and tools would eventually result in perfect measurements that, for a given object, would consistently produce one number. Variability in a particular measurement was considered a result of *measurement error*. Lagrange and Laplace formally incorporated this concept of measurement error into science and measurement. A specific formulation of an *error function* is defined for a Gaussian random variable (to be defined later):

$$erf(\mu) = \frac{2}{\sqrt{\pi}} \int_0^u e^{-x^2} dx \qquad (2.5)$$

The goal of measurement was to completely eliminate error. However, experience and now theory reveal that there is always variability, and therefore uncertainty, to any and all measurements. Hence the earlier goal of error elimination has been modified to one of error reduction and statistical analysis. While there remains a constant goal of error reduction, there is also an imperative to explicitly incorporate variability into all scientific statistical processes. This thinking reflects the evolution of science and scientific measurement from a *deterministic* to a *stochastic* or *probabilistic* process.

There are many sources of measurement variability, including those due to the sample itself, those due to the environment of the sample, and those due to the measurement process. Examples include sample randomness, interfering signals, observational errors, sampling errors, instrument errors, systematic errors, etc. In many cases the variability is unpredictable or random. A numerical quantity associated with unpredictable events or experimental results is defined as a *random variable*. Random variables may be continuous or discrete, and they have three attributes: an estimate (of truth), an error bound, and a probability that the true measurement lies within the error bound of the estimate.

Measurement variability can be directly reflected by a series of repeated measurements of a random

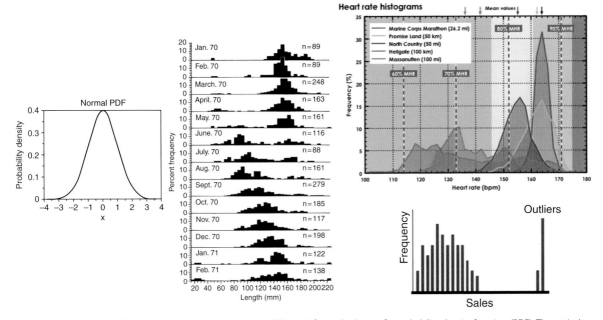

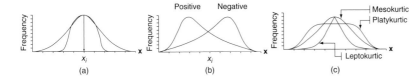

Figure 2.8. A frequency histogram shows measurement variability and forms the basis of a probability density function (PDF). Theoretical normal distribution and experimental samples of fish characteristics, marathon runner's heart rates, and sales volumes, the latter with "outliers." Diamond turbot length courtesy of California Department of Fish and Game. Heart rate by Keith Knipling.

Figure 2.9. PDF parameters: (a) mean and standard deviation, (b) skew, and (c) kurtosis.

variable. This is often graphically illustrated by a frequency histogram showing the relative number of times (frequency) that any particular measurement is made from a sample (Figure 2.8). Such a display directly reflects the *distribution* of the measurements and their frequency of occurrence. If the sum of all frequencies is normalized to 1, then the histogram also reflects the *probability*, P, of making any particular measurement. The data now define a *probability distribution*, with the y-axis giving the probability for any measurement point on the x-axis (probability having values of 0 to 1, with 1 equaling certainty). There is a probability distribution associated with any set of measurements, though it may not be known. The data of a probability distribution can be defined by a *probability density function* (PDF), which provides a statistical description of the probability distribution (of a continuous random variable):

$$P(a \leq x \leq b) = \int_a^b p(x)dx \qquad (2.6)$$

This function allows the calculation of the probability that a random variable x falls within the interval (a,b). A set of measurements from any sample has its unique PDF, and since there are potentially an infinite number of samples, there are an infinite number and variety of PDFs. However, any PDF has the following properties:

$$p(x) \geq 0 \qquad (2.7)$$

$$\int_{-\infty}^{+\infty} p(x)dx = 1 \qquad (2.8)$$

While a PDF describes the complete data set, it is not always available nor is it an easy construct to work with. For this reason, summary measures are often desired. A PDF can be summarized by four parameters: mean, standard variation, skew, and kurtosis (Figure 2.9). These are the *descriptive statistics* of the data. The *mean*, μ, is the best estimate of the true value x or the *expected value*, E(x), of the random variable and is the single most important descriptor:

43

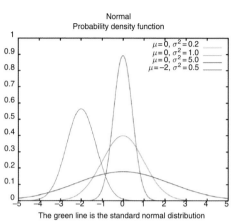

Normal
Probability density function

$\mu = 0, \sigma^2 = 0.2$
$\mu = 0, \sigma^2 = 1.0$
$\mu = 0, \sigma^2 = 5.0$
$\mu = -2, \sigma^2 = 0.5$

The green line is the standard normal distribution

Parameters	μ location (real) $\sigma^2 > 0$ squared scale (real)
Support	$x \in \mathbb{R}$
Probability density function (pdf)	$\frac{1}{\sigma\sqrt{2\pi}} \exp\left(-\frac{(x-\mu)^2}{2\sigma^2}\right)$
Cumulative distribution function (cdf)	$\frac{1}{2} + \frac{1}{2}\mathrm{erf}\left(\frac{x-\mu}{\sigma\sqrt{2}}\right)$
Mean	μ
Median	μ
Mode	μ
Variance	σ^2
Skewness	0
Excess kurtosis	0
Entropy	$\ln \sigma\sqrt{2\pi e}$
Moment-generating function (mgf)	$M_x(t) = \exp\left(\mu t + \frac{\sigma^2 t^2}{2}\right)$
Characteristic function	$\chi_x(t) = \exp\left(\mu i t - \frac{\sigma^2 t^2}{2}\right)$

Figure 2.10. Normal Gaussian distribution. From http://en.wikipedia.org/wiki/Normal_distribution.

$$\mu = E\{x\} = \int_{-\infty}^{+\infty} xp(x)dx \qquad (2.9)$$

In terms of the PDF, the mean is its center of gravity or, in keeping with the previous use of the mapping analogy, the mean is the best estimate of the *location* of the true value along the measurement line. The next important descriptor is the *variance*, σ^2, which is a measure of the spread of the random variable about its mean:

$$\sigma^2 = \mathrm{Var}\{x\} = E\{(x-\mu)^2\} = \int_{-\infty}^{+\infty} (x-\mu)^2 p(x)dx \qquad (2.10)$$

Skew and *kurtosis* further describe the shape of the PDF, with the former being a measure of symmetry about the mean, while the latter is a measure of the convexity of the peak. While there are an infinite variety of PDFs, it turns out that most can be reasonably summarized by a small number of relatively simple PDF models, a few of which will now be illustrated.

Consider weighing a piece of gold with a very sensitive analog scale. Repeated measurements create the PDF illustrated in Figure 2.10. Many types of measurements, particularly those involving continuous numbers, have a distribution such as this that approximates the classical "bell-shaped curve," which is defined as a *Gaussian distribution*. A *normal* Gaussian distribution is mathematically described as:

$$p(x) = \left(\frac{1}{2\pi\sigma^2}\right)^{1/2} \exp\left[-\frac{x^2}{2\sigma^2}\right], \quad -\infty < x < \infty \qquad (2.11)$$

This standard *normal distribution* has a unit area of one and a mean of zero. The mean and variance of a non-normalized Gaussian distribution are defined as:

$$\mu = \int_{-\infty}^{+\infty} xp(x)dx \qquad (2.12)$$

$$\sigma^2 = \int_{-\infty}^{+\infty} (x-\mu)^2 p(x)dx \qquad (2.13)$$

The Gaussian distribution function is fully characterized by just these two parameters. The mean of a Gaussian distribution is the maximum peak height of the curve, about which all other measurements are symmetrically distributed. The variability or spread of the peak is often reported as σ, the *standard deviation* (which reflects the inflection points of the curve), rather than σ^2. The standard deviation is well characterized and encompasses approximately 68% of the measurements. The normal distribution allows easy comparison of many random variables by such statistical tools as the *z*-score.

While many scientific measurements are well characterized by a Gaussian distribution, some important ones are not, such as the decay rate of a radionuclide, which has a *Poisson distribution*, and the width of

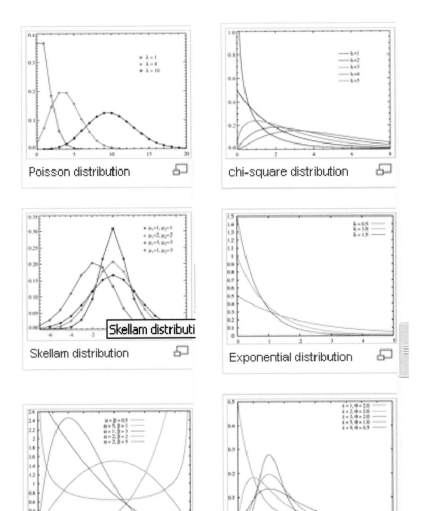

Figure 2.11. Non-Gaussian distributions. All from the www.wikipedia.org articles bearing their names.

an NMR spectral peak, which has a *Lorentzian distribution* (Figure 2.11). Non-Gaussian distributions will be presented where needed for specific applications, but unless otherwise stated this introductory discussion will assume normal Gaussian distributions. Furthermore, the *central limit theorem* states that the sum of a large number of identically distributed independent variables is approximately normal. Therefore in many cases the normal distribution can be used as an approximation of other distributions, further justifying our attention to this particular distribution.

Multidimensional measurements

By the process of detecting a signal and mapping it to a number along a line, a measurement describing one feature or dimension of the sample has been performed. A sample may have many features that one might want to measure, each of which can be considered an additional variable. Consider the environment of a forest that has many descriptive components such as temperature, humidity, oxygen and CO_2 concentrations, wind, etc. (Figure 2.12). A measurement of any single environmental parameter provides a very incomplete description of the forest; the more parameters measured, the richer the description. If each individual measurement of a variable is independent of all other measurements of this same variable, it is a *random variable*. If the measurement of a random variable is independent of the measurement of other random variables, it is an

45

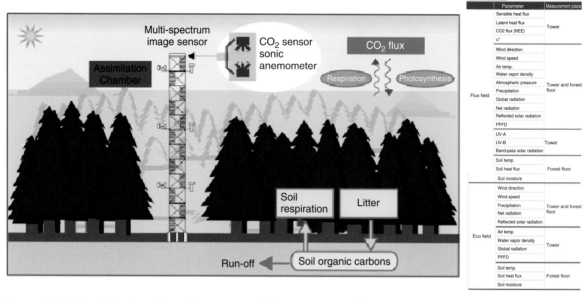

Figure 2.12. Multimodality observations and measurements of a forest. From Center for Global Environmental Research, National Institute for Environmental Studies.

independent random variable. We are often interested in the relationships or functions of two (or more) random variables. Similar to describing a single set of events or random variable by a PDF as in Equation 2.8, the behavior of two sets of events reflected by two random variables x and y can be described by a *joint PDF*, $p(x, y)$, which if normalized satisfies:

$$\int\limits_{-\infty}^{+\infty} \int\limits_{-\infty}^{+\infty} p(x', y') dx' dy' = 1 \qquad (2.14)$$

A number of simple relationships follow, for instance the sum of two random variables, $z = x + y$:

$$\mu_z = \mu_x + \mu_y \qquad (2.15)$$

For statistically independent variables their joint PDF can be expressed:

$$p(x, y) = p(x)p(y) \qquad (2.16)$$

This definition of an independent variable is different from the definition that distinguishes known (independent) variables from unknown (dependent) variables in an algebraic expression. For independent random variables, the variances of the underlying variables also add:

$$\sigma_z^2 = \sigma_x^2 + \sigma_y^2 \qquad (2.17)$$

Each variable reflects one dimension or metric space. Multiple variables can reflect measurements of N

dimensions in an N-dimensional space. Measuring the length of a cube would be a one-dimensional measurement (along a line); measuring the length and width of a cube would a two-dimensional measurement; measuring the length, width, and depth of a cube would be a three-dimensional measurement (Figure 2.13). Three dimensions happen to fully describe physical space, but physical space is just one example of a three-dimensional space. MRI signal characteristics can be described by a 3D space of spin-density, T_1 and T_2, none of which relates to physical space. While often used interchangeably, variable, dimension, and (metric) space may have different definitions in different applications and should always be carefully defined. For instance, in the physics community the dimensions of an object are often limited to mass, length, and time, with dimension being limited to fundamental characteristics of an object. In some mathematical applications, any variable can be considered a dimension in an infinite dimensional space.

If points in a metric space follow the axioms and postulates of Euclid, then it is called a *Euclidean space*. In Euclidean geometry, one dimension defines a line, two independent dimensions define a plane, and three independent dimensions define a 3D space. A Euclidean 3D space describes physical space sufficiently to have allowed Euclidean geometry and its mathematics to model our universe for over 2000 years. Over the past two centuries important non-Euclidean spaces have been defined and have proved essential for better describing certain aspects

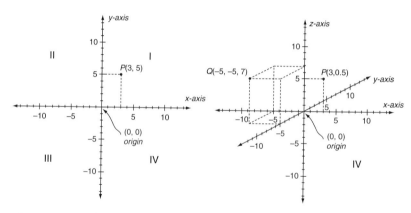

Figure 2.13. Multidimensional measurements (2 and 3) in Euclidean (Cartesian) geometric space. http://en.wikipedia.org/wiki/Cartesian_coordinate_system, by Gustavb.

of nature, particularly the quantum world. For our immediate discussion, Euclidean space will suffice, though later we will introduce other spaces, such as the more inclusive *Hilbert space*.

While there is a fundamental physical difference in m, E, space, and time, there is no mathematical difference. Mathematically, each can be handled as a dimension or metric space. Any component of the universe can be considered a dimension and represented as a series of point measurements along a line. The three spatial dimensions are orthogonally fixed to each other, and at every point in this 3D space, m,E extends in a fourth orthogonal dimension. These four dimensions extend orthogonally along the fifth dimension – time. While perhaps easily expressed mathematically, high-dimensional space is not necessarily intuitive or easy to envision. Nature depends greatly on the uniqueness of the three physical domains, m,E, space, and time; mathematics often ignores the restrictions of these physical domains.

Euclidean geometry and mathematics allow an infinite number of spaces, none of which is required to be of physical space. In this mathematical sense, an object may have many dimensions, some spatial, some not. Most scientific images involve at least four dimensions – one m,E, two spatial, plus a static time point. A cine "3D" image includes all three spatial dimensions, plus at least one m,E dimension, plus a dynamic time dimension. A metric space or dimension is just a series of numbers along a line representing a set of measurements.

All natural dimensions are unknown until observed. A completely naive observer does not know in advance anything about m,E, space, or time. However, in the case of scientific measurements, some of the dimensions are predefined by the observer. Time is usually fixed at specific sampling times. With imaging, physical space is often predefined. That is, the spatial locations of the m,E measurements are predetermined by the imaging device. The imaging device

defines the time and location of unknown m,E measurements. The goal of the imaging system is to make an m,E measurement for every prescribed location within the image. The m,E measurement is therefore *dependent* on its location and time of measurement. In this case the unknown m,E measurement x is a *dependent variable* of the predefined *independent variables* space and time: $(x,y,z)(t)$. Note this second definition of independent variable. In a typical one-dimensional, non-imaging measurement, space and time are not explicitly expressed, and the m,E measurement is simply the dependent variable (x) of the function f or $f(x)$. Likewise for imaging measurements, the independent functions are often not explicitly expressed: the image is simply expressed as the function $g(x)$. The imaging equation, for a deterministic system, can then be reduced to:

$$g(x) = \mathbf{H}f(x) \qquad (2.18)$$

For most scientific imaging, m,E is the dependent variable while space and time are independent variables.

Imaging measurements

Imaging is always multidimensional, involving at least one unknown/dependent m,E dimension or variable; one, two, or three known/predefined/independent spatial variables; and the often-implicit time dimension. A typical "2D" image consisting of one m,E dimension, two spatial dimensions, and one point in the time dimension may be statistically displayed on a printed page or computer monitor (Figure 2.14). However, advanced imaging technology increasingly measures multiple m,E dimensions spatially defined in three dimensions with frequent time sampling. This would be a multidimensional, "3D" image displayed cinematically. The unique and critical aspect of imaging measurements is that they are spatially defined. For each

47

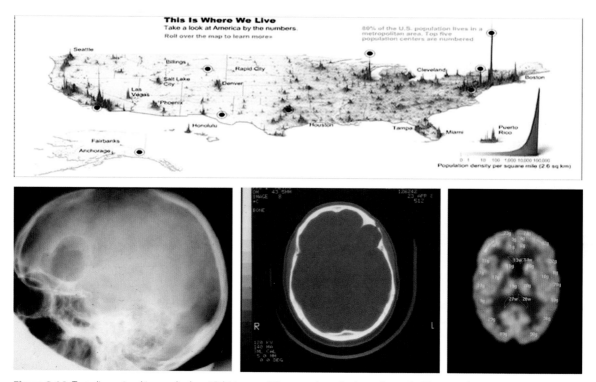

Figure 2.14. Two-dimensional image displays: 3D histogram; 2D gray-scale projection radiograph; 2D gray-scale x-ray CT scan; 2D color-scale PET scan with ROIs. Data from U.S. Census Bureau and LandScan 2003/UT-Battelle, LLC, graphic ©2006 Time Inc. All rights reserved. Reprinted by permission. PET scan courtesy of A. Newberg.

picture element, *pixel*, in a 2D planar image, or volume element, *voxel*, in a 3D volumetric image, at least one m,E measurement is made. Each m,E measurement is an estimate of some true physical value at a specific location and will have appropriate statistical properties associated with it, though this is often not reflected in a displayed image. This important information is, however, available and should be appropriately used in any related quantitative analysis of the image. For a 3D medical MRI, each of the three spatial dimensions would be sampled 128 times at approximately 1 mm intervals, resulting in a $128 \times 128 \times 128$ 3D image that contains 2 097 152 voxels. Using a minimal 8-bit gray-scale display, such a 3D image would contain approximately 16 Mbits of data. Until recently such large data sets provided major technological challenges; however, with contemporary digital tools, large data volumes have become more of a nuisance than a real limitation.

The necessity of making spatially defined measurements in imaging introduces additional opportunities for variability and errors. Obviously there is statistical variability in each voxel's m,E measurement, so a large object within an image scene might be represented by many voxels whose aggregate numbers will form a sample

distribution. For instance, a 1 cm^3 volume of liver imaged at 1 mm isotropic resolution on a CT scan might contain 1000 voxels with HU (Hounsfield unit) mean of 30, SD 5. The measurement variability in this sample will be secondary to actual liver tissue variability (spatial heterogeneity), plus measurement variability with its two potential components, non-random systematic errors or bias, and random noise for each voxel.

In addition, there is the possibility of variability and error in spatially defining or locating the source of the signal measurement. That is, imaging offers the additional opportunity of spatial measurement errors. Spatial errors are due to limitations of imaging systems to precisely define, limit, and report the location of each m,E measurement. An ideal imaging system would make perfect m,E measurements at precisely defined points in the sample (scene/object space U) and accurately transform those measurements and their locations into image space (V). An imaging system's spatial mapping from U to V is usually not perfect, and measurements from a single point may get displaced or blurred over adjacent voxels. Spatial error and variability can and should be defined for every imaging system.

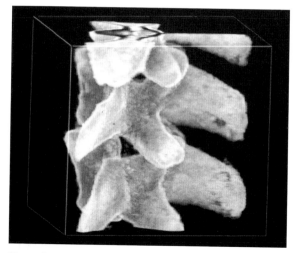

Figure 2.15. High-resolution x-ray CT scan of mouse spine. Courtesy of F. Wehrli.

Imaging systems

Technologically, imaging presents two challenges: first and foremost, how to make not one, but many spatially defined measurements, and second, how to handle and display these data. Different types of imaging systems perform their m,E measurements in unique fashions that sample a particular signal of interest. Spatial localization of the m,E measurements is also system-dependent, though there are some commonalities among imaging methodologies for this purpose. Temporal definition or sampling is limited by how fast individual images can be made. Before describing how specific imaging systems work, let's first examine some general features of any imaging system.

Model imaging system

An ideal imaging system or operator **H** would make a perfect representation of the object; the system would accurately map every m,E measurement of every object point to a geometrically corresponding region of the image. There should be no error in the quantitative mapping of the m,E measurements to numbers, nor should there be spatial errors or distortions of the signal's locations. No system does this perfectly, but well-designed and well-operated contemporary imaging systems do a remarkably good job. A high-resolution x-ray CT image of a mouse has signal (HU) measurement errors of less than 0.5% with spatial accuracy of approximately 200 microns (Figure 2.15).

The complete description of an imaging system is complex, but can be greatly simplified by the use of appropriate models. In engineering terms a system, **H**,

takes an input signal, performs some operation on that signal and produces an output signal, $g(x) = \mathbf{H} f(x)$, as in Equation 2.18. However, all measurements, including imaging measurements, are confounded by signals that do not derive from or accurately reflect the sample. Some of these confusing signals are secondary to the measurement – imaging – system, but are predictable and result in measurement *bias*. While undesirable, such measurement errors can often be retrospectively adjusted or "removed." More problematic is *noise*, which is unpredictable, random, confounds the measurements, and cannot be explicitly extracted from the data. This necessitates a modification to the previous deterministic expression for an imaging system. Noise must be explicitly incorporated into the model, which now is a *stochastic* or probabilistic model:

$$g(x) = \mathbf{H} f(x) + n \qquad (2.19)$$

The input and output signals, including noise, may be continuous (C) or discrete (D). Systems that have continuous input and output numbers are continuous/continuous (CC) systems, and there are correlating DD, CD, and DC systems. As most scenes, patterns, and objects in nature are continuous, CC systems might theoretically be preferred. Furthermore, the underlying mathematics of CC systems is common integral transforms. Hence, for this introduction to imaging systems we will often assume CC systems. Remember, however, that most scientific imaging systems are CD or, even more often, DD. The mathematics of these systems will be presented separately.

An imaging system, defined as the *operator* **H**, transforms or maps the scene or object $f(x)$ to an image $g(x)$. A common mathematical model of the operator **H** is that of a *linear shift-invariant system* (LSIV) (see Appendix 1). In a linear system, if the input consists of a weighted summation of several signals (f_1, af_2, bf_3), the output will also be a weighted summation of the responses of the system to each individual input signal:

$$\mathbf{H}\left[f_1 + af_2 + bf_3\right] = \mathbf{H} f_1 + \mathbf{H} af_2 + \mathbf{H} bf_3 \qquad (2.20)$$

The image of an ensemble of signals will be the same as the sum of individual images of each signal. Infinitesimally small perturbations of the input signal will be reflected by infinitesimally small perturbations of the output signal. The linear model includes a class of relatively simple systems that are tractable and enjoy a number of practical properties. If the input – object, $f(\mathbf{r})$ – and output – image, $g(\mathbf{r}_d)$ – of a linear system are

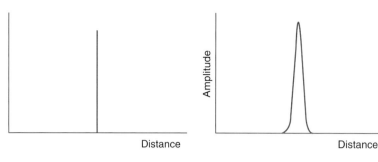

Figure 2.16. Dirac delta function "instantaneous" input function; blurred output function. C. R. B. Merritt.

continuous (CC), then the action of the system can be described by a linear integral transform:

$$g(\mathbf{r}_d) = \int_{S_j} d^q r h(\mathbf{r}_d, \mathbf{r}) f(\mathbf{r}) \qquad (2.21)$$

Abstractly, and more simply, this integral can be expressed as:

$$g = \mathbf{H}f \qquad (2.22)$$

where f and g are Hilbert-space vectors and $\mathbf{H}$ is now defined as a linear operator as in Equation 2.19. With noise, the mapping from object to image space becomes $g = \mathbf{H}f + n$.

Another important and simplifying model assumption is that of shift invariance. In a *shift-invariant* system, the origin of the input signal (in time or space) does not affect the operator, i.e., there is no preferred origin of the system. An arbitrary shift or translation of the input signal results in an identical translation in the output signal:

$$\text{if } f_{xoyo}(x, y) = f(x - x_o, y - y_o)$$
$$\text{then} \quad g(x - x_o, y - y_o) \qquad (2.23)$$

For an LSIV spatial system in q dimensions, the output is given by:

$$g(\mathbf{r}_d) = \int_{\infty} d^q r h(\mathbf{r}_d - \mathbf{r}) f(\mathbf{r}) \qquad (2.24)$$

Shift invariance reduces the complexity of $\mathbf{H}$ and allows the *convolution* operation:

$$g(\mathbf{r}_d) = [h * f](\mathbf{r}_d) = h(\mathbf{r}_d) * f(\mathbf{r}_d) \qquad (2.25)$$

For our immediate purposes only, CC LSIV systems will be considered. In practice, most imaging systems, certainly most biomedical imaging systems, approximate this mathematical and engineering model.

Image quality

As previously noted, the necessity of spatially defining m,E measurements creates additional opportunities

for error. In particular, there is opportunity for error in defining or reporting the location of a signal. A metric is needed for this type of imaging error, which we will now define. Start with a signal source from a very small region of the sample, a *point source* or *point impulse*. A point source can be considered a very (infinitely) large signal from a very (infinitely) small spatial region. Mathematically this can be modeled as a *delta function* defined as:

$$\delta(x - x_0) = 0 \quad \text{if } x \neq x_0 \qquad (2.26)$$

From an imaging perspective, this function can be depicted as a very large signal $f(x_0)$ at a single point, x_0, along the spatial dimension x in object space U (Figure 2.16). An ideal imaging system would perfectly transform the magnitude of this signal to a single point along the spatial dimension x in image space V. However, no real imaging system does this. Instead, the image signal function $g(x)$ is extended or blurred over a number of adjacent points in image space. This distorted signal is commonly called the *point response function* (PRF), *impulse response*, or under certain circumstances is equivalent to the *kernel* of the imaging system. Using the definition of $\mathbf{H}$ as a continuous linear operator and the sifting property of the delta function, the PRF can be represented as.

$$h(\mathbf{r}_d, \mathbf{r}_0) = [\mathbf{H}\delta(\mathbf{r} - \mathbf{r}_0)(\mathbf{r}_d)]$$
$$= \lim_{k \to \infty} [\mathbf{H}d_k(\mathbf{r} - \mathbf{r}_0)](\mathbf{r}_d) \qquad (2.27)$$

The PRF reflects the spatial blurring of the system and defines limits of its spatial resolution. This blurring occurs along any sampled spatial dimension; the PRF can be depicted as blurred points, lines, or balls in 1-, 2-, or 3D images, respectively (Figure 2.17). The PRF could vary with the location of the source within the object, but not in the case of an LSIV system. Therefore, in a two- (spatial) dimension LSIV system, the four-dimensional PRF is reduced to a two-dimensional *point spread function* (PSF).

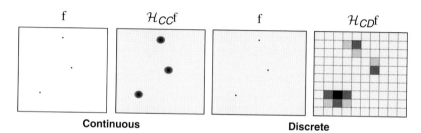

Figure 2.17. Image operator performance metrics: point spread function (PSF) and point response function (PRF) of continuous input function and continuous and discrete output functions. C. R. B. Merritt, after Barrett HH and Myers KJ, *Foundations of Image Science*, Wiley, 2004.

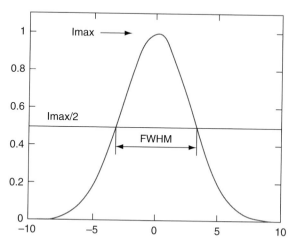

Figure 2.18. Full width at half maximum (FWHM), the distance between the points on a PSF intensity curve that are half of the maximum signal, is a common metric of spatial resolution. C. R. B. Merritt.

the imaging system itself. If the point source and PRF are known for all points in an object and image, then the imaging system **H** can be completely defined, though this is seldom feasible:

$$\text{Imaging formula:} \quad g(x) - f(x) = \mathbf{H}f(x) - f(x) \tag{2.29}$$

$$\text{Solve for } \mathbf{H}: \quad \mathbf{H} = f(x) - g(x) \tag{2.30}$$

Real imaging systems

In this section representative components of specific imaging systems will be briefly presented for the purpose of illustrating some general principles of imaging methodology. In subsequent chapters common contemporary biomedical imaging systems will be more fully described. Before we consider each of these factors individually, it is important to review the limits of our discussion. Scientific images for our purposes consist of measurements of nature (broadly defined) that explicitly reflect at least one and usually two spatial dimensions of the sample. The signals detected are of some form of energy, though such signals may be indirectly related to mass. At some point the images are to be observed by the human visual system. Given these constraints, let us now briefly examine some specific elements of imaging systems.

For any imaging system there are key factors that should always be well defined and understood. The physical nature of the m,E signal to be detected is obviously important, as it is the basic measurement to be made. Intimately related to the signal is the source of the signal. While signal is necessary for imaging measurements, it alone is not sufficient in terms of providing useful information. After all, it is the sample, i.e., the patient, not the signal that is of primary interest. Critical to the information content of an image is how the signal relates to the sample. What does the signal tell us about the sample? Two critical aspects of the signal/sample relationship are the signal

The PRF defines the spatial resolution of the system, but a full PRF is difficult to obtain, much less display, and more practical descriptions of the *spatial resolution* of imaging systems are often used, particularly the *full width at half maximum* (FWHM) of the PRF. Using the histogram display of Figure 2.18 for a one-dimensional image, the FWHM of a particular point *x* is simply the width of the intensity/location histogram at half the maximum height of the peak, or:

$$\delta_{FWHM}(x_0) = x_{d+} - x_{d-} \tag{2.28}$$

PRFs are often well approximated by a Gaussian distribution, and can be easily extended to multiple spatial dimensions. In terms of spatial resolution, FWHM is commonly taken as the smallest dimension that can be resolved by a particular imaging system, but great care should be taken when using this limited measure.

While the PRF can be used to describe how well the imaging system **H** did its job of transforming the signal $f(x)$ from object space to the corresponding signal $g(x)$ in image space, the PRF, in conjunction with the input function, can also be used to describe

Table 2.1. m,E signals

Electromagnetic (EM) radiation
  Wave-like
    Radio waves
    Microwaves
    Infrared
    Visible light
    Ultraviolet
    Low-energy x-rays
  Particles
    Neutrons
    Protons
    Heavy ions
    High-energy x-rays
    Gamma rays
  Quasi-static fields
    Geomagnetic
    Biomagnetic
    Bioelectric fields
    Electrical impedance
Non-EM energy
  Waves
    Seismic
    Water
    Ultrasound
    De Broglie

There are many types of physical signals measured by contemporary imaging systems, a few of which are categorized in Table 2.1. The two most common imaging signals are (1) *electromagnetic radiation*, described by particle and wave characteristics, and (2) non-electromagnetic energy, usually having wave-like characteristics. High-energy physics makes measurements of and with atomic particles and high-energy, short-wavelength electromagnetic radiation, whereas biomedical imaging usually involves signals from longer-wavelength, lower-energy electromagnetic radiation. The latter are less likely to significantly alter the sample, while the former are more likely to damage or even destroy the sample. The most common biomedical imaging signals are electromagnetic radiation in the forms of x- and gamma rays, visible light, infrared light, and radio waves. Quasi-static electrical and magnetic fields are used to create corresponding images of organs such as the brain. Various forms of mechanical waves provide a number of signals appropriate for imaging, such as ultrasound, which is the major biomedical non-electromagnetic imaging signal.

Imaging, at least non-invasive imaging, requires that the measurement energy exit the sample in order to reach a detector. This requirement implies and requires that the energy flows or propagates not only from its source to a detector, but also through and beyond the sample. The movement or propagation of energy is termed *radiation*, and imaging generally requires some form of radiation. Scientific samples can emit their own radiation or they can reflect, scatter, or transmit radiation from an external source. The goal of the imaging system is to make measurements based on these emitted, reflected, scattered, or transmitted signals from the sample. The detector in an imaging system responds to the energy radiated from the sample. The detected energy reflects characteristics of the sample; these characteristics are the encoded information about the sample that must be decoded by the system in order to communicate sample information to the observer.

Most, though not all, imaging systems detect some form of electromagnetic (EM) radiation, and thus for introductory purposes we shall use the propagation of EM radiation as a generic model of energy flow. Energy flow can be described in terms of classical electromagnetic theory by the flow of the energy density of an EM field, with:

source and how the signal physically interacts with the sample. The preceding factors relate to m,E measurements, but equally important from the imaging perspective is the spatial localization of the measurements. How are measurements spatially defined? Finally, one needs to define how an actual image recognizable by a human is created from the many individual m,E measurements. In some cases the imaging system directly constructs an image, literally makes a picture. In other cases, the measurement data itself is not something that is recognizable by a human observer, so an image must be *reconstructed*, generally by some mathematical process and a computer. All of these factors contribute to the creation of scientific images, and they can be simply classified as follows: signal, sample, detection, and image. We will now briefly consider each one in turn.

Signal

The m,E signal to be measured might be more appropriately considered a property of the scene or object to be imaged than the imaging system itself. This is certainly true of m,E signals that originate from the object being imaged. However, in many imaging applications, the signal being measured does not originate from the sample, but is imposed on the sample. In this case, the signal is part of the imaging system. In either case the physical nature of the signal is so intimately related to the imaging system that we shall consider it a component thereof.

$$u_e = \frac{\varepsilon_0}{2} E^2 \qquad (2.31)$$

representing the electric field density and:

$$u_m = \frac{1}{2u_0} B^2 \qquad (2.32)$$

representing the magnetic field density.

Using these expressions of the components of the electromagnetic field, both the volumetric density and the flow of energy of an EM field can be calculated:

$$S = \frac{1}{u} E \times B \qquad (2.33)$$

This is the Poynting vector, which gives the density of the flow of energy and its direction. This vector has dimensions of power per unit area and provides a measure of energy flow. Energy density has dimensions of energy per unit volume and describes the energy stored in the electrical and magnetic fields. The propagation of an EM field through space is described by the full development of these formulae. While electrodynamics can fully describe the flow of an energy field, it is often more useful to describe energy transport in terms of quanta of radiation – *photons*. This quantized energy of EM radiation has discrete energy levels, the spacing between levels being equal to:

$$E = h\nu \qquad (2.34)$$

where h is the Planck constant and ν is the frequency of the radiation.

These complex principles of physics can be grossly simplified by considering signal energy simply as propagating particles and waves – streaming balls and flowing waves. Propagating waves can be characterized by velocity, frequency, phase, amplitude, and direction. Propagating particles can be characterized by mass, number, velocity, and direction. These are the basic characteristics of the signal energy. Hence, any interaction of the propagating energy with the sample will result in changes in one of more of these basic signal characteristics.

Each m,E signal has a specific source, but there may be more than one type of physical source for any given signal. For instance, solar nuclear reactions produce many different forms of electromagnetic radiation, including gamma rays, x-rays, infrared, and visible light, all of which can be used to make images. However, for medical imaging, x-rays are generated by a Crookes tube (modified cathode ray tube) whereas ultrasound waves are produced by piezoelectric crystals. The signal source defines the physical nature and spatial origins of the signal. Other than sharing general

Table 2.2. Signal source

Intrinsic signal (passive Imaging)
  Natural
    Infrared
    Magnetic field
    Electric field
  Unnatural
    Infrared
    Visible light
    Gamma rays
Extrinsic (active imaging)
  Radio waves
  X-rays
  Ultrasound

particle or wave characteristics, the exact physical features of different signals are relatively unique and will be discussed in more detail in later chapters.

In terms of both engineering and information content, the source of the imaging signal is critical. Perhaps the most important aspect of this factor is whether or not the signal originates from the sample itself, or whether the signal originates external to the sample. Table 2.2 distinguishes images on this basis. With an intrinsic signal, the energy to be measured is spontaneously emitted from the sample. With *spontaneous emission imaging*, no energy is added to the sample and the examination is therefore, by definition, *non-invasive* and *non-destructive* – at least no more destructive than the sample is to itself. Furthermore, the signal is directly and uniquely reflective of the sample. Hence the source signal itself is of primary interest. Since intrinsic signals contain the information of interest, it is generally preferable that they not otherwise interact with or be modified by the sample or its environment. Ideally the original signal would not interact with any contents of an imaging scene from within which it originated. If the source signal were to interact with other contents of the scene, the detected signal would contain information not only about the source but about other components of the scene as well. While technically an imaging system that detects a naturally occurring intrinsic sample signal does not include a signal source, for practical purposes it does.

Visible light, an intrinsic, emitted signal from the star Betelgeuse, may allow it to be imaged. However, if that light signal is attenuated or blocked by clouds, which become components of the scene presented to an earthbound telescope, then the image will be compromised. The detected light signal reflects both the source (star) and extraneous scene (cloud) information, the former being of primary interest, the latter only a nuisance. Likewise, if the light signal is diffracted by the earth's atmosphere, then the location of the signal source will be inaccurately mapped and the image will have spatial errors. An intrinsic sample signal contains the desired information, and it is preferable that the signal not interact with anything other than the detector, including other parts of the sample itself. Solutions to decrease intrinsic signal corruption from the scene environment include removing surrounding material (vacuum), isolating the sample from extraneous signals (Faraday shield), and placing signal detectors as close as possible to the sample. Images of Mars from the Hubble Space Telescope are superior to those from earth telescopes not only because the detector is located closer to the star but also because it is beyond earth's atmosphere, eliminating atmospheric signals from the scene (Figure 2.19). There are other reasons to have detectors as near as possible to signal sources, as we shall see.

While energy originating from the sample might be preferable for imaging measurements, since it would generally be non-destructive and yield information directly about and only from the sample, such signals are not common in biomedical applications. The intrinsic EM energy of many outer-space objects such as suns, pulsars, etc. is immense and sufficient for direct sample imaging. Emission products from naturally radioactive samples offer very useful signals for a variety of scientific applications, including the characterization and dating of geological and anthropological samples (Figure 2.20). However, such samples are either considered spatially uniform, in which case there is no need for imaging, or are of such low energy content that there is insufficient signal for the multiple, spatially defined measurements required for imaging. Most biological samples do not spontaneously emit energy that is of sufficient strength or nature to allow imaging on the basis of an intrinsic signal source.

A rare example of a biomedical imaging technique that is a function of a natural, intrinsic signal is *thermography*. Thermography is dependent on infrared (IR) signal generated by the natural thermal energy of the body. The thermal energy of the body and the associated IR signal is of very low energy, but it propagates well through space, even the earth's foggy atmosphere. While human retinal photodetectors are not sensitive to IR, IR-sensitive film and solid-state detectors are, and IR imaging is routinely used by the military for "night vision." IR energy is sufficient to penetrate several centimeters of body tissue, varies between different physiological and disease states,

and therefore has been used for imaging superficial disease processes such as breast cancer (Figure 2.21).

The signal content of a sample can be modified by injecting or *labeling* the sample with a signal source that might then be imaged. Artificially labeled samples emit an intrinsic signal, but an unnatural one. Sample labeling is invasive and potentially destructive. However, the distribution and behavior of the introduced signal can reveal important information about the sample. As with a natural intrinsic signal, any interaction with the sample by an unnatural intrinsic signal is generally undesirable, although likely to occur. Biomedical nuclear imaging is performed by injecting a radioactive compound into a sample (such as a patient) and imaging the location and intensity of the energy emitted by the radioactive material. For instance, ^{123}I is a radioactive form of iodine with a half-life of 13.3 hours that is produced by a cyclotron and decays by electron capture, emitting 159 keV photons. These gamma rays have sufficient energy to travel through the body of a patient and be detected by an external *gamma detector*, a nuclear medicine imaging device. In the body, iodine is preferentially metabolized by and therefore accumulates in normal and cancerous thyroid tissue (Figure 2.22). Hence ^{123}I injected into a patient will preferentially concentrate in the normal thyroid gland and in primary and metastatic thyroid tumors. The ^{123}I signal is an artificial internal signal, but its location and concentration are of great diagnostic value. Any alteration to the original signal will compromise the information contained therein. In practice, the ^{123}I signal interacts with adjacent tissues, where it is scattered and absorbed, particularly by bone. Scattered signal limits the spatial accuracy of the image, and absorption falsely lowers the magnitude of the detected signal, in some cases sufficiently to completely mask the presence of a tumor. While some of this signal/sample interaction can be corrected in retrospect by *attenuation correction*, signal/sample interaction results in the loss of information from any internal signal.

Measurement energy need not originate from the sample itself, but can also derive from an external source. If a sample does not have a measurable internal source of energy, the sample might still be imaged by applying external energy to it. The sample is often said to be *irradiated* or *excited* by an external energy source. In this paradigm the source signal is not in itself of primary interest as it is not uniquely reflective of the sample. External signals carry information about their source as well as the sample. The former is usually not

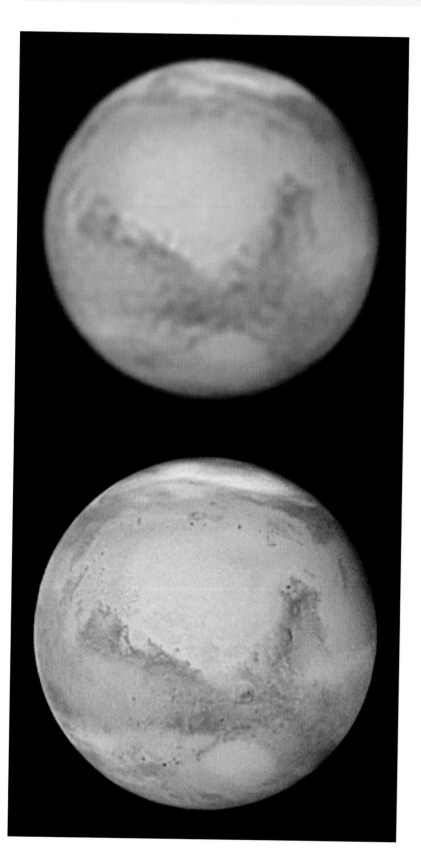

Figure 2.19. Earth versus Hubble telescopic images of Mars. Detector proximity to sample decreases obscuring scene elements, in this case the earth's atmosphere. By Sean Walker of Sky&Telescope. www.skyandtelescope.com/about/3304191.html.

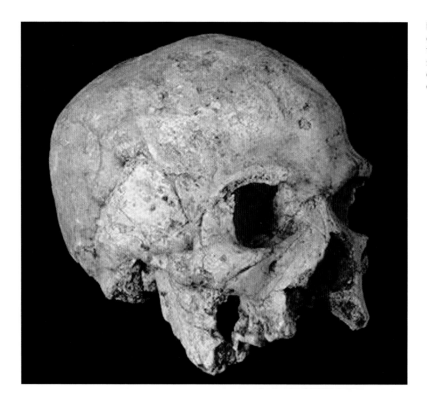

Figure 2.20. Natural radiocarbon dating of thirteenth-century Hofmeyr skull, treated as a temporally uniform, though spatially heterogeneous, sample. Courtesy of Frederick E. Grine, http://en.wikipedia.org/wiki/Hofmeyr_Skull.

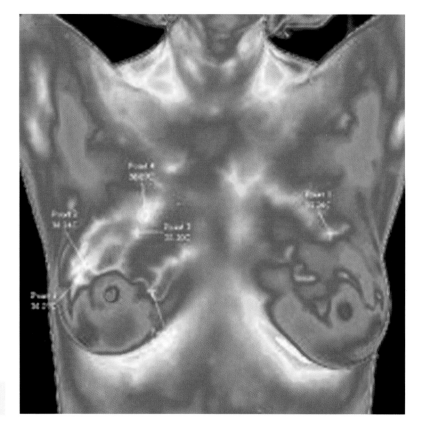

Figure 2.21. Breast infrared thermography based on a natural, intrinsic signal source. Courtesy of Philip P. Hoekstra, III, http://en.wikipedia.org/wiki/Thermology.

of primary interest, the latter is. Hence the decoding of these signals necessitates discriminating the components of the detected signal due to the external source from those due to the sample. Furthermore, signals that originate external to the sample add energy to the sample, are by definition invasive, and may alter, damage, or even destroy the sample.

An imaging system that involves an external signal must incorporate the signal source into the system. Hence a medical ultrasound (US) imaging system must include a US signal source – a piezoelectric crystal (see Chapter 6). A piezoelectric crystal responds to an oscillating electrical current by small physical vibrations that produce longitudinal mechanical waves (high-frequency sound waves of 1–100 MHz). These *ultrasound* signals propagate through appropriate media such as water and soft tissue (but not bone and air) at an average speed of 1480 m/s. These are interesting features, but alone are of little practical value. However, the additional fact that US signals are modified in predictable fashions by different tissues makes US an

important imaging tool, as the modified signal now contains information about the sample. Specifically, the US signal is differentially absorbed, scattered, and reflected by tissue interfaces, which allows the exquisite delineation of solid versus fluid-filled structures such as calcified stones in the gall bladder (Figure 2.23). The physical behavior of US can be modeled as a one-dimensional wave equation, the general solution to which can be written:

$$p(x,f) = \cos\left(\frac{2\pi f}{c}\right)(x - cf) \qquad (2.35)$$

with c being the speed of sound and f the frequency of the US wave form.

Remember that external signals used for imaging do not arise from the sample, and at their sources contain no information about the sample. The practical value of an external imaging signal is dependent on how it interacts with the sample and yields information about that sample. Slow neutrons can be detected as a function of their location and are therefore potential imaging signals. However, they pass through most biological samples without any interaction and are of no practical value for biomedical imaging.

Sample

Signal effect on sample

An important aspect of the signal/sample interaction is how signal energy affects and interacts with the sample

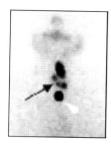

Figure 2.22. ^{123}I gamma camera scan of thyroid cancer.

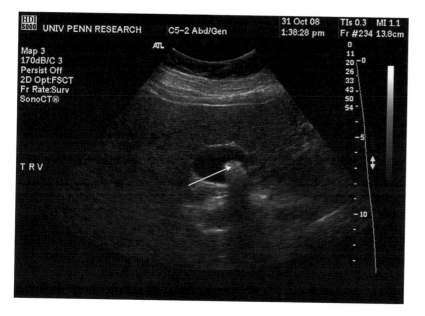

Figure 2.23. Ultrasound of stone within gallbladder.

(Table 2.3). Ideally, for non-destructive imaging, the sample should not be significantly modified by signal energy. In the case of a natural intrinsic signal, no energy is added to the sample, so the sample is unaffected by the imaging measurement. This is different with an extrinsic imaging signal. The interaction of an external signal with a sample necessitates energy transfer. Some intrinsic sample m,E will modify the external signal, which will yield sample information. At the same time, some of the external signal energy will be deposited in the sample. There is always net energy deposition into the sample. In order to be minimally invasive and non-destructive, the external signal should have as little energy as possible and require minimal sample interaction. There should be just enough signal/sample interaction to allow the signal to gain some desired sample information, but not enough to significantly modify the sample. Exactly how much external signal energy might be appropriate depends on the energetic requirements of the measurement, the

fragility of the sample, and analytical requirements. A very fragile sample such as a very thin microscopic tissue section can tolerate only a small of amount of incident light energy before sufficient heat is generated by the signal/sample interaction to completely burn it up.

Mass spectrometry is a chemical measurement that utilizes a very high-energy electron beam that is deliberately designed to exceed the chemical binding energy of molecules such as proteins in order to create smaller chemical constructs such as constituent amino acids that can be individually recognized (Figure 2.24). The sample is deliberately destroyed by the external measurement signal. Although measurements that destroy the sample can be very informative, destructive measurements are not pertinent in this discussion.

There are two common mechanisms by which external irradiation used for imaging can significantly affect biological samples – heating and ionization. These potentially hazardous biological effects are a function of the energy level of the radiation and, to a much lesser extent, the physical nature of the sample. Heating is the main biological effect of EM radiation from $100\,\text{kHz}$ to $300\,\text{GHz}$ ($3 \times 10^{10}\,\text{Hz}$), while ionization is the main hazardous effect above $3.0 \times 10^{16}\,\text{Hz}$ (or $13\,\text{eV}$). In addition, there is an infrequent biological effect – electro-stimulation – which can be induced by EM radiation between $3\,\text{kHz}$ and $5\,\text{MHz}$.

Thermal energy is secondary to friction between moving, vibrating particles. All objects with temperatures above 0 K radiate this energy with a frequency spectrum defined by:

$$M_c = c_1 \lambda^{-5}/[\exp(c_2/\gamma T) - 1]\text{Wm}^{-3} \qquad (2.36)$$

Table 2.3. Signal/sample interactions

Signal effect on sample
 Energy deposition
  Modify
  Destroy
  Safety limits
Sample effect on signal
 Reflect
 Scatter
 Absorb/attenuate
 Modulate
  Wave: amplitude, velocity, frequency, phase
  Particle: mass, number, velocity
Image contrast
 Intrinsic signal
 Extrinsic signal

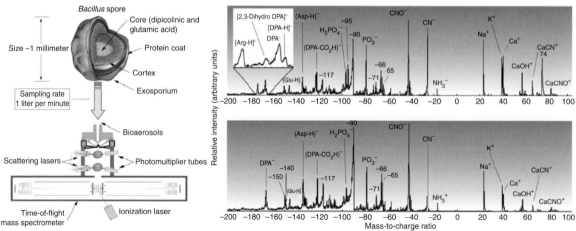

Figure 2.24. Mass spectrometry: destructive measurement. Courtesy of Lawrence Livermore National Laboratory. https://www.llnl.gov/str/September03/Gard.html.

AIRS NIGHTLY AIR TEMPERATURE (F) AT 700mb 20090724-20090726

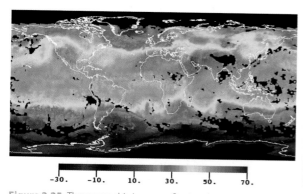
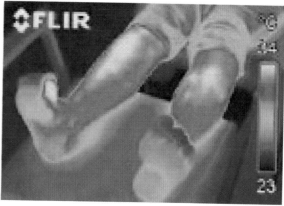

Figure 2.25. Thermographic images reflecting the temperature in the USA and limb perfusion. Map courtesy of NASA/JPL-Caltech, http://airs. jpl.nasa.gov/satellite_feed/Air_Temperature_Night/Air_Temperature_Night_3DayFull.jpg. Limb scan courtesy of Bath Royal National Hospital for Rheumatic Diseases.

For biological tissues, thermal energy is very low, in the μeV, infrared range, and is primarily due to molecular vibrations. Hence infrared imaging can be used to image temperature from a variety of samples, including the earth and people (Figure 2.25). In humans, as well as in other animals, temperature is known to be increased under certain physiologic conditions (exercise) and disease states (cancer). *Heating* increases thermal energy, generally by increasing particulate vibrations. The major biological effect and health hazard associated with non-ionizing radiation is heating – acute heating in particular. The lower energy forms of EM radiation that are commonly used for biomedical imaging, i.e., radio waves, infrared, visible, and ultraviolet light, as well as ultrasound, can not only heat, but also burn and destroy tissue if sufficient intensity is applied. Most mammalian tissue is irreversibly damaged, killed, if maintained at temperatures greater than 50 °C for more than a few seconds. Hence there are exposure limits defined for all of these methods, which are generally well below those which would cause harmful heating and burning. In general these guidelines restrict total body heating to less than 0.08 °C and local (10 g) heating to 2 °C in the body proper and 4 °C in the extremities, levels that are not associated with any tissue damage. Tissue damage from heating is relatively acute, and there are no known chronic or cumulative effects of non-ionizing radiation. While the heating effect may be important in terms of tissue damage, it is not usually important from the imaging perspective, with two notable exceptions. Both infrared and magnetic resonance (MR) imaging can be sensitive to, and actually measure or image, sample temperature.

MRI uses very low-energy EM radiation in the *radiofrequency* (rf) range of 1–200 MHz to measure electromagnetic properties of atomic nuclei in samples such as protein solutions, experimental mouse models, and human patients. This signal/sample interaction only minimally and transiently alters the sample. Thus MR imaging has gained great popularity as a non-destructive imaging examination. Despite the low external signal energy, signal/sample interaction is sufficient to allow the detected signal to contain very important information about the sample (patient), such as whether or not a tumor or stroke is present.

While some measurement signals are of lower energy than others, all can become destructive if introduced in sufficient quantity. The rf signal energy of MR can be increased sufficiently to heat and even burn tissue. Usually benign ultrasound waves can be focused and delivered with sufficient power to kill normal tissue, as well as tumors (Figure 2.26). The small doses of relatively low-energy x-rays of diagnostic studies may cause minimal damage to normal tissue, but higher doses can cause cell death by disrupting DNA and chromosomes. Even sunlight causes sunburn!

Far more important in terms of tissue effect and imaging is ionizing radiation (see Chapters 4 and 5). Ionizing radiation has sufficient energy to alter chemical bonds and atomic structure. Major health hazards associated with ionizing radiation include cataract formation, non-thermal burns, genetic damage, and carcinogenesis. These biological effects can result from immediate, as well as long-term, cumulative exposure. In contrast to heating, which usually is not directly related to the imaging itself, ionization is intimately related to the imaging process. For all of these reasons, more detail of sample ionization is now provided,

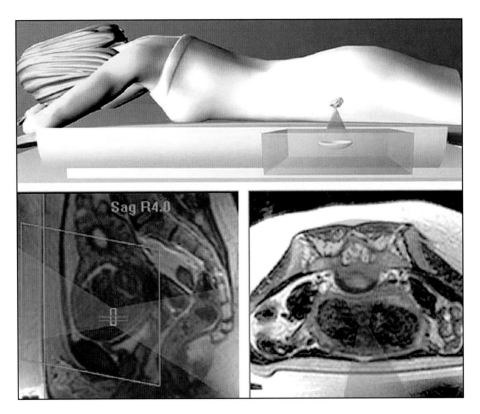

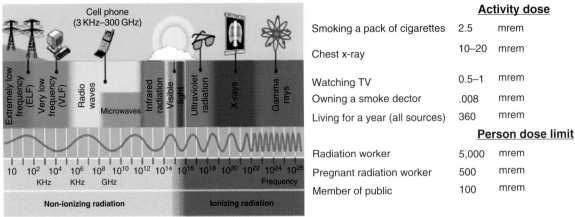

	Activity dose	
Smoking a pack of cigarettes	2.5	mrem
Chest x-ray	10–20	mrem
Watching TV	0.5–1	mrem
Owning a smoke dector	.008	mrem
Living for a year (all sources)	360	mrem
	Person dose limit	
Radiation worker	5,000	mrem
Pregnant radiation worker	500	mrem
Member of public	100	mrem

The U.S. Food and Drug Administration (FDA) have responsibility for assuring manufacturers produce cabinet x-ray systems that do not pose a radiation safety hazard. For most electronic products that emit radiation, safety regulation is divided between FDA and state regulatory agencies. Typically, FDA regulates the manufacture of the products and the states regulate the use of the products. For further information on FDA regulations that apply to manufacturers of electronic products that emit radiation (such as a cabinet x-ray system) see the FDA web site: (http://www.fda.gov/cdrh/comp/eprc.html).

Figure 2.26. MRI-guided US thermal ablation of uterine fibroid. Civilian exposure limits of EM radiation. Ablation images from Suzanne LeBlang, MD, *Improved Effectiveness of MR Guided Focused Ultrasound for Uterine Fibroids with Commercial Treatment Guidelines,* University MRI, Boca Raton, Florida. Used with permission. Radiation charts courtesy of www.HowStuffWorks.com, http://electronics.howstuffworks.com/cell-phone-radiation1.htm.

beginning with a brief, simplified introduction to atomic structure.

According to the Bohr planetary model, an atom consists of a dense, compact *nucleus* consisting of positively charged *protons* and electrically neutral *neutrons* surrounded by a cloud of negatively charged *electrons* in orbit about the nucleus. In the simplest, lowest energy state, there are an equal number of

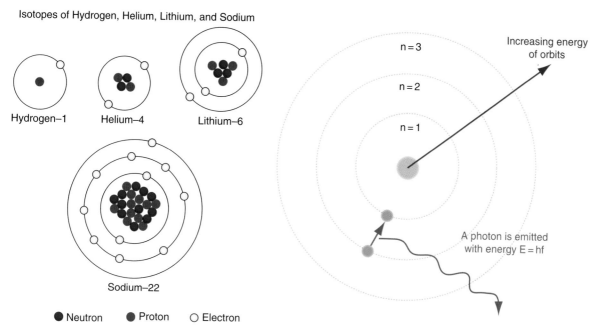

Figure 2.27. Bohr atomic model. C. R. B. Merritt.

equally and oppositely charged protons and electrons (Figure 2.27). In this scenario the protons, neutrons, and electrons are the principal subatomic particles of an atom, all having mass but with the heavier nuclear particles (nucleons) being relatively stationary, while the lower-mass electrons spin rapidly through their orbits. A particular element has a name (carbon) and a discrete number of protons (six) in its nucleus, which is its atomic number (Z). The atomic mass of an atom is the total number of nucleons, as electrons have comparatively little mass. Any unique combination of protons and neutrons defines a *nuclide*. The number of neutrons for a given element approximates the number of protons, but may not be exactly the same. Hence the element carbon always has six protons in a nucleus, but may have from three to ten associated neutrons, resulting in one element having eight possible nuclides ($^{9}_{6}C, ^{10}_{6}C, ^{11}_{6}C, ^{12}_{6}C, ^{13}_{6}C, ^{14}_{6}C, ^{15}_{6}C, ^{16}_{6}C$). Not all nuclides are temporally stable, and those that are not are termed *radionuclides* and commonly called *radioactive*. An unstable *radionuclide* will undergo nuclear rearrangement or *decay*, which results in a more stable nuclide. Nuclear decay occurs over some time period, often defined as the *half-life*, which is the time it takes for one-half of the radioactive nuclei of a sample to decay to a more stable configuration.

Within an atom, the electrons are arranged in a hierarchy of orbits or shells, with the K shell being closest to the nucleus and succeeding shells labeled by sequential letters of the alphabet (K, L, M, N, etc.). Electrons are restricted to specific quantum spin states within a shell, and this results in a maximum number of elections per shell, defined by $2n^2$, where n is the shell number. Different spin states and shells are associated with different energy levels, and the lowest or *ground state* is preferred. In the ground state the lowest orbital shells are preferentially filled. Electrons are *bound* to the nucleus by an electric force termed the *electron binding energy*, in units of electronvolts (eV). An electron's binding energy is dependent on the specific element, decreases as the shell number increases, and ranges from a few eV to several keV. The simplest atom, hydrogen, ^{1}H, has a single electron with a binding energy of 13.6 eV. This is one of the lower binding energies of natural elements.

Electrons do not have to be bound to an atom, but can be *free electrons*. However, free electrons are generally at higher energy levels than bound electrons. Hence it takes energy to create a free electron, and there is a tendency for free electrons to return to the lower-energy bound state. A bound electron can be displaced or ejected from an atom by radiation (particulate or EM) having greater energy than that electron's binding energy. This results in two electrically charged particles or *ions*, the negative free electron and the positive atom minus one electron. By definition, radiation capable of creating ions is *ionizing radiation*, as compared to *non-ionizing radiation*. By convention,

61

radiation with energy greater than 10 eV (just below the relatively low binding energy of the hydrogen electron) is considered ionizing. This is not a hard definition, as ionization can take place at lower or higher energy levels. Furthermore, ionizing radiation can cause atomic effects other than ionization that can have less biological consequences but still affect imaging. What is important is that radiation of higher energy levels, which includes x-rays and gamma rays, can significantly change the basic physical structure of an atom or the chemical structure of a molecule. Such fundamental changes in a sample can lead to numerous side effects, of which the adverse biological effects previously mentioned are of particular concern. On the other hand, some ionization effects can be beneficial in special circumstances. The ionization of chromosomes can lead to DNA damage resulting in cancer or, oddly, the cure of cancer. Regardless, ionizing radiation can significantly alter the sample – and strictly from an imaging perspective this is not desirable. Hence, while ionizing radiation provides an important imaging signal, its beneficial use must always be balanced against its potential detrimental effects.

As for all forms of measurement, energy is required for imaging. If the source of energy is extrinsic to the sample, the applied energy will affect the sample in some fashion. For purposes of biomedical imaging, signal/sample effect should be minimized and energy levels kept below those injurious to the sample. There are safety guidelines for all imaging signals used for medical applications. Medical imaging safety limits are defined in energy units commonly applied to a particular imaging signal type and are based on the *dose*, or amount of energy, to which the patient is exposed. There are often limits for total body dose, as well as sensitive organ dose. It should always be remembered that these safety "limits" are not absolute and should be taken as indicators of potential risk to the patient that have to be balanced against the potential value of the test results – the *risk/ benefit ratio*. While the amount of energy applied to a non-human biological sample is not regulated by governmental agencies or limited by patient safety, there are practical energy deposition limitations related to sample integrity.

Sample effect on signal

To be of scientific value, externally applied energy must be modified by the sample in such a fashion that the detected signal provides information not only about the energy source, but also about the sample. Imaging using an external signal source is the most common form of imaging, the most obvious example being the daily imaging of our surroundings. Most of the things humans see are invisible without their exposure to an external source of visible light such as the sun. Many objects in our environment reflect visible light energy waves that are refocused by the eye's lens onto retinal photodetectors that convert the reflected light energy into electrochemical energy, which the brain uses to process the image data. In order for this process to provide information about the sample, the original light signal must be modified by the sample. For instance, a red beach ball modifies the initial multispectral, "white" light of the sun by absorption and refraction, which results in a reflected red light signal that now carries information about the sample. It is the modified signal (red) resulting from signal/sample interaction that is of interest, not the original signal (white). An imaging system based on intrinsic sample signal does not want any signal/sample interaction to distort the original signal. On the other hand, the information content of an imaging system that uses an external signal source is completely dependent on signal/sample interactions.

There are many different mechanisms through which a signal may interact with a sample, a number of which are enumerated in Table 2.3 and will be detailed in the chapters on specific imaging modalities. The nature of the external signal defines how it might be modified. If the external signal is wave-like, interactions with the sample could result in a change in amplitude, frequency, phase, and/or direction of wave propagation. If the external signal consists of particles, their number, mass, speed, and direction of movement might be altered by the sample. In general, signal/ sample interactions result in absorption of energy by the sample and the requisite *attenuation* of the original signal. In order for the measurement or image to provide information about the sample, the signal change induced by the sample must be detected.

Conventional microscopy depends on an external source of visible light that very thin specimens modify by several mechanisms. Light is absorbed by the sample, which diminishes the brightness of the signal. The original signal is multispectral, having multiple wavelengths (colors). Different tissues preferentially absorb different wavelengths, which results in the original "white" light becoming differentially colored. Spectral differences in the detected light signal reveal

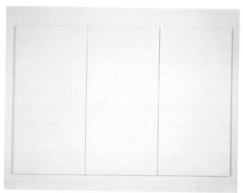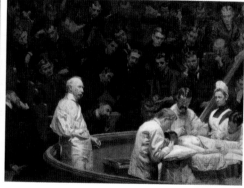

Figure 2.28. Image contrast: spatial homogeneity, "random" spatial heterogeneity, and non-random spatial heterogeneity. Works by Robert Rauschenberg, Jackson Pollock, Thomas Eakins. *White Painting (Three Panel)*, Robert Rauschenberg, (c) Estate of Robert Rauschenberg, Licensed by VAGA, New York, NY. J. Pollock, No. 5, 1948, http://en.wikipedia.org/wiki/Jackson_Pollock. The Agnew Clinic, Thomas Eakins, 1889, is at the Philadelphia Museum of Art.

the encoded sample information. The specimen can also alter the phase of the light signal and, if the microscope is equipped with phase-sensitive optics, phase-contrast images can be made.

Diagnostic x-rays interact with biological tissues in a number of specific ways, including the *photoelectric effect*, *Compton scattering*, and, to a much lesser extent, pair production (see Chapters 4 and 5). In the case of the photoelectric effect, incident photons from the external source (x-ray tube) are completely absorbed by the sample, while with Compton scattering incident photon directions are changed. The net result is attenuation and scattering of the incident x-ray signal. It turns out that the photoelectric effect primarily accounts for differential tissue attenuation, while Compton scattering may limit the spatial resolution and contrast of x-ray imaging. If x-rays interacted similarly with different tissues, x-ray measurements would provide no tissue-discriminating information. Fortunately the amount of signal attenuation varies from tissue to tissue, each tissue having different *linear attenuation coefficients*, which is primarily a function of tissue *atomic mass* or *electron density*. Linear attenuation coefficient, μ, for a specific material or tissue can be defined as:

$$\mu = \frac{n/N}{\Delta x} \qquad (2.37)$$

with n being the number of absorption photons, N the number of incident photons and Δx the relative thickness of the sample (assumed to be small). By appropriate manipulations and integration, this definition evolves into the *fundamental photon attenuation law*:

$$N = N_0 e^{-\mu \Delta x} \qquad (2.38)$$

Where N_0 is the number of incident photons at the surface of the sample. Tissue-specific differences in linear attenuation coefficient result in differential signal attenuation producing the *contrast* in a medical x-ray. Contrast is the relative difference in two signals and provides most of the information content of an image. Images such as Robert Rauschenberg's *White on White* paintings may be of artistic interest, but they have no contrast, no signal heterogeneity (Figure 2.28). Images of this type may have aesthetic value, but provide minimal information content.

The information content of an image is due to variations in the detected signal from different parts of the sample. In the case of an intrinsic signal source, the differential signal contrast is due to local variations in the intensity or concentration of the signal source. For images derived from an external signal source, signal differences are due to locally different signal/sample interactions. These modifications of the source signal must be detected by the imaging system in order to gain information about the sample. If the key information needed from a microscopic study is the phase change of the light signal induced by mitochondria, and the microscope is not equipped with phase-sensitive optics, the needed information will not be provided by the study (Figure 2.29).

Signal propagation

How signals move or propagate from or through a scene and sample is critical for imaging. Table 2.4 outlines common mechanisms of signal propagation. Signal propagation influences how signals will interact with a sample, how measuring devices might be arranged to detect the signal, and how spatial information is incorporated into the signal. As previously noted, all m,E signals have an associated

63

directionality. The m,E signals propagate along a straight path, unless they meet an obstacle in the form of matter. Interaction of energy with mass

results in some combination of signal attenuation and change of direction. Critical to non-invasive measurements, including imaging as presented here, is how the signal escapes the sample. Non-invasive measurements are dependent on signals that escape the sample. Signals that are confined to the sample can only be detected invasively, either by forcing a detector into the sample (endoscope) or by extracting a piece of the sample for measurement by an external detector (biopsy). A signal that does not propagate beyond the sample cannot be non-invasively detected or imaged.

If the signal does exit the sample, the imaging system must be configured to detect the signal along its pathway. Signal sources can be viewed as small

Table 2.4. Signal propagation

Linear propagation
  Intrinsic source – omnidirectional
  Extrinsic source – directed to/through sample
Sample
  Reflected
  Scattered
  Transmitted
    Opaque
    Lucent
    Projection/shadow casting

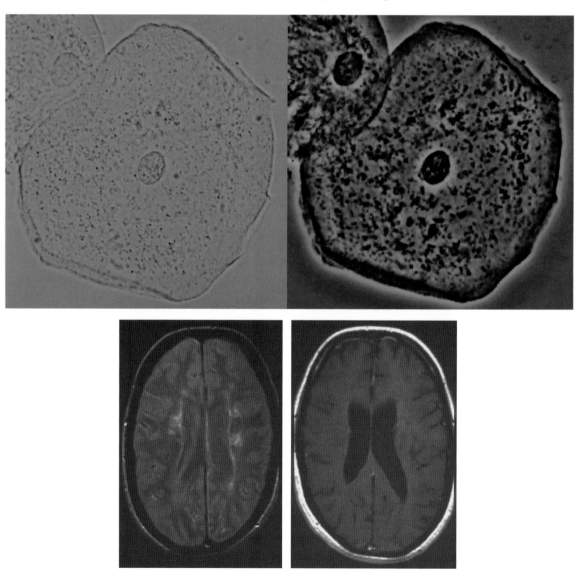

Figure 2.29. Living cells in bright-field and phase-contrast microscopy. Multiple sclerosis: PD and T1-weighted MR scans. Courtesy of G. Overney. http://en.wikipedia.org/wiki/Phase_contrast.

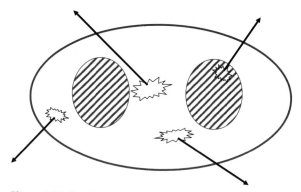

Figure 2.30. Signal propagation from internal sources: photons from radionuclide decay. C. R. B. Merritt.

the source simply due to geometric dispersal of the signal and according to the inverse square law, assuming a point source:

$$I_D \propto \frac{I_S}{4\pi d^2} \qquad (2.39)$$

I_D being the signal intensity at the detector, I_S being the signal intensity at the source, and d being the distance from source to detector. This geometric spread of the signal as distance from the source increases is the reason external signal sources are often placed very close to the sample. Within the sample, as the external signal propagates, it is continuously modified by signal/sample interactions.

From a directional perspective, common mechanisms of signal propagation within a sample can be appreciated by simply thinking of the ways externally imposed energy might interact with an object (Figure 2.31). The impinging energy might be *reflected*, in which case the modified signal would contain information about the reflective surfaces of the object. If the signal cannot penetrate the object, then only superficial surface features can be interrogated by a reflective system, as with optical imaging by the human visual system. If incident energy can penetrate the sample, internal reflective surfaces can be studied, as with ultrasonography.

Incident energy might project itself in a straight line through and/or past the object, in which case it would cast a shadow – *shadow casting* or more technically *projection imaging*. If the object were completely *opaque*, fully blocking the incident energy, only the contours of the object would be outlined by the shadow. If incident energy is sufficiently powerful so as to not only enter but also pass all the way through the sample, the shadow would contain not only surface/contour information, but also information about the interior of the object, unless the sample was completely *translucent*. In this case, the signal does not interact with the sample and there is no shadow; and therefore no evidence of the sample. For example, common radio waves pass through forests without interacting with the trees; hence the forest cannot be imaged by this signal.

Intrinsic signals by definition come from the sample, but so do the signals that are used to create images from systems using an external signal source. The original signal was external to the sample, but it is the modified signal after signal/sample interaction that is needed to make a useful image. These modified signals do come from the sample, despite their origins

energy radiators or point sources. A signal emanates in all directions from a point source, such as decaying radionuclides (Figure 2.30). Most signals tend to propagate in straight lines away from their sources. Hence signals from an intrinsic source that escape a sample will be propagating in all directions. However, signals may interact with their environment, including the sample. When they do so, the energy level and possibly the direction they are traveling will change. When the signal pathway is altered and the signal proceeds at an angle to the original, the signal is *scattered*. A signal scattered by the sample has potential sample information that may be captured in certain types of measurements, such as flow cytometry. However, scattered signal can be very complex and is more often handled by an imaging system as attenuated signal or even noise.

In the case of an external signal source, the signal initially propagates away from the source. Visible light propagates away from the sun or a flashlight, and x-rays from the anode of an x-ray tube. The signal from an external source can propagate in all directions from the source, as does an intrinsic signal. However, for imaging purposes, the signal of interest is that which propagates from the source to the sample. It is only this component of the initial signal that will interact with the sample and, in the process, gain sample information. Hence an external signal that does not hit the sample is wasted and potentially dangerous. Ideally the signal from an external source is carefully focused or *collimated* on the sample, or even better on the signal detectors, so as not to impose on other areas. Many external source signals may be modeled as columns (of energy) extending in a straight line from the source to the sample to the detector. Signals will decrease in intensity as they propagate away from

65

outside the sample. In any case, signal directionality contains spatial information about the sample. Most intrinsic signals emanate in all directions from the sample, and the directions of individual signal elements point away from their source. In general, an external signal propagates along a linear path from the source to the sample and beyond. The signal will exit the sample in a direction that is a function of the original external signal direction and its modification by the signal/sample interaction. The signal might be completely attenuated and not exit the sample. It might be scattered and exit the side of the sample. Or the signal might pass straight through the sample and participate in the shadow cast. In all cases, signal directionality has spatial information about the source and, more importantly, about the sample as well, because of the linear propensities of signal propagation.

Signal detection

Signal detection is first determined by the physical nature of the signal being measured (Table 2.5). The measurement system must be sensitive to the form of the m,E of interest. If the thermal energy of a sample is

Table 2.5. Signal detection

Detector
  Signal sensitivity
  Efficiency
    Serial/parallel

to be measured, then the measurement device, the *detector*, must be able to measure this type of signal, such as a solid-state infrared detector for temperature measurement. Detectors are generally sensitive only to a single type or small range of signals. An infrared detector cannot effectively measure x-rays. However, a particular signal may be detectable by more than one type of detector. X-rays can be detected by analog silver photographic film, a cloud chamber, a Geiger counter, or the more recently developed solid-state digital x-ray detectors (Figure 2.32).

Detectors basically function as energy transducers. A detector must respond to the signal of interest by producing a new signal that represents some characteristic of the incident energy. For non-invasive, non-destructive imaging, only detectors placed outside the sample are of interest. This requires that the signal, usually some form of radiant energy, propagate beyond the sample. Radiant energy detectors produce responses such as an increase or decrease in electric potential or current flow or some other perceivable change, such as exposure of radiographic film. The basic physics of signal capture by different detectors will be detailed with each modality.

The performance of a detector is critical to the overall performance of an imaging system. Since it is often desirable to require minimal signal for the measurement, detector efficiency is critical. *Detector efficiency*, E_d, is measured by the percentage of incident signal, I_S, that is detected, I_D:

Transmission

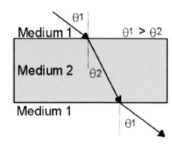

Reflection

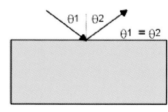

Figure 2.31. Signal sample interactions: reflection, absorption, scatter, and transmission. C. R. B. Merritt.

Scattering

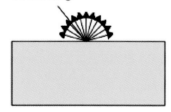

Absorption

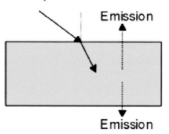

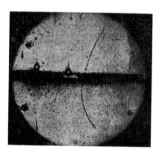 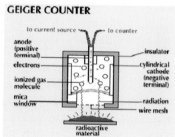 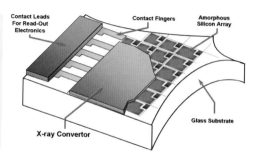

Figure 2.32. Ionization detectors: cloud chamber, Geiger counter, solid-state detector. Cloud chamber from Anderson CD, *Physical Review* 1933; **43**: 491. Geiger counter http://en.wikipedia.org/wiki/Geiger-M%C3%BCller_tube. Detector courtesy of A. Maidment.

$$E_d = 100 \frac{I_D}{I_S} \qquad (2.40)$$

If a particular gamma detector can count all of the incident photons, it has 100% efficiency, while a different detector that detects half of the incident photons has only 50% efficiency and is half as efficient as the first detector. Ideally a detector would measure and report only the true signal from the sample. Unfortunately, detectors are not perfect, and they report "false signal" or *noise*. Detector noise is measurement error, is ubiquitous in all measurement systems, and adds to measurement error or variability. Importantly, noise contains no information specific to the sample, but, if sufficiently large, can obscure the information contained in the true signal. Hence, an overall measure of detector performance is *signal-to-noise* (SNR, *S/N*):

$$S/N ratio = \frac{S}{N} \qquad (2.41)$$

This measurement is most simply made by dividing the signal (*S*) from a *region of interest* (ROI) placed over an important part of the sample by that from another ROI outside the sample, but within the field of view (FOV) of the image, where there is presumably only noise (*N*). A very efficient but noisy detector may capture all the available true signal, but obscure that signal with its own noise. Much of modern imaging technological development has involved detectors, occasionally inventing detectors that measure novel signals (Roentgen's x-ray) or more frequently improving detectors for previously detectable signals, such as the more convenient charge-coupled devices (CCD) for optical imaging and the more efficient gamma-ray detectors for positron emission tomography (PET) scanners.

If the signal is intrinsic to the sample and this signal encodes the desired information about the sample, then the detector must be sensitive to this original signal. A radioactive sample emitting 511 keV x-ray photons from positron decay must be imaged by detectors sensitive to this specific type of EM radiation.

In the case of an external signal source, the detector must be sensitive to the signal modification induced by the signal/sample interaction that contains sample information. While an extrinsic signal source sets some restrictions on the detector, it is the modified signal, reflecting sample properties, that is of primary importance. In many imaging systems, the basic physical nature of the detected signal is very similar, if not identical, to the incident signal. In conventional projection radiography, the detected signal is mostly photons emitted by the original signal source, the x-ray tube. The detected signal is identical to the incident signal minus that absorbed or scattered by the sample. If the detector measures a 70 keV photon, it is likely that the photon is unchanged from its source. There are many photons leaving the x-ray tube that do not reach the detector, and this accounts for image contrast. In systems such as this, detector design is heavily predicated on the signal source.

In fluorescent imaging, the incident, exciting light for quinone typically has a wavelength of 350 nm, but because the emitted light is of lower energy, its wavelength is slightly longer, 450 nm (Figure 2.33). In NMR spectroscopy the external, irradiating rf signal excites a set of nuclei, but no element of this incident energy will be detected by the NMR receiver coil. Granted, the rf signal subsequently detected may be very similar to the incident signal, but it is fundamentally a different signal emitted from the sample as the excited nuclei relax. It will typically have a similar, but distinctly different spectral bandwidth. The NMR rf detector of such a system must be sensitive to the emitted signal, containing sample information, which is not the same

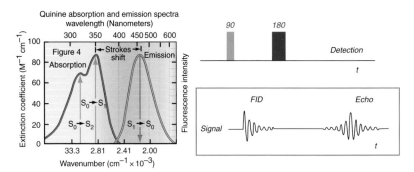

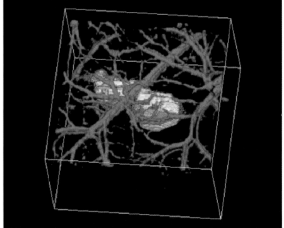

Figure 2.33. Signal differences between external signal at its source and at the detector: fluorescence excite/emit spectra; MR rf excitation pulse and detected rf signal. Stokes shift with permission from M. W. Davidson, http://www.olympusfluoview.com/theory/fluoroexciteemit.html. Rf signal from http://en.wikipedia.org/wiki/Spin_echo.

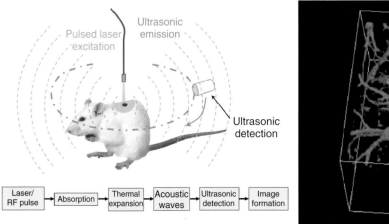

Figure 2.34. Photoacoustic imaging. From http://en.wikipedia.org/wiki/Photoacoustic_imaging_in_biomedicine.

as the original source signal. However, the bandwidths of the exciting and emitted rf signals are sufficiently similar that in most cases the same rf coil is used for transmission and reception.

Photoacoustic imaging goes even further in separating the energizing and detected signal, using completely different energy forms for irradiation and detection. In photoacoustic imaging, the sample is irradiated with non-ionizing optical energy (infrared, visible, rf, or microwave) that interacts with the sample in such a fashion that an acoustic signal is generated and detected (Figure 2.34). These hybrid techniques combine the high signal contrast due to the differential electromagnetic (EM) absorption of different tissues with the high spatial resolution of ultrasound. Pulsed EM energy is deposited as uniformly as possible throughout the imaging object, causing a small amount of thermal expansion. One clinical hypothesis is that cancerous masses preferentially absorb EM energy and therefore heat, thus expanding more quickly than neighboring healthy tissue. The

expanding (and contracting) tissues are internal acoustic sources, creating pressure waves which are detected by ultrasound transducers surrounding the object. The initial signal is EM radiation, the phenomenon of interest is tissue heating, and the detected signal is US, which carries spatial information. Needless to say, such hybrid images are not only technically sophisticated but difficult to interpret, much less model. As with most imaging techniques, their future will depend on technical developments and empirical testing.

Signal detectors

After the signal itself, the sample and its environment influence the nature of the detector. For non-destructive imaging, the detector itself cannot intrude on the sample, or it becomes an invasive procedure. Therefore the detector must not only be able to detect the m,E signal of interest, but it also has to sample the signal external to the sample. This requires knowledge of the signal/sample interaction and how the signal escapes the

Table 2.6. Detector arrangement

FOV
  Internal signal source
    Side
    Around
  External signal source
    Front
    Side
    Behind
    Around

sample. The detector must be physically located somewhere along the signal pathway. Imaging detectors must be arranged such that they can receive signals emanating from the sample (Table 2.6). The arrangement of imaging detectors partially defines the *field of view* (FOV), the spatial area from which the detector(s) can detect signals; where the detector(s) will "look." A FOV may be one-, two-, or three-dimensional, reflecting the detection of signal along a line, across a plane, or of a volume. Remember, by our definition, signal from a single point does not compose an image, though technically such a measurement implicitly, if not explicitly, has a spatial component. One-dimensional images have minimal spatial information and are infrequently a goal on their own. Most scientific images are two- or three-dimensional, preferably the latter, as nature, including most biomedical samples, has three important, finite spatial dimensions.

The FOV defines the scene that will be imaged, and it should obviously include the *sample* – the object of interest, the portion of nature in which the scientific imager is interested. It must be emphasized that, in contrast to many non-imaging measurements, that which is to be measured is not explicitly defined in advance of making the imaging measurements. Rather, a scene is defined by the FOV, within which may be the sample. In most cases specific patterns or objects within an image are defined after the fact. This key fact of imaging will be discussed in greater detail in Chapter 3 and Section 3, on image analysis.

As previously noted, signals with useful information about the sample must emanate from the sample, even those signals that originated outside of the sample. Hence all detectors must "face" the sample. This can be accomplished by placing a single detector outside the sample, with its sensitive face pointing towards the sample. The FOV will be determined by detector size, as well as by any focusing mechanisms between it and the sample. If the detector is small and tightly focused, then its FOV will be small and perhaps signals from only a

portion of the sample will be detected. A large detector or a detector with a divergent focusing system will have a larger FOV, perhaps larger than the sample. An array of multiple detectors can also increase the FOV.

Geometrically it is obvious that a 1 : 1 correspondence between the spatial distribution of an external signal and the FOV of the detector is not required. Light emanating from our sun irradiates half the earth and more, while a single person's FOV is an infinitesimally small fraction of that area. Sunlight beyond the FOV of an individual is useless (for imaging purposes) for that individual, but obviously not to others. In contrast, the incident and detected (reflected) ultrasound beams are almost spatially identical. An imaging system with tightly aligned source and detected signal is termed a *narrow-beam* system, while the external source signal of a *broad-beam* system extends well beyond the detector FOV. If the external, exciting signal can be harmful to the sample or environment, a narrow-beam system is desirable so as to minimize any harmful exposure.

FOV is one factor in the ultimate spatial resolution of an imaging system. Within an imaging system there are numerous contributors to spatial resolution, FOV being an important one affecting both absolute and relative spatial resolution. More attention is often paid to the former, so let us start there. Unless performing a "single voxel" measurement (which is generally not desirable and hardly an image by our definition as it would not reflect spatial heterogeneity), a FOV is subdivided into individual image elements (pixels for 2D, voxels for 3D images). For a 2D image, this process is most commonly implemented, and illustrated, by dividing a square FOV into a matrix of isotropic (equal-sized) pixels. The geometric resolution, R_g, of the **image**, not the system, can be found by dividing the FOV of the image by the number of contained picture elements, P:

$$R_g = \frac{FOV}{I_e} = \frac{FOV_{sq}}{P_x P_y} = \frac{FOV_{cu}}{P_x, P_y, P_z} \qquad (2.42)$$

For example, a 2D image with a square FOV of 10×10 cm and a 100×100 isotropic pixel matrix has 10 000 square pixels, 1 mm on a side. This geometric resolution, or more properly pixel resolution of 1 mm, defines the maximum spatial resolution of the image, but does not define the actual spatial resolution of the system and can therefore be very misleading. The previously described PSF is the far more complete description of a system's absolute spatial resolution.

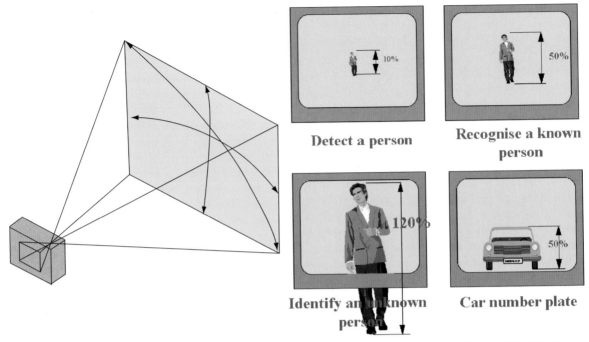

Figure 2.35. Field of view (FOV) defines the dimensions of the recorded scene and is adjusted to the object of interest. C. R. B. Merritt.

While absolute spatial resolution is important, it does not necessarily convey practical value. Higher spatial resolution is not always better. The practical value of spatial resolution has to take into account not only theoretical system resolution, but also the size of the sample, SNR, and imaging time. The reciprocal relationships between SNR, spatial resolution, and imaging times are important to remember. *In general, SNR decreases linearly with spatial resolution and increases with the square root of imaging time*:

$$S/N \propto Vol\sqrt{t} \qquad (2.43)$$

Let us now consider sample size. The FOV defines how big an image scene will be. Though important, this concept is not usually explicitly defined, and for want of a better term I shall call it *relative resolution*, which is the size of the FOV in relation to the size of the sample or object(s) of interest (Figure 2.35). Relative resolution is important in terms of how big a sample or what portion thereof can be imaged and at what spatial detail. At the simplest level, if one wants to make a single image of a large sample, a large FOV is required, at least as large as the sample. A 2 cm FOV is adequate for a MR image of a mouse's brain, but not a human's. On the other hand, if only an image of a human cochlea is desired, a 2 cm FOV is fine.

Given similar matrix size, a large FOV image of a small sample will result in a "relatively" lower resolution image than a small FOV image. The former will spread fewer pixels or voxels over a defined portion of the sample than the latter. In this case, not only will the absolute geometric resolution of the small FOV image be greater, but its relative resolution will also be greater. On the other hand, a large FOV image of a large sample (human) might have the same relative spatial resolution as a small FOV image of a similar, but smaller sample. The two different FOVs will spread the same number of pixels over anatomically, but not geometrically, equivalent objects (kidney). For many applications, the relative spatial resolution is as important as, or more important than, the absolute resolution.

Image formation

The ultimate means by which spatial information is incorporated into an image is a result of appropriate geometries of the signal source, sample, and detectors, and/or spatial modulation of the signal (Table 2.7). Geometric spatial encoding tends to be relatively simple, while spatial signal modulations can be very complex, though sublime. The rectilinear gamma scanner is a good example of a simple imaging system based on geometric encoding of spatial information (Figure 2.36). This device remarkably resembles an ancient pantograph and has been superseded by more efficient methods, but its underlying principles are informative. The sample in this case is a patient who has been injected with a radioactive compound, ^{99m}TcPhosphate, which accumulates in bone tumors and produces an intrinsic, though artificially introduced, gamma-ray signal source. The detector is a 1 cm diameter scintillation crystal that converts gamma rays into faint, brief flashes of light that, in turn, induce an electrical current in the detector assembly. The amplitude of the electrical signal is proportional to the intensity of light flashes, which are in turn proportional to the number and energy of gamma rays reaching the detector. The detector assembly is directed towards the sample and *collimated* such that only gamma rays traveling orthogonal to the crystal face will be detected. In most cases the detected gamma rays will have traveled

in a straight line from the radionuclide in the patient to the crystal. The basic geometry of linear energy propagation from a source to a focused and aligned detector is the mechanism for encoding spatial information in this simple system. Therefore the detector's FOV for an individual measurement is a 1 cm rectangular column extending from the crystal face through the sample. The signal intensity measured is a sum of the total number of gamma emissions along this column that are directed at the detector. Given that it is a continuous signal and detector, this is a CC system measuring the line integral of the number of emissions (or other linear signals) along the column (Figure 2.37):

$$F(x) = \int_{-\infty}^{+\infty} dx f(x) \qquad (2.44)$$

A measurement at one detector position is a collapsed one-dimensional image; as the emissions at all points along the line are summed together, their individual information is lost. After the integration, or summation, there is no spatial information along the axis of the line. This is our first example of *partial volume effect*. Signal information from small pieces, partial volumes, within the FOV (in this case, points along a line) are subsumed within the single measurement.

Spatial encoding by this type of geometry is that of *projection imaging*. The encoding of spatial information through projection imaging is dependent on the rectilinear propagation of energy. This is the case for human vision, in which spatial information is conveyed by the rectilinear propagation of light from a light source or

Table 2.7. Image formation

Spatial encoding
  Geometric
    Projection
    Scattering
  Non-geometric signal modulation
Spatial decoding
  Direct/indirect
  Computer
    Graphic display
    Reconstruction
      Forward/inverse solution

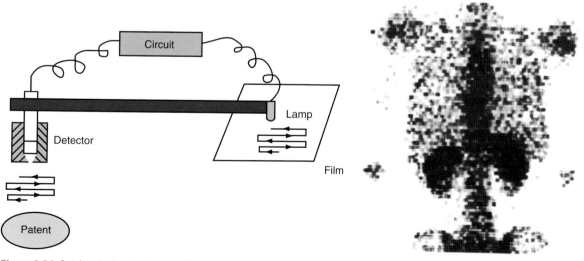

Figure 2.36. Serial projection imaging; rectilinear gamma camera. Diagram from http://en.wikipedia.org/wiki/Rectilinear_scanner.

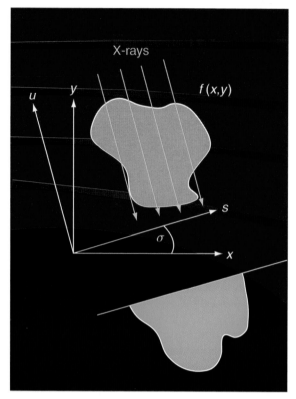

Figure 2.37. 2D x-ray CT projections: collection of linear line integrals across the sample at varying angles through the sample. C. R. B. Merritt.

reflective surface to the retina. In this example from nuclear imaging, a signal generated along one spatial dimension is projected along a line to the detector.

The signal with m,E and spatial information is encoded, but subsequently must be decoded for presentation to an observer. The scintillation detector is attached to a mechanical arm, the other end of which holds a small printing device that makes a mark on a sheet of paper, the darkness of the mark being proportional to the electric current created by the detector. The detector is positioned over the patient and makes a measurement of gamma-ray signal intensity that is recorded on a sheet of paper by the printing device. However, this one-dimensional measurement is of little value. More spatial information is desired and additional spatial dimensions are needed. This goal is achieved by simply moving the detector and measuring the signal from another location. The detector/printer assembly is moved to the right 1 cm by a motor drive, and another line integral measurement is made and recorded, and so on. When the detector has passed beyond the left side

of the patient, it is moved 1 cm caudad and then traverses back across the body, left to right. This process is repeated in a zigzag manner until the detector has been positioned over and made measurements of the entire body. The result is a direct image of radioactivity in the body that closely relates to the presence and locations of bone metastases. Though not very pretty, no further manipulation of the data is needed for the image to be easily appreciated by a human observer. The recorded data directly form an image.

The m,E detector of this system is a scintillation detector that differs little in function from a Geiger counter used for non-imaging measurements. However, this detector has been integrated into a system that now allows it to make many localized measurements and report these measurements in a spatially coherent fashion so that one may appreciate the spatial distribution of the signal. The spatial information in this crude system is directly and only related to the geometry of signal propagation and the detector. A few details warrant attention. Since the signals, gamma rays, are continuously emitted from the entire body, this measurement system using a single, small detector is very inefficient. For an individual measurement, the detector's small FOV excludes all but a very small proportion of the available signal (broad-beam configuration). While the detector efficiency might be good, the system efficiency is not. Such *serial* collection of data is generally inefficient in terms of sample signal dose and demands long imaging times. Spatial resolution is largely determined by the detector size and hence will be relatively low, at best 1 cm. The large crystal size, with reasonable collimation, will further compromise spatial resolution by detecting photons arising from tissue surrounding the facing 1 cm column. The final spatial resolution of such an instrument is reflected by a FWHM of approximately 1.5 cm. Fortunately advances in technology have dramatically improved nuclear imaging system sensitivity and spatial resolution.

To increase efficiency, more than one detector might be used simultaneously. A human retina simultaneously uses approximately 20 million cone detectors for color vision. The Anger gamma camera is based on this concept, being a "multidetector" scanner that is based on a large sodium iodide crystal fused to an extensive array of collimated photomultiplier tubes (Figure 2.38). The result is in effect several hundred scintillation detectors simultaneously collecting signals from a large volume of the body, faster and at

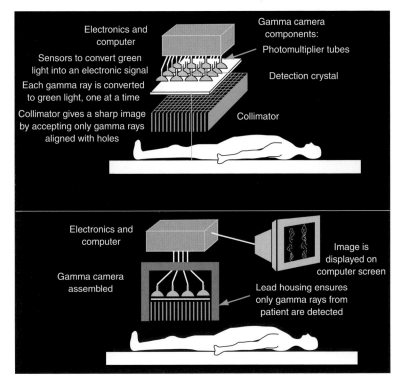

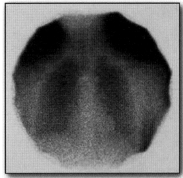

Figure 2.38. Parallel imaging: Anger gamma camera. Diagram used with permission from Douglas J. Wagenaar.

higher resolution than the more primitive single-detector rectilinear scanner. Additional detectors can be used to increase efficiency (by making parallel measurements), to increase FOV (more detectors directed over larger area), to increase spatial resolution (more, smaller detectors covering the same FOV), or to add angular views. Of course an array of many detectors completely surrounding a self-emitting sample would be very efficient, capturing signals traveling in all directions and providing many viewing angles. Multidirectional detector systems are not only desirable, but a requisite for PET imaging.

For geometric systems dependent on external signals, the signal source and direction of signal propagation heavily influence the position and configuration of detectors. If an external signal is reflected by the sample, the detector must be on the same side of the sample as the source. This is the case for US imaging, where the same piezoelectric crystal that emits the external signal is sensitive to the returning, reflected US signal (Figure 2.39). If an external signal passes through the sample, the detector must be on the opposite side from the source. This is shadow casting, and the detector must be in position to "catch" the shadow. This is a very common configuration, as with optical microscopy and radiography (Figure 2.40). In all these examples, whether the signal is reflected or transmitted through the sample, the spatial information is encoded by the linear propagation of the signal onto appropriately positioned detectors, and in most cases the detected signal directly forms an image.

Non-projection spatial signal modulation

While many contemporary imaging techniques take advantage of signal directionality to geometrically encode spatial information, some do not. There are many ways that a signal may be modulated in order to carry information. After all, a wave-like signal has amplitude, frequency, phase, and directionality that can be used to carry information. Radio waves are modulated in a variety of ways to carry sound information – AM, amplitude modulated; FM, frequency modulated (Figure 2.41). In many imaging methods, amplitude modulation, for example by attenuation, is reserved for m,E measurement. Signal directionality is frequently used for spatial encoding. MRI makes use of frequency and phase modulation of an rf signal to encode spatial information. The simplest MRI spatial encoding is frequency modulation.

73

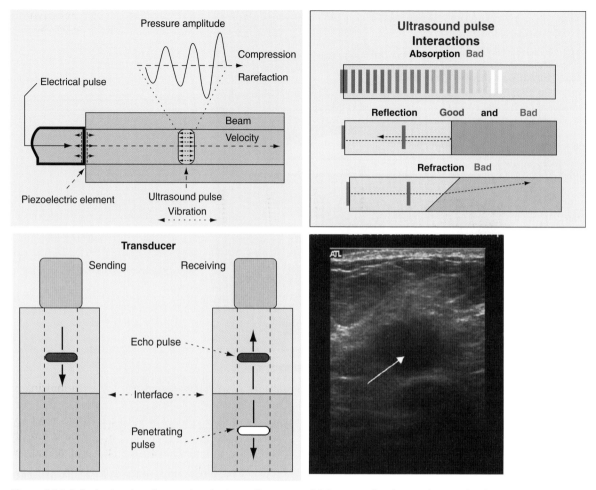

Figure 2.39. Reflective imaging: ultrasound mechanics and breast cyst. C. R. B. Merritt, after drawings by Sprawls Educational Foundation, used with permission.

MRI is one of the most sophisticated imaging techniques, whose exquisite details require significant space and effort to appreciate; we shall discuss this further in Chapter 7. For brevity and simplicity, let us elaborate on the previously presented Bohr atomic model by having all the nuclear elements spin about their own axis, with nuclear pairs spinning in opposite directions. From the perspective of the whole nucleus, nucleons spinning in opposite directions will cancel each other out. However, nuclei with odd atomic number or mass will have unopposed spins that will impart a small, net angular momentum or *spin* to the whole nucleus. Since nuclei are electrically charged (positive), those spinning nuclei with net angular momentum will have an associated magnetic field and can be considered as minute, spinning dipole magnets (Figure 2.42). The direction of the dipole moments will tend to be randomly oriented unless influenced by an external EM field. MRI utilizes a strong, external magnetic field, the B_0 field, to *polarize* the sample, aligning the nuclear magnets either parallel or antiparallel, with the former slightly predominating, to the imposed, static external magnetic field. This results in a net magnetic field, M, pointing along the B_0, or z, direction. The polarized sample is then irradiated with a carefully crafted external rf signal, the B_1 field, that *perturbs* or *excites* the nuclei, temporally aligning them orthogonal to the B_0 and B_1 fields. When this excitation signal is terminated, the nuclear spins will return to their previous energy levels and realign with the B_0 field through a process called *relaxation*. During relaxation a component of the net magnetic field, M, will rotate, or precess, in the x,y plane inducing an rf signal that can be detected by a sensitive, external rf receiver. It is almost as if the nuclei are made temporarily "radioactive." Indeed they are, but

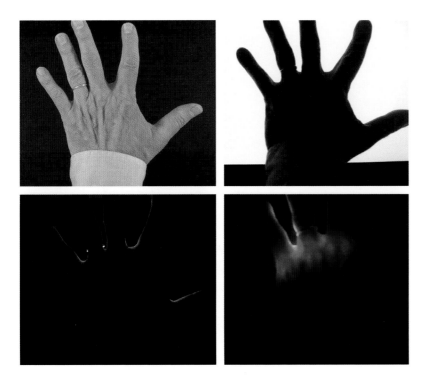

Figure 2.40. Projection imaging with visible light: reflection, shadow casting, transmission.

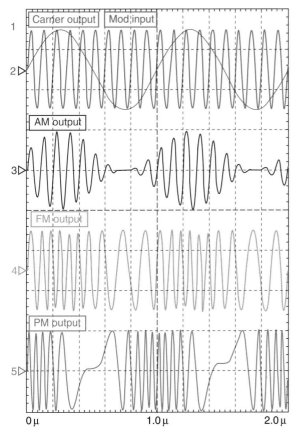

Figure 2.41. Rf signal modulation. Courtesy of Aubraux.

the emitted EM signal is of very low, non-ionizing, rf energy level.

Importantly, the relaxing nuclear spins rotate or *precess* at the *Larmor frequency*, w_0, which is directly proportional to the local magnetic field B and the gyromagnetic ratio γ:

$$\omega_{Larmor} = \gamma B \qquad (2.45)$$

MRI takes advantage of this physical feature to encode spatial information. During the relaxation time, a second weaker graded magnetic field, B_g, is imposed across the sample (Figure 2.43). This results in nuclei on one (right) side of the sample being in a higher magnetic field than those on the other (left) side. Hence the right-sided nuclei will spin faster and emit an rf signal of higher frequency than those on the left side. Right/left is spatially encoded by rf frequency. The spatial encoding does not rely directly on the directionality of either the exciting or the detected rf signal, but on spatial modulation of the frequency of the detected signal by transiently imposed magnetic field gradients. MRI spatial encoding can involve all three spatial dimensions, using a combination of rf pulses and orthogonal magnetic field gradients to modulate the frequency and phase of polarized atomic nuclei. The detected rf signal is in the so-called *time*

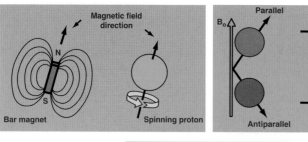

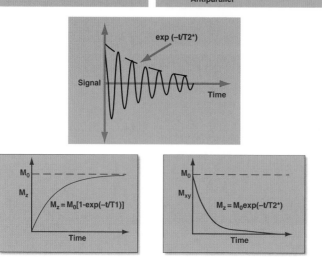

Figure 2.42. Nuclear magnetic resonance: nuclear spins, rf excite/detect signal, T1 and T2 exponential decay. C. R. B. Merritt after K. Maher's diagrams on http://en.wikibooks.org/wiki/ Basic_Physics_of_Nuclear_Medicine/ MRI_&_Nuclear_Medicine.

$M_z = M_0[1-\exp(-t/T1)]$

$M_z = M_0\exp(-t/T2^*)$

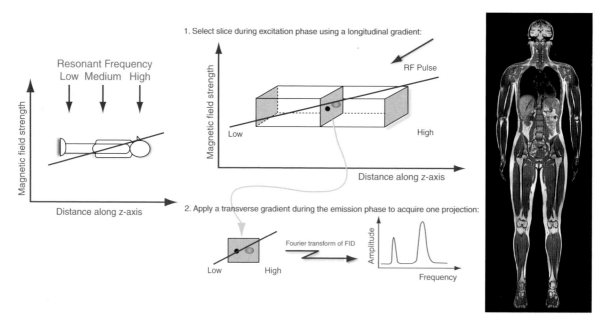

Figure 2.43. Magnetic resonance imaging; frequency and phase spatial encoding; T1-weighted whole body scan. C. R. B. Merritt after K. Maher (see Figure 2.42).

domain and resembles a complex radio signal as observed on an oscilloscope (Figure 2.44). The rf signal does not directly create an interpretable image. An MR image must be *reconstructed* by a computer algorithm, usually based on the Fourier transform, which takes a digitized sample of the time-domain signal and converts it into an image interpretable by a human.

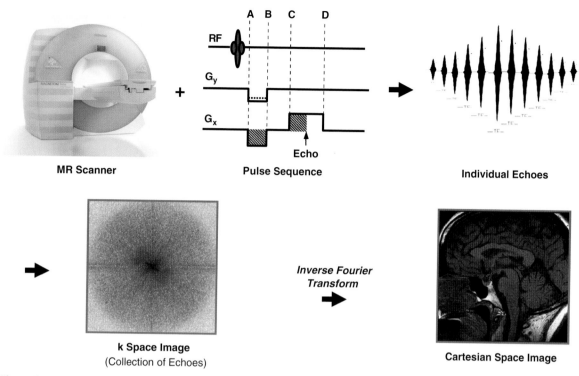

MR Scanner

Pulse Sequence

Individual Echoes

k Space Image
(Collection of Echoes)

Inverse Fourier Transform

Cartesian Space Image

Figure 2.44. Final MR image dependent on initial *k* space image being reconstructed into a Cartesian image by inverse Fourier transform. Scanner courtesy of Siemens Healthcare.

Direct/indirect image formation

A distinguishing feature of spatial encoding methods is whether or not an intuitively interpretable image is directly reflected by the data. Ordinary people require a conventional Cartesian display of *x, y, z* (right/left, up/down, front/back) spatial dimensions. In a *direct image*, the spatial component of the data is inherently organized in this fashion. The data are the image. Traditional imaging systems such as photographic cameras produce results that are directly perceived by humans as an image with obvious, conventional spatial information. Most such systems use geometric encoding of spatial information, and the data directly "constructs" an image. Image *reconstruction* is necessary for data in which the spatial component is not intuitively interpretable. In *indirect imaging*, the data are not an image; the data must be reconstructed into an image.

The issue of direct versus indirect imaging can often be posed as forward and inverse problems. Solution of a forward problem entails determining unknown effects (lung cancer) based on observations (image data, chest x-ray) of their cause (chest). Solution of an inverse problem entails determining unknown causes (chest

CT slice) based on observations of their effects (2D projections through the chest). In the latter case, the sample, which is now the CT slice, is determined from the known measurements, the projections. Expressed another way, in a forward problem the question is known, but not the answer; while in an inverse problem the answer is known, but not the question. With a CT scan the projections are known, but the slice from which they derive is not. The slice is the desired image, and it must be reconstructed using an inverse solution. Unfortunately, inverse problems are often *ill posed*, in contrast to a *well-posed* problem. The Hadamard criteria for a well-posed problem are: a solution exists, the solution is unique, and the solution depends continuously on the data. In many inverse imaging problems, these conditions may not be met and adjustments to the data must be made, often called regularization, i.e., smoothing.

Traditional radiography is a direct imaging system that is completely analog with little need for numbers and requiring no computations for construction or reconstruction of an image. In a simple x-ray system, an x-ray tube produces a "beam" of x-rays that is

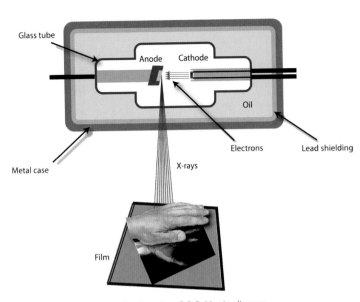
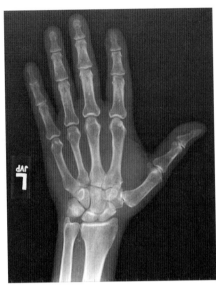

Figure 2.45. X-ray projection imaging. C. R. B. Merritt diagram.

directed at the sample (in Roentgen's case, his wife's hand). The x-rays are of a particular wavelength/energy, and the amount of x-rays produced is a function of the electrical current in the tube and *exposure time* (length of time a sample is exposed to an external signal). The x-rays propagate towards and through the patient. For simplicity's sake, this external signal can be modeled as an array of very small parallel beams (Figure 2.45). The x-ray beams interact with the sample through several types of physical events that generally result in differential absorption of the x-ray signal and deposition of energy into the sample. Some tissues absorb more x-rays than others, such as bone, which has very high electron density and is therefore relatively *radiodense*. Some of the individual rays will be blocked, while others pass through the body with minimal attenuation. The x-rays that pass through the body can be detected by an *analog* detector, such as a 14×17 inch piece of photographic film that is positioned directly behind the patient, in relationship to the x-ray tube. The photographic film includes a thin layer of a silver compound, the chemical structure of which is changed by energy absorbed from incident x-rays. This is a *parallel* imaging system, as many line integrals of signal are simultaneously detected. This greatly improves efficiency, as compared to *serial* detection. The entire 2D (right/left, cranial/caudal) projection image is created in less than 50 ms. The exposed x-ray film contains a *latent* image that is not visible to the naked eye. However, after the film is developed, those portions of the film

that were exposed to more x-rays will appear relatively dark, while those exposed to fewer x-rays will be relatively bright. The developed film contains an image that can be easily and directly perceived and recognized by a human observer. The right side of the patient is on the right side of the film, up is up, etc. The bones are bright, while soft tissue is gray, and air-containing structures, such as the lungs, are dark. The image is immediately viewable and intuitively appreciated by most human observers; the bones look like a skeleton.

This CC imaging system can easily be converted into a CD system by substituting for silver film an array of solid-state detectors. This simple change, however, has many operational implications. First, the detectors are digital and their output is discrete numbers. If for no other reason, a computer with digital graphical software is required to both create and present the image. This seemingly trivial conversion from a continuous analog imaging system to a discrete, digital imaging system was actually a revolutionary change for radiography. However, the basic digital image is still directly interpretable by a human observer.

Whether analog or digital, a 2D projection radiograph contains spatially explicit information from only two of three spatial dimensions, and the third dimension can be very important. In order to appreciate all three dimensions from projection data, the sample must be viewed from multiple angles. A stationary detector or fixed array of parallel detectors can view a stationary sample from only one angle. For a three-dimensional object, this is very

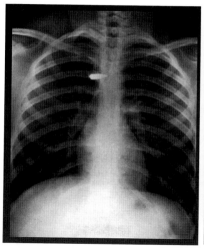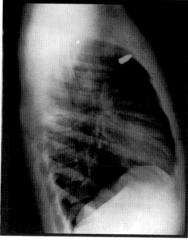

Figure 2.46. Frontal and lateral 2D projection views of 3D object: chest with bullet.

limiting (Figure 2.46). However, it is possible to modify conventional 2D projection imaging in order to appreciate the third spatial dimension. In order to obtain more views of the sample, either the detector or the sample can be rotated in relation to the other and additional images made at each new position. For a solid sample, a common and minimal number of angular views is two projections, front and side, 90° apart.

This is a very important and practical approach, but it does not provide detailed information about the third dimension. Tomography, exemplified by x-ray computed tomography (CT), takes advantage of many different one- or two-dimensional viewing angles and a *reconstruction algorithm* to make a 3D image. The simplest CT scanner makes a series of transverse line scans using an external x-ray tube on one side of the patient and a collimated x-ray detector on the opposite side of the patient (Figure 2.47). The aligned tube and detector traverse the patient similar to the rectilinear gamma scanner. However, rather than incrementing the tube/detector assembly in a cranial/caudal direction to create a 2D projection image (which is quite feasible), the assembly is rotated one degree and a second set of line scans are obtained. This is repeated through a minimum of 180 degrees. The resultant collection of 2D projections do not form a directly interpretable image, but with an appropriate computer reconstruction algorithm, this projection data can be converted into a 2D Cartesian slice through the sample. Any single image is only a 2D slice, with the third dimension represented by a series of slices. Importantly, objects that are superimposed on conventional 2D projection images are now

separated in the slice. Furthermore, tissue contrast within the slice is much greater than on conventional projection images. In order to make a CT image, the original, continuous CT signal must be discretized and fed to a reconstruction algorithm that creates a digital image, which is displayed by computer graphics. This is a CD system. Spatial information is initially encoded as with any projection imaging via signal/detector directionality. However, an individual projection is not intuitively interpretable, and an appropriately stacked series of projections is called a *sinogram*. This perfectly good, but not intuitively comprehensible, spatial information in individual projections of the sinogram must be reconstructed by a computer algorithm that converts or *transforms* 2D projection data into a conventional image. This conversion of sinogram spatial information into Cartesian spatial information can be performed by two different mathematical approaches, iterative or algebraic. In the iterative approach, which was originally used by Hounsfield in the original CT scanner, voxel values within the image are literally guessed at until a reasonable match to the data is found (Fig 2.48). This methodology was quickly complemented by algebraic solutions such as *back projection* using the *inverse Radon transform*, which converts projection data into a conventional image matrix:

$$\lambda(p, \phi) = \int_{\infty} d^2 r f(\mathbf{r}) \delta(p - \mathbf{r} \cdot \hat{\mathbf{n}}) \qquad (2.46)$$

Two spatial dimensions are serially sampled by line integrals at multiple angles, creating projections that are then indirectly reconstructed into an image, which

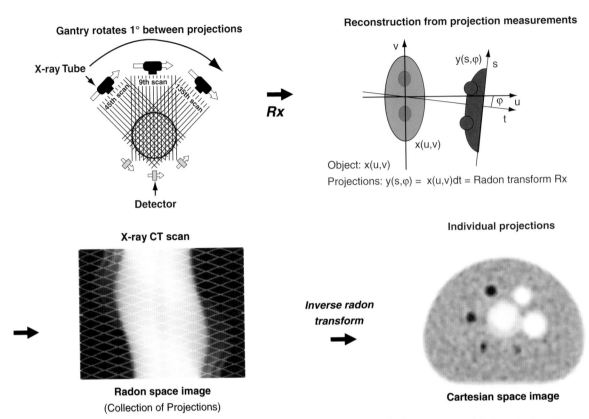

Figure 2.47. X-ray CT tomography: multiple angular projections result in sinogram image that is reconstructed into Cartesian image by inverse Radon transform. C. R. B. Merritt.

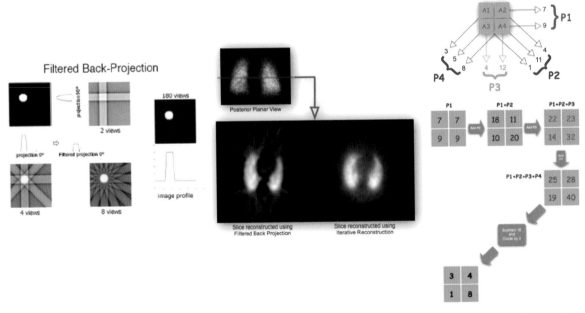

Figure 2.48. Tomographic reconstructions using analytic or iterative methods. Projections courtesy of J. S. Karp. Diagram C. R. B. Merritt after K. Maher (see Figure 2.42).

is a 2D slice through the sample. The third dimension, represented by a series of slices, is defined by x-ray beam and detector collimation. The images are discrete, digital, and quantifiable.

References

1. Kelvin WT. *Popular Lectures and Addresses*. London: Macmillan, 1891.

2. Stevens SS. On the theory of scales of measurement. *Science* 1946; **103**: 677–80.

3. International System of Units (SI). The NIST Reference on Constants, Units, and Uncertainty. www.physics.nist. gov/cuu/Units/units.html.

General reading

Barrett HH, Myers K J. *Foundations of Image Science*. Hoboken, NJ: Wiley-Interscience, 2004.

Bushberg JT. *The Essential Physics of Medical Imaging*. Philadelphia, PA: Lippincott Williams & Wilkins, 2002.

Prince JL, Links JM. *Medical Imaging Signals and Systems*. Upper Saddle River, NJ: Pearson Prentice Hall, 2006.

Rosner B. *Fundamentals of Biostatistics*. Belmont, CA: Thomson-Brooks/Cole, 2006.

Salsburg D. *The Lady Tasting Tea: How Statistics Revolutionized Science in the Twentieth Century*. New York, NY: W. H. Freeman, 2001.

How to analyze an image

R. Nick Bryan and Christopher R. B. Merritt

Having defined the universe and nature, introduced concepts of imaging portions thereof, and outlined how to make such an image, let us now address the issue of how to analyze an image. Imaging is not necessarily science. The ancients imaged the heavens for eons, but performed no science. Instead, they fantasized animals and mythical creatures in the heavens and created the constellations (Figure 3.1). The ancients practiced non-scientific astrology, not scientific astronomy. Perhaps the first example of modern scientific imaging was Galileo's discovery and description of the moons of Jupiter in 1610 (Figure 1.25). Galileo used a new imaging tool, the telescope, which improved the imaging capabilities of the naked eye by increasing spatial resolution. This technology allowed him to image previously invisible, small, faint objects in the vicinity of the even-then known planet of Jupiter. At this point Galileo had performed novel imaging, but not science. He had a choice as to what to do with this new information. He could have mythologized the images he saw and empirically filled the telescopic sky with more fantastic creatures. Fortunately, he chose the heretofore unorthodox scientific approach. Instead of imagining monsters, he used his new imaging tool to make localized measurements of energy (visible light) in the spatial vicinity of Jupiter over time (several weeks). He exquisitely displayed these observations with simple images – drawings. Importantly, he then applied the scientific method to first hypothesize and then prove mathematically that these faint light signals were from four previously unknown moons. This extraordinary example of scientific imaging not only expanded our knowledge of planetary space, but also fundamentally changed our concept of the universe and mankind's role in it. Galileo performed scientific imaging by making rigorous spatially and temporally defined observations of m,E that led to an explanatory hypothesis, a hypothesis that in turn was rigorously proved and then used to predict future celestial events.

The universe as we have described it consists of collections of m,E distributed heterogeneously through three-dimensional space that evolves with time. It is this universe, or portions thereof, that interests scientists. Scientists seek information about the universe, nature. An image is a corresponding display of measurements of m,E made as a function of spatial location and time. An image is the most robust representation of a piece of the universe. An image depicts only a portion of the universe, a scene, within which the object(s) of interest, or sample, is located.

Imaging as communication

As previously noted, imaging is simply a form of communication. Communication is the transfer of information. Specifically, imaging is humans' primary means of communicating spatial information. Imaging is the natural language of space. A basic theory of communication, focusing on information transfer, is well documented in the works of Shannon [1]. In Shannon's model, an information source passes a message to a transmitter, which creates a signal that flows to a receiver that passes the message to its final destination – an observer (Figure 3.2).

The signal is generally confounded by unwanted noise, a signal that does not accurately reflect the sample. As applied to our discussion, the information source is a piece of the universe, which contains the information about which we are interested. This information is encoded in measurements made by a detector that sends a signal, confounded by noise, to a receiver, some type of visual display unit. Finally, an observer decodes the message in order to make a decision.

Introduction to the Science of Medical Imaging, ed. R. Nick Bryan. Published by Cambridge University Press. © Cambridge University Press 2010.

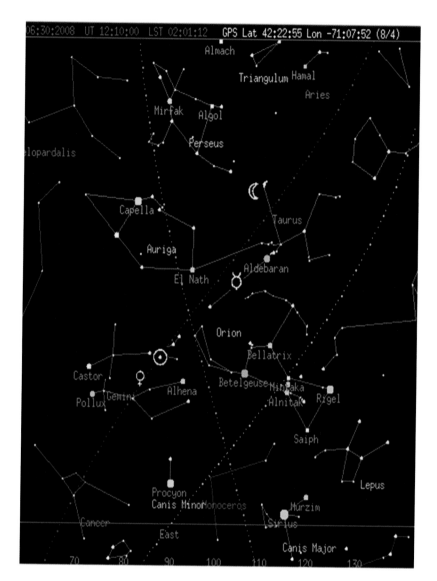

Figure 3.1. Non-scientific imaging of constellations. From http://wiki. openmoko.org/wiki/Orrery.

Information transfer through a contemporary medical image communication system is represented in Figure 3.3. In the case of mammography, the information source is the patient's breast; the imaging system consists of an x-ray tube and digital detector that encodes information about electron density in 2D images that are displayed (decoded) by a computer graphics program for observation and analysis by an observer. The observer might be a human or a computer. The final product is a report containing a clinical decision based on the image, i.e., the presence or absence of cancer. The quality of this decision depends on how accurately the imaging system describes the physical state of the tissue in the patient's breast.

Information

What is the nature of the information that one would like to communicate with a scientific image? We have already indicated that scientists are interested in the spatial distributions of m,E over time, but more specifically, scientists are interested in non-random, ordered collections of m,E. Unordered, random distributions of m,E have no structure, are unpredictable, reveal no underlying patterns, and are not generally of

83

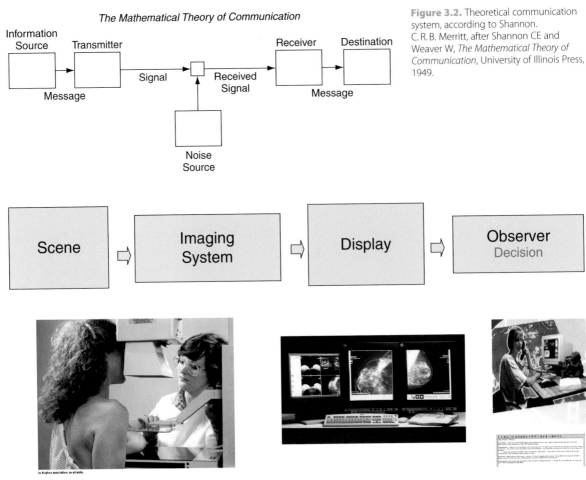

The Mathematical Theory of Communication

Figure 3.2. Theoretical communication system, according to Shannon. C. R. B. Merritt, after Shannon CE and Weaver W, *The Mathematical Theory of Communication*, University of Illinois Press, 1949.

Figure 3.3. Contemporary biomedical communication system, mammography. Photo 1 courtesy of National Cancer Institute, www.cancer.gov/cancertopics/pdq/screening/breast/Patient/page3.

scientific interest. Randomness is ultimately boring, repetitive nothingness. Order, on the other hand, accounts for predictable patterns, identifiable objects – the aggregates of nature that engage the interest of scientists. Scientific images strive to communicate nature's order, particularly nature's spatial order. It is natural order that one wishes to communicate with a scientific image.

How is this non-random information expressed, quantified? Though originally defined in terms of heat machines, thermodynamics offers a clue to defining information. The first law of thermodynamics states that energy is conserved. The second law of thermodynamics states that nature tends towards disorder. According to this law, as promulgated by Boltzmann, the natural state of the universe is disorder. Things left alone become disorganized, random in nature. Order requires energy for its creation and maintenance. A

measure of disorder is *entropy*, which is a reflection of randomness. Highly organized structures have low entropy, while high entropy reflects lack of organization or order. Scientists are generally interested in low-entropy states, like biological systems, which are highly ordered and require energy for self-maintenance.

Entropy was originally defined as:

$$\Delta S = Q/T \qquad (3.1)$$

with entropy (S), temperature (T), and heat (Q). Entropy represents the probabilistic state of a system, with high-entropy states having many possible states with relatively low probabilities for any particular state, while low-entropy states have high probabilities for few possible states. Rewording Richard Feynman, disorder can be measured by the number of ways that a system might be arranged and still look similar from the outside [2]. The logarithm of that number of ways is entropy.

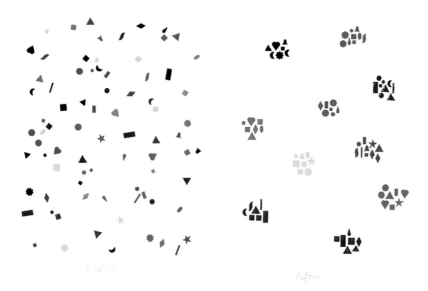

Figure 3.4. Less ordered (high entropy) and more highly ordered (low entropy) states. C. R. B. Merritt.

Shannon expands this physical concept of entropy as a measure of disorder to define information in probabilistic terms that can be quantified similarly to thermodynamic entropy. *Information* as defined by Shannon is semantically confusing and is not the same as *meaning*. Consider a message as a unit of information expressing a particular state of a system. A particular message has meaning, which might be highly specific or gibberish. In distinction, information is a measure of the number of options that exist for the message: how many states of the system might exist. The more options one has in selecting a particular message, the more information there is related to the system. Information, "relates not so much to what you *do* say, as to what you *could* say. That is, information is a measure of one's freedom of choice when one selects a message" [1]. There are few options for a message to describe a highly organized, non-random system, pattern, or object. The message might have great meaning, but the system has low entropy and low information content. A highly structured system has relatively few highly probable states.

The information related to a signal depends on the orderliness of the system from which it is derived and can be measured as units of entropy. A system may exist in a state, *i*, with a probablility, *p*. Entropy is determined by the number of possible states, *i*, and the probability, *P*, of being in any particular state:

$$H = -\sum p_i \log p_i \qquad (3.2)$$

The overall entropy, H, of an information source is an average of the entropy, H_i, of all possible states, P_i, of a system weighted by the probability of the various states:

$$H = \sum P_i H_i \qquad (3.3)$$

While the mathematics may be dense, the concept is straightforward. Scientifically interesting parts of the universe consist of statistically likely accumulations of m,E that can be measured and encoded in signals that contain information about the non-randomness of the sample. Images include the spatial components of this information. Scientific observers look for non-random spatial patterns in images, such as the structured spatial and color groupings in the "after" image of Figure 3.4. Such scenes are organized, have low entropy, and contain little information (but great meaning). On the other hand, the spatially randomly distributed colored symbols in the "before" image of Figure 3.4 have high spatial entropy and information content (but little meaning to most people). Using Feynman's explanation of entropy, the highly ordered visual scenes, if randomly perturbed, would not look the same, while the already random color images would look the same after even more random shuffling.

Noise

Noise is a constant confounder of measurements with a unique aspect in imaging measurements, as one actually sees the noise in the image (Figure 3.5).

85

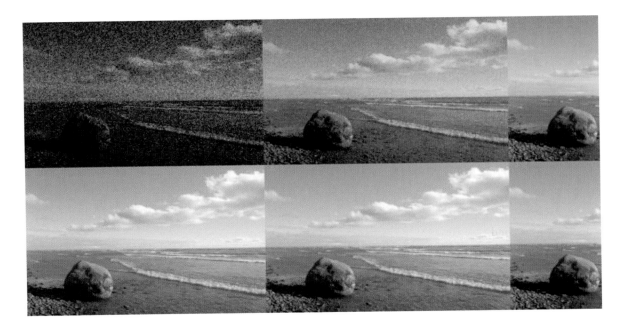

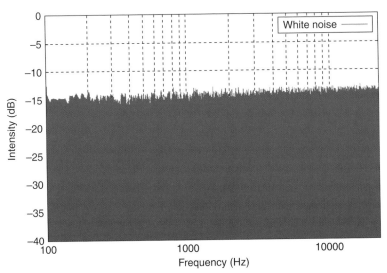

Figure 3.5. Visualization of noise: superimposed in an image of colored strips; frequency histogram of noise. From http://en.wikipedia.org/wiki/Image_noise and http://commons.wikimedia.org/wiki/Category:White_noise.

Noise is a signal that does not relate to the sample. In Shannon's model, the received signal is not the same as the transmitted signal. Noise comes in two forms: non-random and random. In the case of non-random noise, a transmitted signal always produces the same received signal. The result is termed *distortion* or *bias* of the system and can potentially be corrected. If no two transmitted signals produce the same received signal, the signal function has an inverse that can be applied to the received signal to correct the distortion.

If the transmitted signal S does not always produce the same received signal E, then the latter can be viewed as a function of the transmitted signal and a second variable, the noise N:

$$E = f(S, N) \qquad (3.4)$$

Just as the signal may be considered as a random variable, so may noise, and both can be treated stochastically. If a noisy system is fed by a single source, there are two statistical processes at work, one involving S and the other involving N. In terms of entropy, one can calculate that of the source $H(x)$, the received signal $H(y)$, their joint entropy $H(x,y)$, and the conditional entropies $H_x(y)$ and $H_y(x)$. In the case of a noiseless system:

$$H(x) = H(y) \qquad (3.5)$$

If the system is noisy, it is generally not possible to reconstruct the original signal from the received signal with certainty by any operation on the latter. Any received signal containing noise results in ambiguity or uncertainty about the original signal. In essence, information has been lost by the system by the introduction of noise. The uncertainty in the received signal is defined by the conditional entropy $H_y(x)$, which can also be used to estimate the amount of additional information needed to correct the received message, i.e., how much additional information is required to make up for the lost information due to noise. For practical purposes, signals, including images, from noisier systems have lost more information than those from less noisy systems.

Noise in images often results in a mottled, black-and-white, salt-and-pepper appearance. A histogram of noise reveals random fluctuations of the signal intensity as a function of location, reflecting no central tendency and, for practical purposes, conveying no information about the sample (Figure 3.6). As with all methods of measurement, imaging strives to maximize the true signal, which contains information about the sample while minimizing noise. The *signal-to-noise* ratio (SNR, *S/N*) is a basic measure of image quality and is simply:

$$S/N = signal/noise \qquad (3.6)$$

SNR in an image is determined by averaging signal intensity within similar-sized regions of interest (ROIs) inside and outside the sample (background). High SNR is desired; SNR of 0 has no information and infinitely high entropy. For many applications, SNR of 5 or greater is considered a minimum for satisfactory analysis. The information content of an image consists of a sample's non-randomness encoded in the signal that has not been obscured by random noise. The observer attempts to extract meaning from the image by identifying low-entropy components.

While SNR is an important measure of image quality and potential information content, perhaps as important for many image analysis tasks is *contrast-to-noise* ratio (CNR). In many imaging applications, the primary task is to differentiate individual components of an image. Components of images are obviously of many different types, including physical entities such as planets, oceanic flow patterns, or chemical spectra. For immediate, simplistic purposes we shall call different components of an image *objects*. *Object* as defined here does not imply any particular physical state, merely different non-random components of an image, including non-random patterns. The performance of object discrimination is dependent upon different objects having different signal characteristics from each other. Differential object signals produce *contrast* (Figure 3.6). Contrast, C, is the difference in signal between two objects:

$$C = S_1 - S_2 \qquad (3.7)$$

Visible light in conjunction with the human visual system allows blue sea to contrast with white sand. In the case of radiography, contrast is a result of differential absorption of x-ray photons due to differences in tissue electron density.

While contrast is important, its practical merit lies in relationship to noise. Intrinsic contrast is due to the difference in m,E between two objects in a sample, but images are results of measurements of m,E. Hence the intrinsic contrast between the objects is confounded by noise. Noise always decreases the relative contrast between two objects. Hence, in practice, contrast-to-noise (CNR, *C/N*) is the usual operational unit, defined as:

$$C/N = \frac{S_1 - S_2}{N} \qquad (3.8)$$

CNR in an image is determined by averaging signal intensity in similar-sized ROIs placed within two objects in the sample and another ROI outside the sample (Figure 3.7). The calculation of CNR requires

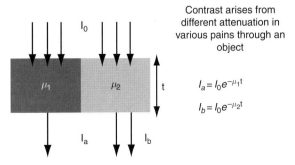

Figure 3.6. Contrast: difference in detected signal between two objects, in this case due to differential attenuation of x-rays. C. R. B. Merritt.

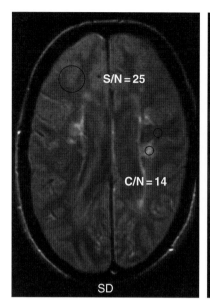 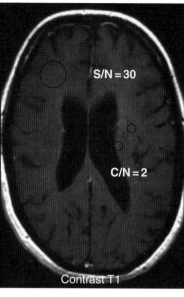

Figure 3.7. SNR (*S/N*) (of normal brain) and CNR (*C/N*) of multiple sclerosis plaques to normal brain on spin-density and T_1 magnetic resonance images.

the explicit definition of objects, at least two in this case. This is not a trivial task, and one that we will return to later. High CNR is desired; CNR of 0 does not allow differentiation of the specified objects. An image might have high SNR for two objects, but no CNR. Noise influences CNR and SNR similarly in that greater noise decreases both. Hence it is always desirable to minimize noise.

Observers

Traditionally and historically, scientific image observers have been humans, like Galileo. While most image observers are still human, there is increasing use of the computer as a stand-alone observer or, more frequently, a combination of human and computer as the observer. The observer plays the final, critical role in the experimental paradigm as he/she/it takes all available data related to the experiment, draws a conclusion, and makes a decision. The final, practical, and even theoretical value of a scientific experiment is the validity of the decision made by the observer. But any observer has a limit as to how good a decision can be made, given the available data. That limit defines the performance of an *ideal observer*. The concept of an ideal observer is Bayesian; ideal and Bayesian observers are synonymous. An ideal observer utilizes all available statistical information to maximize task performance, as measured by Bayes' risk or some other related measure of performance (see Appendix 3). The ideal or Bayesian observer defines the upper limit for

any observer performance. Specific characteristics of an ideal observer include: (1) no observer noise, (2) presence, knowledge, and maintenance of a decision threshold, and (3) all the information necessary to calculate the probability of the observation (data), given the hypothesis to be tested ($\mathrm{pr}(g|H_j)$). The latter condition is very demanding and includes descriptions of the objects to be classified, complete information about the measurement (imaging) process, and noise statistics. As with all Bayesian analysis, an ideal observer uses not only *a posteriori* information, but also *a priori* information; that is, not only data from specific observations or experiments, but any additional task-related information. We will return to the ideal observer later, but remember this important concept: a limit to observer performance can be defined.

Let us now take a brief look at the most common, real, generally non-ideal observer – a human being.

Human observers

Imaging devices generally make measurements of a sample, some aspect of m,E, which cannot be directly observed. As a requisite first step this raw data must be converted to an appropriate format for the observer. For human observers, the image must be perceptible by the human visual system. This requires converting the m,E observations into corresponding visible light signals that can be detected by the retina. Usually this is done by converting the detected signals into numbers (measurement) and then assigning specific light

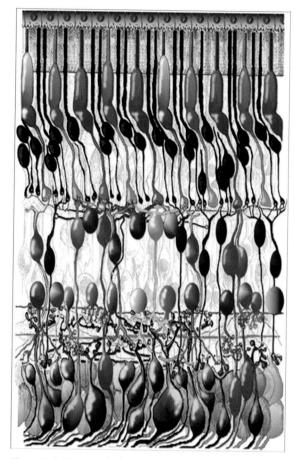

Figure 3.8. Human retinal organization, with rod and cone light receptors for scotopic and photopic vision respectively. http://webvision.umh.es/webvision/anatomy.html.

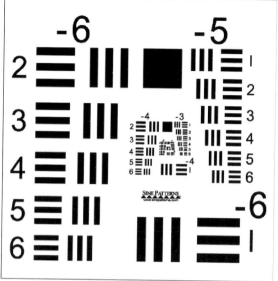

USAF - XL (40" x 40" on photographic paper)

Figure 3.9. Spatial resolution metric: line pairs (lp) per millimeter. USAF diagram, photo courtesy of Electro Optical Industries.

signals to sets of numbers. There are two photodetector systems in the retina, one subserving *scotopic* vision, and the other *photopic* vision (Figure 3.8). Scotopic vision is dependent on rhodopsin-containing *rod* detectors that are sensitive only to *luminance* or light intensity. By this visual system, humans perceive only shades of gray (approximately 256 from black to white). Rod vision is very sensitive, down to the level of one photon of light, and hence predominates at low light levels. On the other hand, scotopic vision has relatively low spatial resolution, about 1 lp/mm (lp/mm = the number of pairs of alternating black and white lines displayed within one millimeter: Figure 3.9). Photopic vision is dependent on three types of iodopsin-containing cones, each type sensitive to different wavelengths (colors) of light, specifically red/orange, green, and blue (commonly referred to as

RGB). Photopic vision is several orders of magnitude less sensitive to light energy, but can distinguish more than a million different colors with spatial resolution approximately 5 lp/mm. These two light-detection systems are differentially distributed in the retina, with rods more sparsely and widely distributed, and cones more concentrated in the posterior retina, particularly in the *fovea*, where approximately 6000 densely packed cones subserve the very highest spatial resolution in the central 1 degree of the visual field. This accounts for the greater spatial resolution of color vision and the lack of central dark vision.

The scotopic and photopic light-detecting systems allow perception of images in either black and white (gray scale) or color format. An image measurement must be converted to and displayed as either a shade of gray or a color (Figure 3.10). A typical human can differentiate approximately 256 shades of gray or a million different colors, to each of which one or a range of measurement numbers can be assigned. However, approximately one in 10 persons will lack one of the sets of cones, and hence be able to discriminate fewer colors. Such *color blindness* is most common in males and most frequently involves the lack of red- or green-sensitive cones (Figure 3.11). There is an intuitive relationship between increasing numerical magnitude and

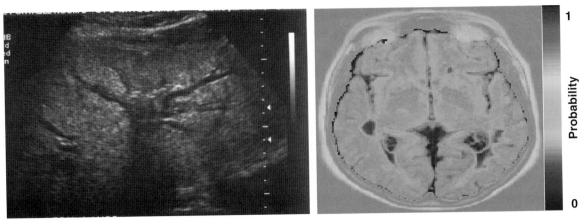

Figure 3.10. Gray-scale ultrasound image of the liver; color-scale image of the probability of ischemic disease of the brain.

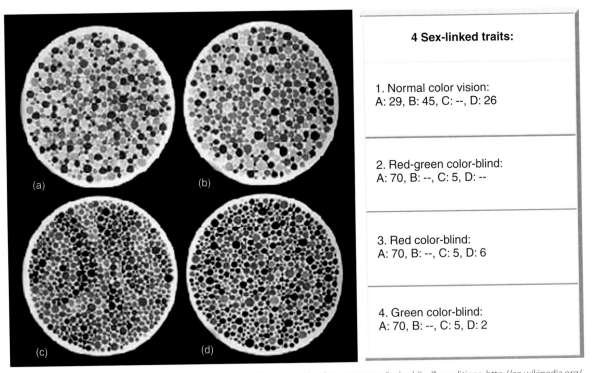

4 Sex-linked traits:
1. Normal color vision: A: 29, B: 45, C: --, D: 26
2. Red-green color-blind: A: 70, B: --, C: 5, D: --
3. Red color-blind: A: 70, B: --, C: 5, D: 6
4. Green color-blind: A: 70, B: --, C: 5, D: 2

Figure 3.11. Test patterns to distinguish normal color detection versus the three common "color blind" conditions. http://en.wikipedia.org/wiki/Ishihara_color_test.

increasing brightness on a gray-scale image. While color images offer a greater dynamic range for numerical representations, there is a less intuitive appreciation of the ordinal relationship between numbers and color. It is important that scientific images are accompanied by a reference scale that explicitly defines what numbers the shades of gray

or colors in the image represent. This is particularly important for color images.

Not only must an imaging system map m,E signals to a format compatible with the observer, but the spatial components of image data must also be appropriately presented to the observer. For intuitive appreciation by human observers, spatial information is

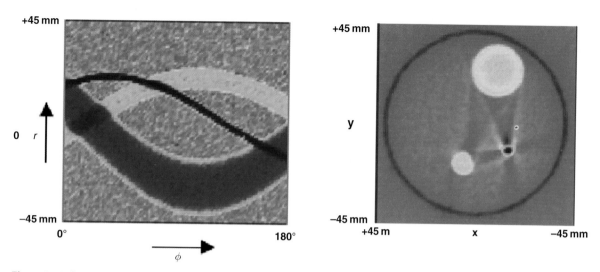

Figure 3.12. Sinogram and Cartesian spatial displays of x-ray CT phantom containing three rods of different size and radiodensity. Courtesy of Siemens Healthcare.

generally presented in a traditional two- or three-dimensional (2D, 3D) Cartesian coordinate system. Computer algorithms have more flexibility in how spatial data is presented and, in fact, do not directly operate on spatial data in a Cartesian space. For instance, spatial information from a 2D CT slice may be presented as a series of angular projections, as in a sinogram (Figure 3.12). This presentation is not interpretable to most people; however, a 2D Cartesian display of the same data is intuitively appreciated. The spatial information is identical in both presentations, but human perception demands the latter. These two steps in image data processing – gray-scale or color encoding of m,E measurements and Cartesian display of spatial information – are general requirements for image displays for human observation.

A pragmatic challenge to imaging is the effective presentation to the human observer of multidimensional data. All scientific measurements are multidimensional. Images always include at least one m,E dimension, two spatial dimensions, and the time dimension. Many images are even more complex, with additional spatial and non-spatial dimensions. Most display formats are physically confined to two spatial dimensions – right/left, up/down – so-called *flatland*. Common display formats superimpose a gray or color scale for the m,E signal dimensions on the two spatial dimensions of the page or electronic display. Edward Tufte deals extensively with graphical opportunities to maximize the expressive capability of these flat displays to represent three or more dimensions, spatial or metric [3] (Figure 1.22). While any

display should preserve the integrity of scientific data, it cannot be denied that there is an aesthetic component to the presentation of image data. Effective images not only present scientific data, but also actively engage and assist the observer in extracting information. Poorly designed images can distort the scientific data and/or obscure information by awkward, ugly, or distracting presentations. Many dimensions can be incorporated into flatland in a fashion that creates compelling and highly informative illustrations, as with Minard's graphic of Napoleon's Russian campaign (Figure 3.13). This figure presents six dimensions – two spatial, three non-spatial, plus time – on a flat, two-spatial-dimensional piece of paper.

The explicit representation of spatial information is a particular challenge in that many scientific samples have three real spatial dimensions that must be compressed into the two physical spatial dimensions of paper or monitor. The first step in the determination of the number of spatial dimensions incorporated into an image involves the imaging process itself, as outlined in the previous chapter. Spatial dimensions may be compressed or reduced by the imaging system and associated spatial transforms. The three physical spatial dimensions of a patient are reduced to two spatial dimensions in a chest film by the projection transform of radiography. Given an image with more than two spatial dimensions, there are a variety of techniques that guide pseudo-3D displays and take maximum advantage of human psychophysics.

91

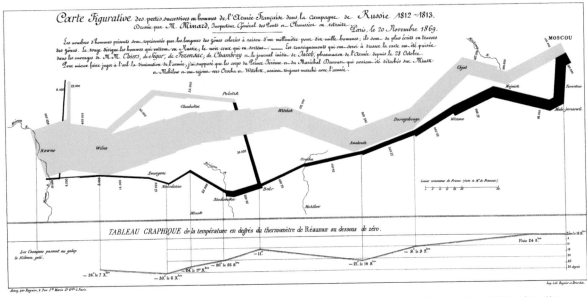

Figure 3.13. Charles Minard's graphic of the Grande Armée during Napoleon's Russian campaign. By Charles Minard 1869, at http://en.wikipedia.org/wiki/Charles_ Joseph_Minard.

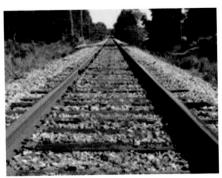

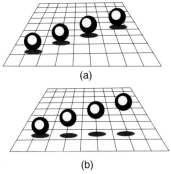

(a)

(b)

Figure 3.14. Fixed position, monocular clues to depth: convergence, shadowing. Kersten D, Mamassian P, Knill DC, Moving cast shadows induce apparent motion in depth. *Perception* 1997; **26**(2): 171–92. Used with permission.

Human 3D imaging is dependent on two physical aspects of the observer: (1) whether one is viewing with one or two eyes and (2) whether one is viewing from a fixed or moving position. There are four clues to depth in monocular viewing from a fixed viewpoint (Figure 3.14):

Relative size	Near objects larger than far objects
Image overlap	Near objects overlap far objects
Haze	Far objects have lower contrast and lower color saturation, and appear bluish
Modeling and texture	Highlights and shadows are lost in far objects

A changing viewpoint brings into play *parallax*, through which near objects seem to move in the opposite direction to head movement, while far objects seem to remain stationary. While in daily life parallax provides powerful clues to depth, it is obviously much less important for printed images, where the number of viewpoints is limited. There is much more opportunity for the use of parallax with dynamic video displays. *Accommodation*, the refocusing of the lens to near and far objects, is also viewpoint-dependent, but plays a relatively small role in depth perception.

Binocular vision adds two more depth clues: *ocular convergence* and *stereoscopic fusion*. The former relates to the inward rotation of the eyes to maintain focus on nearer objects. The latter is a much more subtle process that takes place in the visual cortex and takes advantage of the slightly different views of an object by each eye because of the ocular separation of 6–7 cm. The visual cortex somehow compares the two images and interprets the differences between them in terms of depth. This is called *stereopsis*, which is a mental

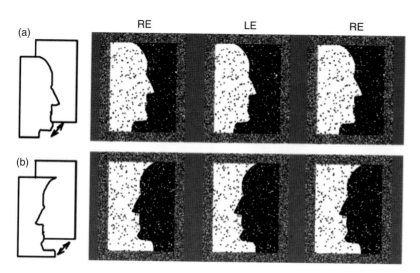

Figure 3.15. Stereopsis requires binocular vision for additional depth perception. Burge J, Peterson MA, Palmer SE. Ordinal configural cues combine with metric disparity in depth perception. *Journal of Vision* 2005; **5**(6): 534–42. © Association for Research in Vision and Ophthalmology. Used with permission.

process that must be developed, and which approximately one in 20 individuals lack. True stereoscopic imaging can be facilitated by a variety of devices, including special lens or mirror arrangements and video monitors with or without special glasses (Figure 3.15). A fundamentally different way to display all three spatial dimensions is *holography*, which requires special imaging equipment. Holography will not be discussed here, but it does offer another means of 3D visualization.

In general, digital computer displays offer more opportunities for effective display of multiple spatial dimensions than hard-copy displays. The short video clip, *Imaging My Brain*, displays two m,E dimensions (CT and T1 MR), three spatial dimensions, plus time (Figure 3.16).

There are two common physical means of presenting images to human observers – *hard copy* or *soft copy*. For over 600 years, paper has been the most common hard-copy medium, though for medical imaging translucent film has been used more frequently. Soft-copy presentations are performed by electronic monitors. Until recently, there had been much discussion about the quality of image display with hard copy versus soft copy. New electronic monitors, particularly LCD monitors with high luminosity, are equal to, if not better, than high-quality printed material (Figure 3.17). Electronic displays offer many other advantages over hard-copy displays, and most scientific imaging is now displayed using high-resolution computer monitors, with hard copy reserved for publication and convenience purposes.

Beyond the basic necessities of physically presenting scientific images in black and white or color with appropriate spatial presentation, human image analysis quickly becomes very complex and is intimately related to *visual psychophysics*. There is a large literature on this topic, which explains how the human visual system performs different tasks under a variety of conditions. Though too vast a topic to be fully addressed here, a few salient points will now be presented. Visual psychophysics involves the extraction of information from image displays related to signal properties, spatial attributes, as well as dynamic temporal information. Some of the more basic visual attractors (those aspects of an image that catch the observer's attention and are presumably important in information extraction) are relative brightness and high-frequency information, either spatial (edges) or temporal (movement) (Figure 3.18).

Key features of human psychophysics can be anticipated by recalling evolution. Visual systems evolved to foster the survival of species, and they tend to differ between species that are predators versus those that are predatory targets. For instance, predatory species tend to have forward-looking eyes with smaller but overlapping visual fields in order to better spot, then rapidly and accurately track, potential targets. Target species tend to have laterally looking, non-overlapping eyes with maximal visual fields to spot predators coming from any direction. From an evolutionary perspective, the human visual system can be viewed as predatory in type. All biological visual systems (as well as other sensory systems) contain elements that attempt to distinguish objects from their background in order to identify those that require more urgent attention and eventually classify them as target, friend or foe, dangerous or beneficial. These visual tools of self-preservation are the same ones we

93

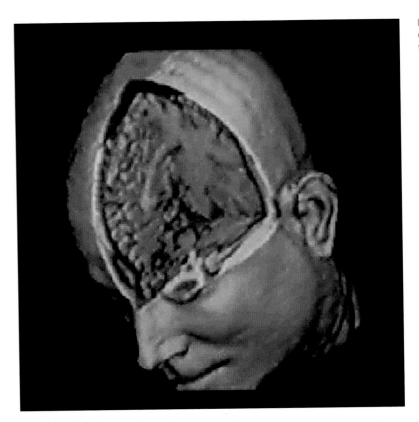

Figure 3.16. *Imaging My Brain*: video clip displaying a combination of six spatial, signal, and temporal dimensions.

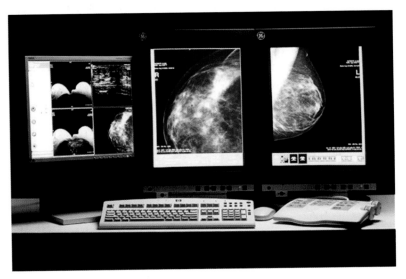

Figure 3.17. High-resolution electronic digital monitors (4 megapixel spatial, 12-bit gray-scale resolution) used for mammography images.

now use for scientific image analysis. It should be emphasized that information extraction focuses on identifying non-random signal patterns from the sample. Noise will obviously compromise and, if severe, obscure sample signal. Predators such as lions, which

could potentially prey upon humans, might have very low visual entropy during daylight, making them easily identifiable. However, this visual entropy can be increased by darkness (loss of signal) or blowing dust (noise). The human observer's task is to extract

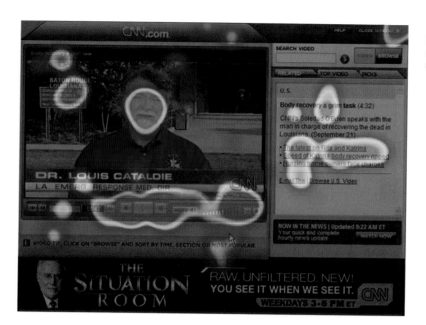

Figure 3.18. Human spatial attractors: brightness and high spatial frequency. Courtesy of Jakob Nielsen, www.useit.com/alertbox/video.html.

key information from very complex and often noisy visual signals. In the case of self-preservation in the jungle, the task is to find the lion; in the case of medicine, it is to find the cancer – another human predator.

Human vision has evolved into an extraordinary and complex system that does a superb job of analyzing visual information. A key feature of the visual system is that it performs its task not by holistically analyzing the "complete picture" as we perceive it, but by breaking the image down into smaller, simpler components that are separately analyzed in "channels." As we have seen, decomposition of the image begins in the retina where multispectral white light is decomposed into three color channels – red, blue, and green (RGB) – and a separate intensity channel. The detected light signals are promptly encoded in complex electrochemical signals that are almost immediately modified in the retina via ganglion cells with surround-inhibition characteristics (Figure 3.19) so as to accentuate certain features such as edges. The neural signals from the retina proceed via the optic nerve through the optic chiasm. This is the structure where the right and left halves of the visual fields are split, each half of the visual field being primarily processed by structures of the opposite side of the brain, the first being the lateral geniculate nuclei (LGN) or bodies (Figure 3.20). In the LGN, neural signals are further divided between two neural pathways,

commonly called the parvocellular (P) and magnocellular (M) systems, which process different image features. Specifically, the M pathway is insensitive to color, has high contrast sensitivity, is responsive to lower spatial frequencies and higher temporal frequencies, and tends towards transient responses. The P pathway is color-sensitive, has lower contrast sensitivity, is responsive to higher spatial frequencies and lower temporal frequencies, and gives sustained responses (Figure 3.21). These two visual pathways, commonly called the "what" and "where" pathways, are microscopically segregated in the primary visual cortex into physiologically, metabolically, and histologically distinct sets of neurons that further modify the neural signals and pass this channelized information downstream to the secondary visual association areas in the parietal and temporal lobes. In terms of process, the chief characteristic of the visual system is its deconstruction of the original image data into specific functional pathways that are processed relatively independently in the brain (Figure 3.22). The world as we "see" it does not exist in any single region of the brain beyond the retina. Low-level visual tasks, such as motion detection, are relatively well understood, but higher-level tasks such as identifying complex shapes like cancerous tumors are not. While division of work apparently optimizes analytical processes, it creates a central dilemma for neuroscience, the so-called "binding problem." How are the outputs of these disparate

95

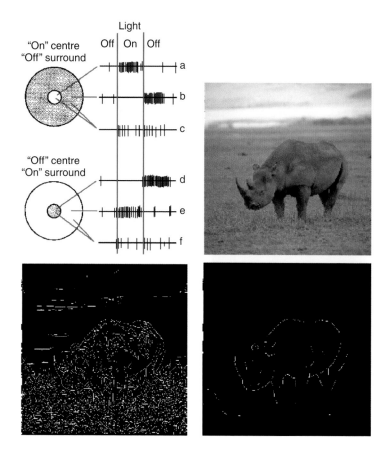

Figure 3.19. Human visual digital image edge enhancement. Visual processing with surround-inhibition mechanism for edge enhancement. Receptive field of ganglion cells courtesy of M. Mann, after Hubel DH, *Scientific American*, 1963, www.unmc.edu/physiology/Mann/mann7.html. Rhino images courtesy of N. Petkov and M. B. Wieling, University of Groningen, http://www.cs.rug.nl/~petkov/.

channels recombined into a single, common perception? How do the individual features of a bouncing red ball, whose temporal, signal, and shape features are separately analyzed, evolve into a single conscious perception?

Human visual search

The process of human visual search for patterns or objects in an image is incompletely understood, but there appear to be certain underlying procedures. First, the visual system searches for areas of non-randomness and low entropy, where there tends to be high information density (in the general, not Shannon terminology). These tend to be image regions that have high frequencies in either the signal, spatial, or temporal domains. A classic example revealed by eye-tracking experiments is the preferential gaze time along edges, regions of high spatial frequency. There appear to be at least two different subsequent

analytical steps: (1) definition of a new pattern (*pattern recognition*) and (2) comparison to previously known patterns (*pattern matching* or *classification*). How an individual chooses a particular approach for a specific task is not clear. Cognition and memory probably play critical roles in both processes, with cognition more involved in pattern recognition and memory more important in pattern matching. In pattern learning, a new non-random pattern is initially identified and then stored, first in short-term and subsequently in longer-term memory. In pattern matching, a non-random pattern is identified and compared to the many previously memorized, stored patterns in search of a match. When a match is made, the newly perceived pattern is assigned the appropriate attributes of the stored pattern, which then influences subsequent decision making. For a newly defined pattern, a set of unique attributes have to be assigned to it for future reference. In the case of pattern matching, previous patterns somehow facilitate the first step of non-random pattern identification. This matching process can be very efficient for common patterns and there may be little or no conscious component. Facial recognition is probably the strongest pattern-

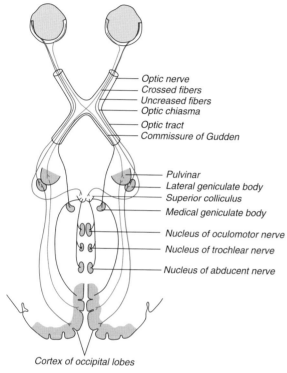

Optic nerve
Crossed fibers
Uncreased fibers
Optic chiasma
Optic tract
Commissure of Gudden

Pulvinar
Lateral geniculate body
Superior colliculus
Medical geniculate body

Nucleus of oculomotor nerve

Nucleus of trochlear nerve

Nucleus of abducent nerve

Cortex of occipital lobes

Figure 3.20. Human visual system, with multiple parallel image processing pathways. From *Gray's Anatomy.*

matching utility of the human visual system (Figure 3.23). Facial pattern recognition is thought to be partially "hard-wired," with critical anatomic components in the posterior temporal lobe, but also very dynamic, with the capacity to learn new faces from infancy through life. Many aspects of "professional" image analysis, such as radiological interpretation of x-rays, utilize pattern recognition and/or matching. It has been documented that a skilled, experienced radiologist needs to view a chest x-ray no more than five seconds in order to determine whether the image is normal or abnormal, and only a few seconds more to assign the image pattern to a specific disease category if the pattern closely resembles those of previously seen diseases. The radiologist is barely conscious of the process. However, this is a learned facility that requires exposure to many, generally hundreds, of examples of a particular pattern, i.e, normal chest x-ray (Figure 3.24). Experienced baseball hitters probably use similar pattern-learning and matching techniques. To hit new pitchers, or new pitches from a familiar pitcher, the batter has to engage a pattern-learning mode. This is a psychophysically more complex mode involving additional visual, cognitive, and motor components that restrict the type of swing the batter can make. The batter must observe as much of the baseball's trajectory as possible, learn and memorize its path, and finally react to the object moving at 150 km/h. A short, relatively late swing is most likely to result in a hit under these circumstances. Maximum

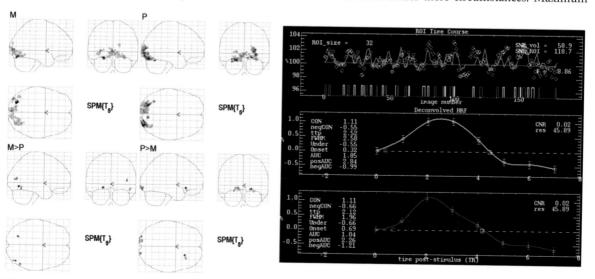

Figure 3.21. Parvocellular (P) and Magnocellular (M) visual pathways for separate processing of "what" and "where" data. (Talairach maps and fMRI BOLD responses.) Liu C-SJ, Bryan RN, Miki A, Woo JH, Liu GT, Elliott MA. Magnocellular and parvocellular visual pathways have different blood oxygen level-dependent signal time courses in human primary visual cortex. *American Journal of Neuroradiology* 2006; **27**: 1628–34, September. Used with permission.

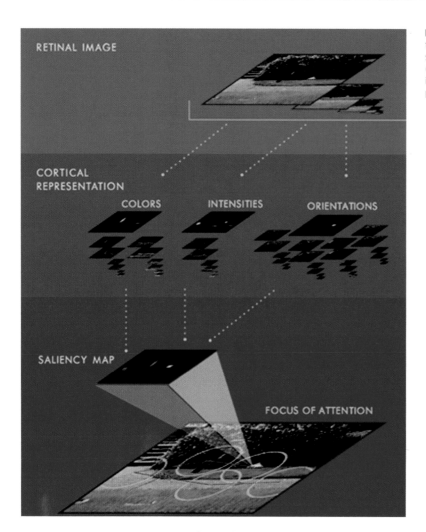

Figure 3.22. Human image analysis through image deconstruction and separate, parallel processing channels. © 2000 University of Southern California, iLab and Professor Laurent Itti. Used with permission. http://ilab.usc.edu/bu/theory/.

observation, much thought, slow response: pattern learning. On the other hand, facing a known pitcher and pitch, a batter observes the ball leaving the pitcher's hand, performs a quick pattern-matching operation, decides that the pitch is a fast ball over the outside corner, makes an early decision to make a vigorous swing at that anticipated spot and hits a home run (Figure 3.25). Minimal observation, no thought, quick reflexive response: pattern matching.

For computerized displays there are a variety of image data manipulations that may be used to modify displays and improve human appreciation and information extraction. These processes can be called *computer-aided visual analysis* (CAVA) (see Chapter 12). CAVA operations include *preprocessing, visualization, manipulation,* and *analysis.* These digital operations take place in image space. Pre-processing is used to "enhance" features of image data. Visualization operations involve viewing and assisting human comprehension of patterns and objects within a scene. Manipulations alter specific patterns and objects within a scene. Analytical operations quantify information, particularly about specific patterns and objects. It should be stressed that these digital operations add no additional information to the data; they may, however, aid information extraction.

Pre-processing operations include such things as the suppression of noise and artifacts and the enhancement of edges (Figure 3.26). Visualization operations include the display format, such as a montage display of multiple images, versus a cine or stack view (Figure 3.27). Two- and pseudo-three-dimensional displays use surface- or volume-rendering techniques for improved visualization. More sophisticated operations include the explicit extraction of patterns and

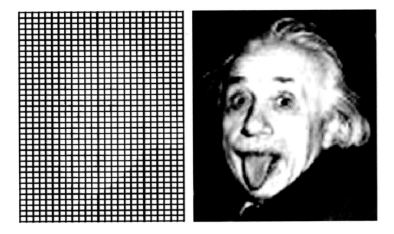

Figure 3.23. Facial recognition: a powerful form of pattern recognition that operates well under high noise and spatial variability. Efficient 3D reconstruction for face recognition. Jiang D, Hu Y, Yan S, Zhang L, Zhang H, Gao W. *Pattern Recognition* [Special Issue on Image Understanding for Digital Photos], 2004.

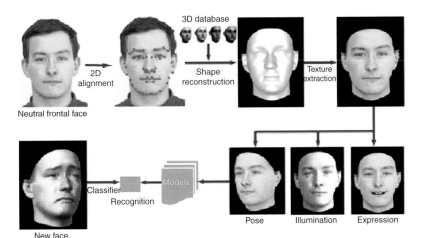

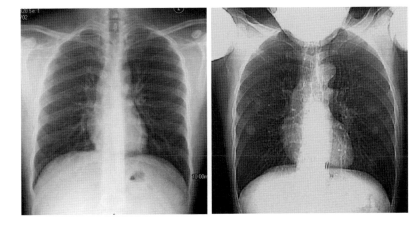

Figure 3.24. Normal and abnormal chest x-rays require 5 seconds for a trained observer to correctly classify/diagnose.

objects from complex scenes via relatively simple processes such as maximum intensity projection (MIP), or via more sophisticated object classification or segmentation algorithms (Figure 3.28). The first two CAVA operations (pre-processing and visualization) are intended to optimize image data for subsequent observation tasks – by human or computer. The second two CAVA operations

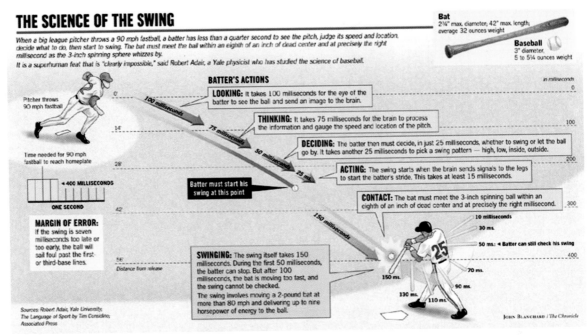

Figure 3.25. Pattern learning applied to hitting a baseball. Graphic by John Blanchard, © *San Francisco Chronicle*. Used with permission.

(manipulation and analysis) may have their own intrinsic purposes, which may or may not relate to subsequent observer operations.

Task performance

Image quality is obviously critical for effective communication via images. Image quality is usually evaluated in two fashions, technical and task-based. At a technical level, image quality relates to the fidelity of the information transmission system. Technical evaluation of image quality should objectively document a system's performance by such criteria as SNR, CNR, and spatial resolution criteria as PSF, FWHM, MTF, etc. These criteria are usually based upon measurements of components of sample images, often of well-defined phantoms. They reflect specific components of system performance, but they do not directly reflect the information content or effective transmission of information by the system. The latter is generally evaluated by measures of *task performance* (See Chapter 11). The key questions that should be addressed include the following: (1) what information is desired, (2) how will that information be extracted, (3) what objects will be imaged, and (4) what measure of performance will be used? Task performance is based upon the desired information – the task – and

the extraction mechanism – the observer. The ultimate measure of image quality is how well an observer performs an image-dependent task.

The most general task of the observer is to extract non-random patterns from image data. These patterns may be very complex and diffuse, such as the pattern of the Gulf Stream, or they may represent a more well-defined object such as the kidney. In many cases complex patterns or objects may be simplified by more tractable models. Random signals are unpredictable and convey no meaningful information about the sample. The sample itself has random, stochastic components that are affected neither by the imaging system nor by the observer. Noise is a random signal that arises from the measurement system and the observer. Not only does noise convey no information about the sample, but it can also obscure the true signal and hinder information extraction. The basic imaging task is to recover the non-random component of the sample.

Classification tasks

There are two specific types of tasks that observers may undertake – *classification* and *estimation*. Classification tasks require the explicit identification of patterns and objects, often followed by the assignment of the patterns/objects into specific categories or

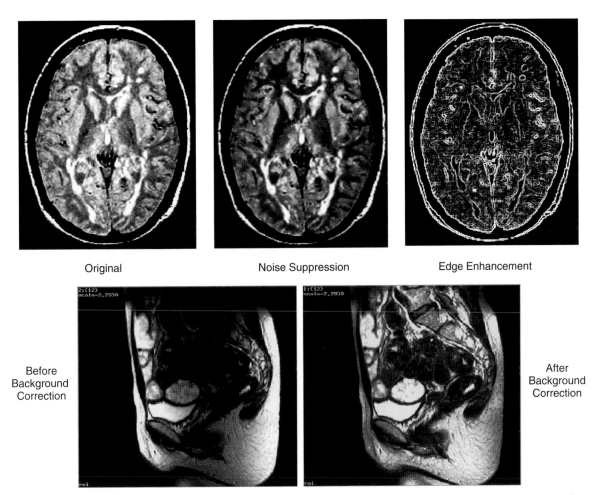

Original   Noise Suppression   Edge Enhancement

Before
Background
Correction

After
Background
Correction

Figure 3.26. Pre-processing of digital image data, an early step for improving human observer performance or subsequent computer analysis. Courtesy of J. Udupa.

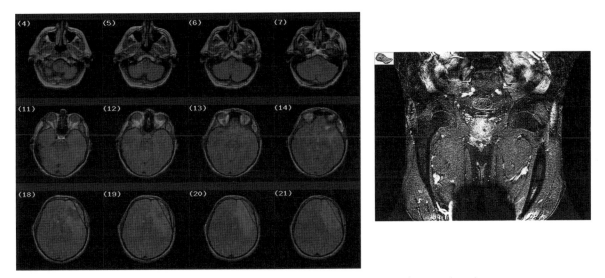

Figure 3.27. Common visualization modes for sequential cross-sectional images: montage and cine–stack mode.

Table 3.1. Classification task definitions and formulae

Accuracy	The likelihood that an observer is correct with respect to an established reference standard
Agreement	The likelihood of one observer giving the same response as another observer
Reliability	The likelihood of one observer giving the same response as a large number of other observers
Sensitivity	The percent of true positive
Specificity	The percent of true negative

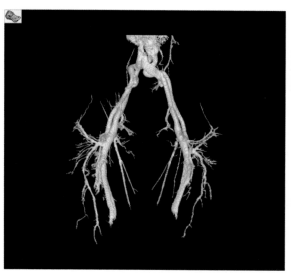

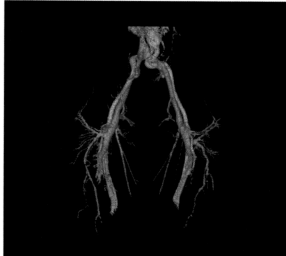

Figure 3.28. Object classification using "fuzzy connectedness" classification of blood vessels. Courtesy of J. Udupa.

groups. Typical classification tasks include the identification of relatively discrete physical objects such as cars, trees, and anatomic structures, as well as more amorphous objects such as clouds and temporal patterns such as ocean flow. The performance of classification tasks is measured by how well an observer classifies a pattern or object as compared to some accepted standard. Classification metrics typically use the chi-square (χ^2) statistic with measures of merit such as *sensitivity, specificity, false positive, false negative, accuracy,* etc. (Table 3.1).

A weakness of classical χ^2 statistics for human-observer classification tasks is that it does not take into account the bias of the observer and ignores the intrinsic reciprocity of sensitivity and specificity. *Receiver operating characteristic* (ROC) analysis is a more robust analytical method to evaluate classification task performance. The ROC curve is a plot of the *true positive fraction* (TPF) against the *false positive fraction* (FPF), as the decision criterion is varied from lenient to strict (Figure 3.29). This produces a whole family of sensitivity/specificity pairs at the

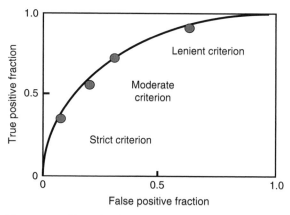

Figure 3.29. Object classification metric: ROC analysis. Courtesy of H. Kundel.

same level of intrinsic observer accuracy, but with different decision bias. ROC parameters include the *area under the curve* (AUC), *specific operating point* (SOP) (the true positive fraction at a specified false positive fraction), and index of detectability. In general, the AUC reflects the overall performance of the

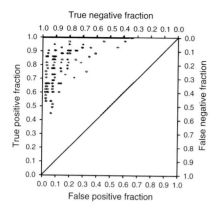

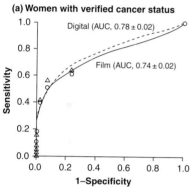

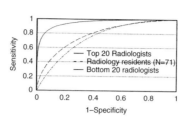

Figure 3.30. ROC analysis of human observer (radiologists) performance on classifying normal versus abnormal mammograms and chest x-rays. Notice the synonymous axis labeling. Beam CA, *et al.* Variability in the interpretation of screening mammograms by US radiologists. *Arch Intern Med* 1996; **156**: 209–13. ©American Medical Association, all rights reserved. Potchen EJ, *et al.* Measuring performance in chest radiography. *Radiology* 2000; **217**: 456–9. Both used with permission.

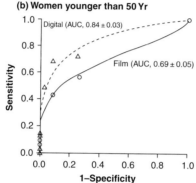

Figure 3.31. ROC analysis of analog versus digital mammography systems. Pisano ED, Gatsonis C, Hendrick E, *et al.* Diagnostic performance of digital versus film mammography for breast-cancer screening. *N Engl J Med* 2005; **353**: 1773. Used with permission.

system, and the greater the AUC the better is system performance.

Sources of error and variation in imaging systems include signal production, signal processing, and observer perception and decision. Surprisingly, signal production is usually a small component of error in well-designed imaging systems, and signal processing is usually a small component with good-quality control procedures. Most often, observer perception and decision contribute the largest component to error and variability in classification tasks. The ROC of reader variability in radiographic mammography is shown in Figure 3.30. The variability is primarily due to the radiologists, the observers. Observer performance can be improved by training and experience, as demonstrated in this example by poorer performance by radiology trainees as compared to that of the best trained and experienced radiologists, although it is interesting to note that the residents rank at approximately the same level as the poorest performing radiologists. Most importantly, the ROC curve shows the efficiency of information extraction from the images

by the observing radiologist as judged by task performance. Observer performance, as reflected by the AUC from ROC analysis, is also a function of the sample. This is demonstrated by the recent comparison of conventional analog film-screen mammography with newer digital-detector mammography systems (Figure 3.31). There is no significant difference in task performance in a sample population that is dominated by women with fatty breasts in which there is high CNR between cancer and normal breast tissue. However, digital systems perform better than the analog system in a sample population dominated by women with dense breast tissue in which there is less CNR between normal and cancerous tissue. In this case, the difference in the AUCs is due to the imaging system, not the observers. Thus ROC analysis can be used to evaluate imaging systems, observers, or both. When performing an ROC analysis, one always wants to clearly define what component of the imaging process is being evaluated.

ROC analysis does not take into account prior information about the sample, such as prevalence of

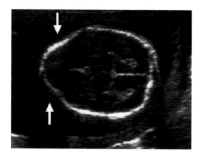
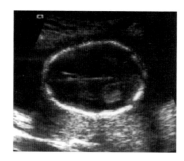

Figure 3.32. Effect of disease prevalence on sensitivity and specificity versus positive and negative predictive values. Thomas M. The Lemon sign. *Radiology* 2003; **228**: 206–7. Used with permission. Table courtesy of H. Kundel.

"Lemon" sign   Normal

Population	Selected	Community
Sensitivity	0.93	0.93
Specificity	0.986	0.986
Disease prevalence	0.061	0.001
Positive predictive value	0.812	0.061
Negative predictive value	0.995	0.999

a population state, i.e., a disease. The application of Bayesian analysis to imaging methodology in the clinical setting is very important, as illustrated by the report on the ultrasound "lemon sign" of the Arnold–Chiari malformation that showed a difference in the ROC AUC in a small, skewed patient population in a specialty care hospital where there was a relatively high prevalence of this condition (Figure 3.32). However, the prevalence of this disease in the general population is known to be low and, as a result, this particular test would not perform satisfactorily as a screening test. Positive and negative predictive values (PPV, NPV) do take prior information about disease prevalence into account. In this example, the PPV is unacceptably low for a screening test. If applied in the general population, most patients having this image feature would not actually have the disease; the false positive rate is too high.

Image analysis involves the extraction of information from an image. Classification tasks are often driven by or lead to *feature extraction*. Feature extraction involves the identification of specific characteristics of patterns or objects in an image. Information is extracted in the form of specific qualitative or quantitative features defined by human observers or (semi-) automatically via computers. Based on these explicitly defined and identified features, a decision is made; an object is classified. Intuitive pattern matching is dependent on

feature extraction in poorly understood ways that result in a simplistic summarization that some feature(s) in an image match some previously learned pattern. There often are no explicitly defined features identified in the image, though on close questioning the observer may be able to provide specific features he/she used in performing the task. On the other hand, an observer might, in advance, explicitly define features required for classification of an object, such as color, shape, or change in time, and then document their presence in a conscious process of object classification. In such cases, explicit feature extraction is involved. Traditional feature extraction by human observers has too often used vague verbal descriptors such as *few, too many to count, medium-sized, ovoid, irregular, dark* to describe such basic object features as number, size, shape, signal intensity, and internal architecture when describing a lesion such as a breast cancer (Figure 3.33). This is due to the lack of a rigorously defined, descriptive lexicon, and the limited descriptive capabilities of the human visual system. New, better defined, descriptive lexicons such as RadLex for medical images, as well as more use of basic workstation quantitative tools, are improving information extraction. Each extracted feature, manually or automatically defined, can be evaluated in terms of its unique classification task performance by sensitivity and specificity and incorporated into an overall ROC curve (Figure 3.34).

Manually extracted features

- Enhancement type
  mass/non-mass
- Shape
  round/oval/irregular/stellate
- Size
  linear/volume
- Margin
  smooth/lobulated/irregular/spiculated
- Intensity
  high/medium/low/minimal
- Internal characteristics
  rim/internal septations

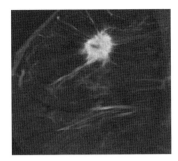

Figure 3.33. Object classification based on human-observer feature extraction. Courtesy of M. Schnall.

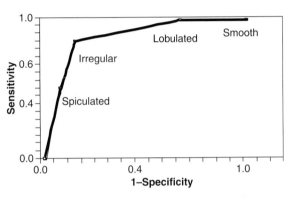

Figure 3.34. ROC analysis based on manually extracted features. Courtesy of M. Schnall.

Estimation tasks

Estimation tasks may involve pure description or hypothesis testing. The former require quantitative measurements that can be summarized by traditional descriptive statistics and therefore have the usual types of *measurement errors*, including random variance, imprecision, as well as systematic bias in accuracy as defined in Chapter 2. While human observers often perform well on classification tasks, they frequently do not do well on estimation tasks. This is because of the limited quantitative capabilities of the human visual system. Humans are not very good at generating numbers from visual observations. In fact, when asked to estimate such things as brightness, size, or position, most humans cannot reliably produce more than five ordered steps, with ill-defined intervals, e.g., mild, moderate, severe; tiny, small, moderate-sized, large, humongous; Grade 1, 2, 3, 4, 5. An estimation task is dependent on a preceding classification task. Before one can estimate some value of an object, one must have defined the object, and this critical step is one of classification.

Estimation tasks involving hypothesis testing are simply the determination of whether the descriptive statistics of two different populations are different from each other. For estimation-based hypothesis testing, one starts with two estimates, perhaps the average, μ, temperature of two groups of patients with streptococcal infection, one group treated with aspirin and another with a new anti-inflammatory drug, and then tests to determine if the averages are different. With such a continuous variable one might perform a *t-test*. While the unaided human visual system can reliably produce only five ordered quantitative estimates, a human equipped with a measuring tool can produce a much more finely graded set of measurements. Traditional analog measuring devices such as rulers, compasses, etc. were applied to hard-copy images, yielding numbers with much greater precision than five crude grades. Very creative, and often tedious, analog measuring techniques were developed for specific applications, such as weighing cutouts of tracings of image objects as an estimate of area of volume. Fortunately the transition to digital images and computer workstations has greatly increased the ease of performing quantitative measurements, and their quality. Such measurements often come under the region of interest (ROI) rubric, in which a human manually defines a particular part of an image and then, with simple digital tools, makes basic measurements related to the ROI such as the following: mean/SD of signal intensity; length, width; area or volume, etc. (Figure 3.35). Manual ROI analysis is still dependent on human object classification, with its attendant weaknesses, and quantitative accuracy is now limited by pixel or voxel resolution. The simple quantitative advances resulting from the transition to digital

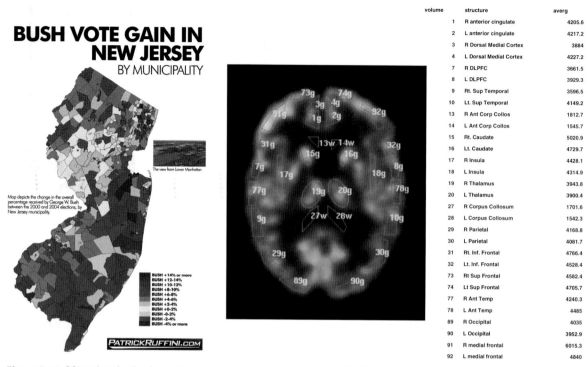

volume	structure	averg
1	R anterior cingulate	4205.6
2	L anterior cingulate	4217.2
3	R Dorsal Medial Cortex	3884
4	L Dorsal Medial Cortex	4227.2
7	R DLPFC	3661.5
8	L DLPFC	3929.3
9	Rt. Sup Temporal	3596.5
10	Lt. Sup Temporal	4149.2
13	R Ant Corp Collos	1812.7
14	L Ant Corp Collos	1545.7
15	Rt. Caudate	5020.9
16	Lt. Caudate	4729.7
17	R Insula	4428.1
18	L Insula	4314.9
19	R Thalamus	3943.8
20	L Thalamus	3900.4
27	R Corpus Collosum	1701.6
28	L Corpus Collosum	1542.3
29	R Parietal	4168.8
30	L Parietal	4081.7
31	Rt. Inf. Frontal	4766.4
32	Lt. Inf. Frontal	4528.4
73	Rt Sup Frontal	4582.4
74	Lt Sup Frontal	4705.7
77	R Ant Temp	4240.3
78	L Ant Temp	4485
89	R Occipital	4035
90	L Occipital	3952.9
91	R medial frontal	6015.3
92	L medial frontal	4840

Figure 3.35. ROI analysis: localized quantitative analysis of election returns and FDG-PET uptake. Map by Patrick Ruffini. PET scan courtesy of A. Newberg.

imaging dramatically improved the scientific power of imaging, but much more lay ahead.

Computer observers

Traditionally, scientific observers have been humans. However, computers are being increasingly used, either alone or in conjunction with the human observer, to extract information from image data. As previously noted in the discussion of human observers, a major challenge in image analysis is the extraction of patterns or specific objects. This is a classification problem that can be approached by a variety of computational techniques, from the simplest use of *threshold* and *maximum intensity projection* (MIP) tools to sophisticated voxel-based statistics, machine learning, artificial intelligence, and vector analysis. A typical example would be the delineation of neuropathological lesions such as multiple sclerosis or ischemic lesions in cerebral white matter. The human eye is very good at qualitatively identifying these lesions, but very poor in quantifying their size or location. The intimate relationship of the classification task to an estimation task cannot be overemphasized. An estimation task is dependent on a preceding classification task. In order to determine the mean value of an object, the object must have been accurately defined – that is, classified.

Threshold and MIP analysis are two of the simplest digital image analysis tools used in classification tasks. Threshold analysis is dependent strictly on signal intensity, reflective of the m,E measurement. The threshold operation is simply setting a range of signal-intensity numbers to define an object (Figure 3.36). The threshold range, which has until recently been empirically set by a human observer viewing an image as a binary gray/color scale, is varied until only the desired object, or best estimate thereof, is displayed. All the pixels/voxels within this numerical range are classified as "object," while all others are not. The accuracy of threshold classification is directly related to CNR of the object to be classified. With very high CNR, this simple operation can perform very well; unfortunately this is not usually the case. However, as with any classification or measurement tool, its accuracy can, and should, be determined by appropriate statistical tests, such as ROC analysis. MIP-based object classification is primarily a visualization refinement of thresholding. Rather than a fixed range of threshold values, the computer identifies the

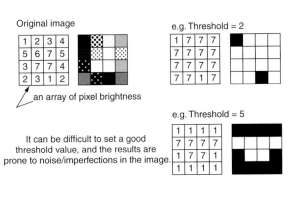

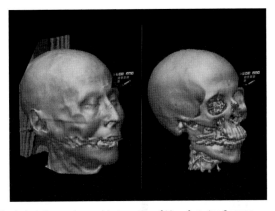

Figure 3.36. Object classification based on voxel thresholding. Tables from Hugh Jack, *Integration and Automation of Manufacturing Systems*, available at http://claymore.engineer.gvsu.edu/~jackh/books/integrated/pdf/integratedbook.pdf. Used with permission. Images courtesy of J. Udupa.

pixels having maximum signal intensity along a ray or line projected through a plane (slice), and these, and only these, pixels are classified and displayed as "object" (Figure 3.37). Once again, the value of this operation is highly dependent on the CNR of the object of interest, a CNR of greater than 30 generally being desired. In medical imaging, MIP is often used for imaging of bone on CT or contrast-enhanced blood flow on CT or MR.

More sophisticated computer algorithms can extract image features, similar to previously discussed human-observer processes (Figure 3.38). Computer-extracted features can be evaluated by ROC analysis, individually or as a group, just like those extracted by human observers (Figure 3.39). There are many statistical features that computers can use to classify patterns and objects. There are usually no specific rules as to which feature-extraction algorithm will perform the best for a particular application, and every extraction algorithm must be validated against other algorithms and some independent estimate of truth in order to determine its practical value (see Chapter 14).

A far more sophisticated and powerful approach to computerized image analysis is *statistical parametric mapping* (SPM), which is the application of the general linear model to each voxel to test a two-state hypothesis [4]. This approach has been most frequently used for time-varying signals, as in functional neuroimaging to identify regions of the brain that statistically differ in their signal intensity between two task states, often referred to as a control and a test state. This methodology is sensitive to very small changes in signal intensity and does not require any *a priori* definition of regions of interest. This statistical testing

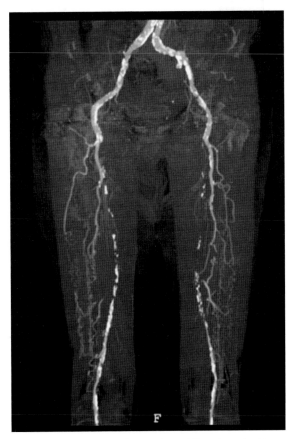

Figure 3.37. MIP display of arteries using MR angiography data. Courtesy of Philips Healthcare.

of voxel signal intensity is simply the imaging version of defining the probability density functions of image data in two different states, and then using statistical inference to define those voxels that differ in the two states.

Case 3

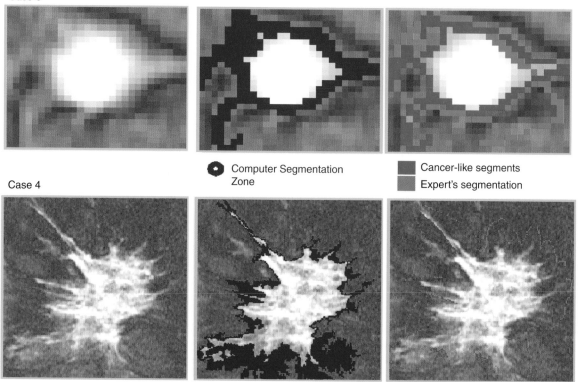

Case 4

Figure 3.38. Automated computer feature extraction. Courtesy of M. Schnall.

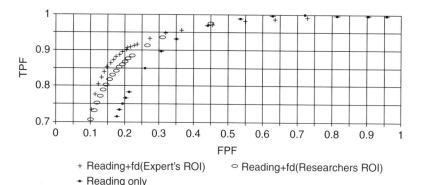

Figure 3.39. ROC analysis based on computer-extracted feature, fractile dimension (fd), with and without additional human classification. Courtesy of M. Schnall.

A typical example of this methodology is the identification of brain regions uniquely activated in scene recognition or sentence memory tasks (test state) versus random visual or auditory noise tasks (control state) (Figure 3.40). The actual signal intensity differences between these task states is less than 2% and is not appreciable by direct observation. One of the main challenges to the use of this methodology is the determination of appropriate statistical thresholds for the classification of activated voxels. Recall that a 128×128 image has over 10 000 pixels. If each pixel were treated as an independent variable, a statistical test using a $p = 0.05$ threshold would, by chance alone, result in approximately 500 pixels being falsely identified as active. On the other hand, use of the typical Bonferroni correction (alpha (p) value divided by the number of hypothesis: α/n) for multiple tests would reduce this number of false-positive pixels to less than

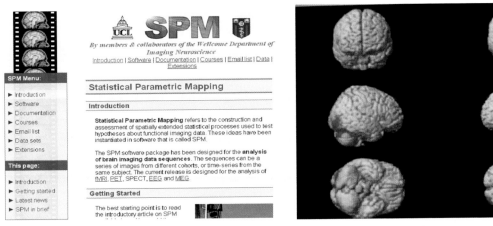

Figure 3.40. Functional MRI identification of a scene-based visual task using SPM, a voxel-based image analysis program. www.fil.ion.ucl.ac.uk/spm/.

one. However, such a correction is clearly excessive and excludes most true-positive pixels. Sensitivity can be increased by changing the statistical threshold, at the usual expense of decreasing specificity. In this example, note the "activated" areas meeting the less strict statistical criteria that lie outside the brain. While there are guidelines to threshold setting, empirical validation is often required. Images that are published are often dramatic summary images of the experiment, images that fully reveal neither the underlying data nor the nuances of the analysis. Such images should be recognized for what they are – compelling and potentially informative summary images that should be viewed with typical scientific skepticism. Inspection of the underlying data is always important. If one can lie with statistics, it is even easier to deceive with images!

SPM can be viewed as a computer form of pattern matching, though without a pattern being explicitly defined in advance of the experiment. The defined pattern, the pattern to be matched to, is the control state. The null hypothesis is that the test state is the same as the control state. SPM simply compares the pattern of signal intensities in the test state to that of the control state, and if the two patterns match the null hypothesis is accepted. Though the end result might be considered a form of pattern matching, the actual process considers only individual voxels, not their aggregate pattern. This is also an example of image analysis in which the term "pattern" is more appropriate then "object" to define that which is of interest. Task-activated regions of the brain are not discrete objects by any usual definition, nor are they random events. They are non-random patterns of brain activity.

Another approach to object classification that has been used to classify brain tissue as normal or abnormal on the basis of multimodal signal intensities is a mathematical/statistical tool based on vector analysis, a support vector machine (SVM). In this approach, an attribute vector based on four independent signals is calculated for every voxel (Figure 3.41). An expertly defined training set is used to calculate the probabilistic attribute vectors of abnormal versus normal tissue (Figure 3.42). The trained algorithm is then applied to unknown cases for tissue classification. This is another computer version of pattern matching, with the requisite training being definition of the attribute vector of the pattern or object of interest. In this case, it is not obvious whether these abnormal areas of the brain are patterns or objects. While physically there might be a difference, there is no difference from an imaging viewpoint: both pattern and object (as well as noise) are represented simply as a signal as a function of location.

Many such classification schemes have been shown to have equivalent or better precision than manual human extraction, with comparable accuracy as well (Figure 3.43). The quantitative advantage of this technique for cross-sectional as well as longitudinal studies has been demonstrated.

Spatial analysis

Spatial variability, such as anatomic variability in clinical imaging, presents significant analytical challenges. In order to quantitatively compare m,E signal measurements from spatially similar voxels, spatial variability must be removed. Physical space identities must be brought into correspondence in image space. This can

109

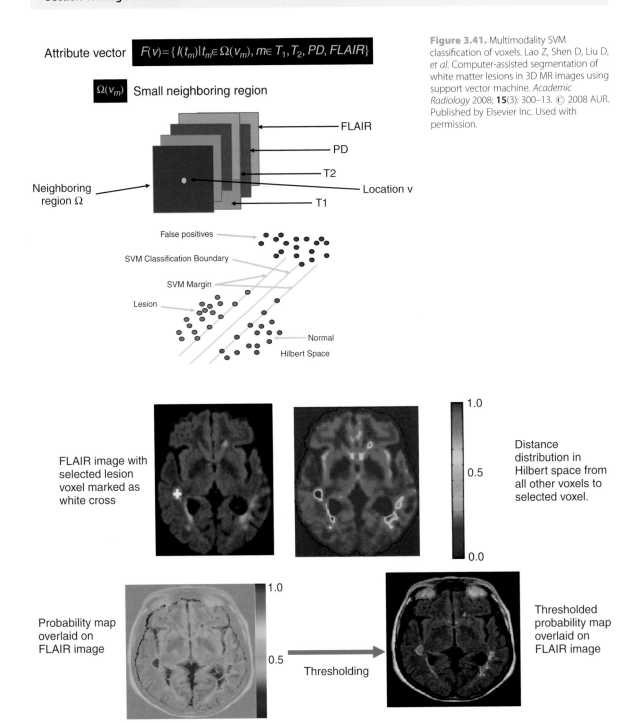

Attribute vector $F(v) = \{I(t_m) | t_m \in \Omega(v_m), m \in T_1, T_2, PD, FLAIR\}$

$\Omega(v_m)$ Small neighboring region

FLAIR
PD
T2
Location v
T1

Neighboring region Ω

False positives
SVM Classification Boundary
SVM Margin
Lesion
Normal
Hilbert Space

Figure 3.41. Multimodality SVM classification of voxels. Lao Z, Shen D, Liu D, *et al.* Computer-assisted segmentation of white matter lesions in 3D MR images using support vector machine. *Academic Radiology* 2008; **15**(3): 300–13. © 2008 AUR. Published by Elsevier Inc. Used with permission.

FLAIR image with selected lesion voxel marked as white cross

1.0
0.5
0.0

Distance distribution in Hilbert space from all other voxels to selected voxel.

Probability map overlaid on FLAIR image

1.0
0.5
Thresholding

Thresholded probability map overlaid on FLAIR image

Figure 3.42. Probabilistic tissue classification based on SVM attribute vector. Same source as Figure 3.41.

be performed with sophisticated warping or morphing algorithms that reshape individual images to match a standard template (Figure 3.44) (see Chapter 12). Humans accomplish this same task by spatial labeling, an operation by which a specific location in one image is given a name corresponding to the same area in a closely corresponding, previously spatially labeled image. This process is obviously dependent on previous labeling of spatially comparable images. Common examples of such spatially labeled images are maps and atlases. Any

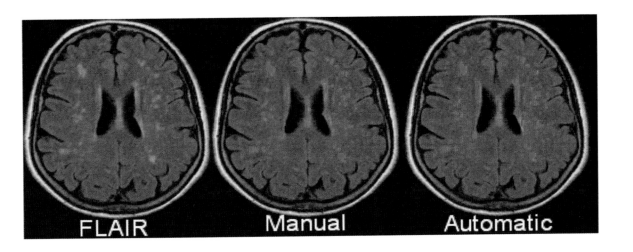

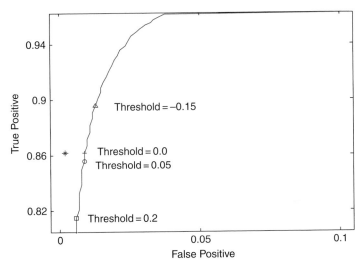

*Single operating point of expert human observer

Figure 3.43. Automated computer versus human-observer classification of ischemic tissue voxels based on multimodality MRI. Same source as Figure 3.41.

spatially labeled image may be used as a *template*, here defined as a special form of match pattern that permits spatial labeling or comparison. In the case of brain imaging, this is often performed by spatially transforming an individual brain to that of an atlas template, such as the Montreal Neurological or Talairach brain atlases, which are defined within a 3D Cartesian coordinate framework (Figure 3.45). Spatial normalization allows comparison of the signal intensity of anatomically identical voxels between subjects. This methodology also allows the registration of anatomic atlases to individual brain scans for anatomic labeling or ROI definition.

Spatial normalization not only allows anatomic labeling and group analysis of signal intensity, but

also allows individual and group analysis of morphological variability. The morphological tools that allow spatial normalization also provide the basis for quantitative morphological analysis. This methodology was creatively and tediously developed by Darcy Thompson for the analysis of morphological (structural) variation between species (Figure 3.46) Appropriate warping algorithms create a *deformation* field that quantitatively defines the spatial variation of an individual or group from a template (Figure 3.47). Deformation fields of groups of individuals can be "averaged" and otherwise quantitatively analyzed in fashions previously impossible. A morphologic group average can be used for inter-group comparisons.

111

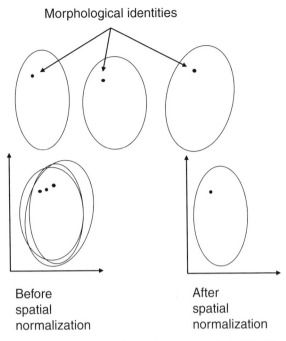

Morphological identities

Before spatial normalization

After spatial normalization

Figure 3.44. Spatial normalization brings morphological identities into spatial correspondence by registration to a standard template. Courtesy of C. Davatzikos.

Quantitative morphometrics now allows evaluation of very small spatial differences among individuals and groups. Subtle changes detected by this technique cannot be appreciated by the human eye (Figure 3.48). However, as with SPM-type analysis of voxel signal intensity, the sophisticated geometric transforms and associated statistics that are used for these morphometric analyses should be carefully considered and skeptically viewed. The methodology has produced well-validated and replicated results showing differences in the anatomy of the right and left cerebral hemispheres, and gender differences of the corpus callosum. More subtle differences related to cognitive decline and schizophrenia are now being reported, the validity of which remains to be determined.

Technology assessment

Imaging is a major field of scientific methodology; as such it is also a technology. The ultimate measure of any technology's performance is how well it performs the task it was designed to do. Specific task performance varies by scientific field and topic. Recall that we have

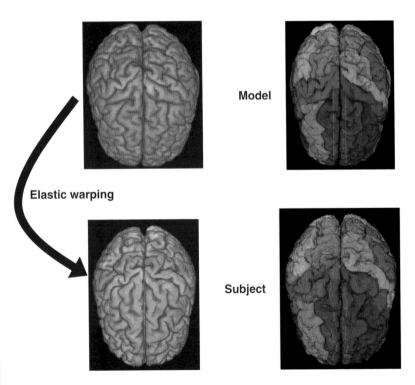

Model

Elastic warping

Subject

Figure 3.45. Atlas registration to individual or group image data for anatomic labeling and ROI analysis. Courtesy of C. Davatzikos.

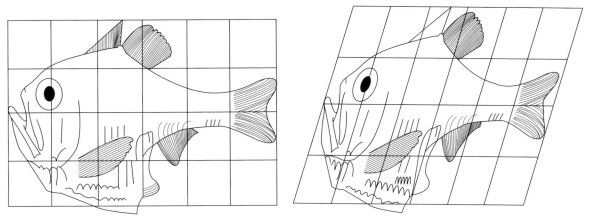

Figure 3.46. Morphometrics: quantitative spatial analysis as originally described by Darcy Thompson. By D'Arcy Wentworth Thompson, *On Growth and Form*, 1917, Cambridge University Press. http://en.wikipedia.org/wiki/D%E2%80%99Arcy_Wentworth_Thompson.

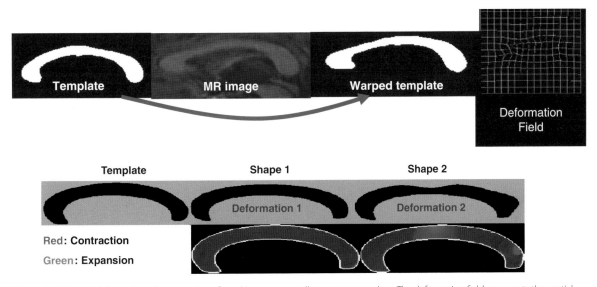

Figure 3.47. Local deformations from warping of an object, corpus callosum, to a template. The deformation field represents the spatial difference between the sample and the template. Courtesy of C. Davatzikos.

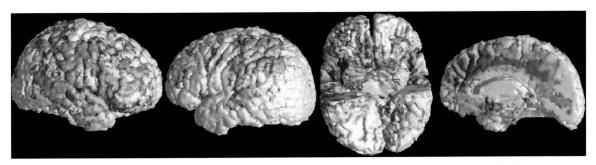

Figure 3.48. Voxel-based morphometric analysis showing subtle volume loss of the brain over four years in normal elderly subjects. Courtesy of C. Davatzikos.

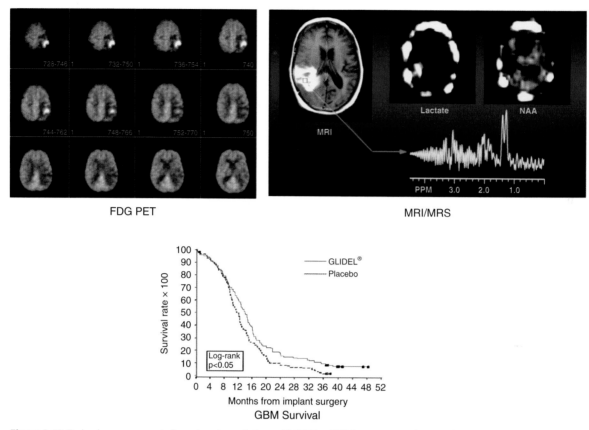

FDG PET

MRI/MRS

Figure 3.49. Technology assessment of new imaging techniques, FDG PET and MRS, requires correlation with clinical outcomes, which in the case of malignant brain tumors has not changed despite new diagnostic tests and therapies. Graph from www.rxlist.com/gliadel-drug.htm.

defined the main task of scientific imaging as *communication*, the passing of information from one entity, or person, to another for the purpose of influencing behavior. Somewhat uniquely, the task of imaging is to communicate spatial information. Weaver, in his introductory note to Shannon's monograph on communication theory, presents three levels of communication against which task performance might be evaluated [1]:

Level A How accurately can the symbols of communication be transmitted? The technical problem.

Level B How precisely do the transmitted symbols convey the desired meaning? The semantic problem.

Level C How effectively does the received meaning affect conduct in the desired way? The effectiveness problem.

The technical problem is concerned with the accuracy of transference from sender to receiver of the symbols of communication. The semantic problem relates to

the degree of approximation between the interpretation of meaning by the receiver as compared to the intended meaning of the sender. The effectiveness problem concerns the success with which the meaning conveyed to the receiver leads to the desired conduct on his or her part. This is a very practical view of communication, the ultimate quality measure relating to human behavior and its impact on daily life.

For the case of medical imaging, Fryback and Thornbury have elaborated on Weaver's points and defined six steps for the specific assessment of imaging technology on the basis of its performance in the field of clinical medicine, the ultimate goal of which is to improve the health of mankind [5]. One can imagine similar technology assessment criteria for other fields with different goals.

(1) *Technical.*   Can I see it?
(2) *Diagnostic accuracy.* How well can I see it?
(3) *Diagnostic thinking.* Is there any impact on diagnosis?

(4) *Therapeutic.* — Does it change therapy?

(5) *Outcome.* — Does the therapy change patient outcome?

(6) *Societal.* — Does the method have a high *cost/benefit ratio*? Is it cost effective?

The practical assessment of imaging systems should follow the task-performance steps of technology assessment. Simply having a new technology that improves diagnosis, or even possibly changes therapy, does not necessarily lead to improvement in patient outcome or societal benefit. For instance, MRI with MRS plus PET imaging of glioblastoma has certainly improved both the sensitivity and specificity of the diagnosis (Figure 3.49). The improved diagnosis has changed therapy, with smaller craniotomies, less residual tumor, and smaller radiation treatment ports. However, the five-year survival rate of this disease has not changed. This is because diagnosis and tumor delineation is not the limiting factor in treating this disease; the problem is the lack of effective therapy. Contemporary imaging of brain tumors might meet Fryback and Thornbury's first four performance criteria, but fall short of the last two – improving patient outcome and benefiting society. Though terribly demanding, the last two are the ultimate criteria for evaluating biomedical image quality.

References

1. Shannon CE, Weaver W. *The Mathematical Theory of Communication.* Urban, IL: University of Illinois Press, 1998.

2. Feynman RP, Leighton RB, Sands ML. *The Feynman Lectures on Physics.* Reading, MA: Addison-Wesley, 1963.

3. Tufte ER. *Envisioning Information.* Cheshire, CT: Graphics Press, 1990.

4. Statistical Parametric Mapping (SPM). Wellcome Trust Centre for Neuroimaging. www.fil.ion.ucl.ac.uk/spm/.

5. Fryback DG, Thornbury JR. The efficacy of diagnostic imaging. *Med Decis Making* 1991; **11**: 88–94.

General reading

Grenander U, Miller MI. *Pattern Theory: from Representation to Inference.* Oxford: Oxford University Press, 2007.

Saxby G. *The Science of Imaging: an Introduction.* Bristol: Institute of Physics, 2002.

Tufte ER. *Beautiful Evidence.* Cheshire, CT: Graphics Press, 2006.

Wandell BA. *Foundations of Vision.* Sunderland, MA: Sinauer Associates, 1995.

Suleman Surti and Joel S. Karp

Physics

The modern structure of an atom was first described in 1932 by Niels Bohr with the shell model. In this model, the electrons revolve in stable orbits, or shells, around a positive core, the nucleus. The nucleus, which consists of positively charged protons and electrically neutral neutrons, is the source of gamma rays used in nuclear imaging. In terms of size, the atom is of the order of 10^{-8} cm while the nucleus is about five orders of magnitude smaller at 10^{-13} cm. The most successful model used to describe the nucleus is a shell model analogous to the shell model of the atom, except instead of electrons we now have protons and neutrons. The shell model of the nucleus has been used to describe the discrete energy levels present in nuclei depending upon the physical state of the protons and neutrons.

The nucleus has two fundamental forces which determine its stability, the repulsive Coulomb (electromagnetic) force between the same-charge protons, and an attractive strong nuclear force between all neutrons and protons. The strength of these two forces depends upon the number of neutrons (N) and protons (Z) present in the nucleus. We find that in stable light nuclei the number of neutrons and protons is about the same, whereas in heavier nuclei the number of neutrons to provide nuclear stability is larger than the number of protons.

Nuclear medicine imaging involves injecting patients with a radiotracer tagged with an unstable nucleus that decays into a more energetically stable state, towards a more favorable N versus Z combination as determined by the nuclear stability curve. The emitted radiation is detected and used to characterize the radiotracer distribution within the body. ^{99m}Tc is the most common tracer used in single photon emission computed tomography (SPECT), emitting 141 keV gammas, while ^{18}F-FDG is the most common tracer used in positron emission tomography (PET), resulting in two 511 keV gammas. Figure 4.1 shows examples of nuclear medicine images: a bone scan acquired with planar camera with ^{99m}Tc-MDP, a cardiac scan acquired with a SPECT camera and ^{99m}Tc-sestamibi, and a whole-body glucose scan acquired with a PET camera and ^{18}F-FDG.

Signal source

A nucleus in an excited energy state (parent nucleus) will decay into a lower-energy or ground state (daughter nucleus) with the emission of excess energy in the form of electromagnetic radiation, specifically gamma radiation. In this decay the number of protons and neutrons remains unchanged and the emitted energy spectrum of the gamma rays is discrete in nature, corresponding to the discrete energy levels of the shell model of the nucleus (Figure 4.2a). Generally, in single photon imaging, the gamma rays emitted by the decay of the excited nucleus represent the signal measured by the detector.

In the beta decay process, an electron or a positron (anti-particle of electron with a positive charge) is absorbed or emitted, respectively, leading to a conversion of a proton into a neutron or vice versa. In the positron emission decay, the positron travels a short distance in the surrounding tissue until it combines with an electron to form a very short-lived particle called the positronium. Most of the time, the positronium will decay into two almost coincident 511 keV energy photons or gamma rays (Figure 4.2b). In positron emission tomography (PET), the two coincident 511 keV photons represent the signal measured by the detector.

Introduction to the Science of Medical Imaging, ed. R. Nick Bryan. Published by Cambridge University Press. © Cambridge University Press 2010.

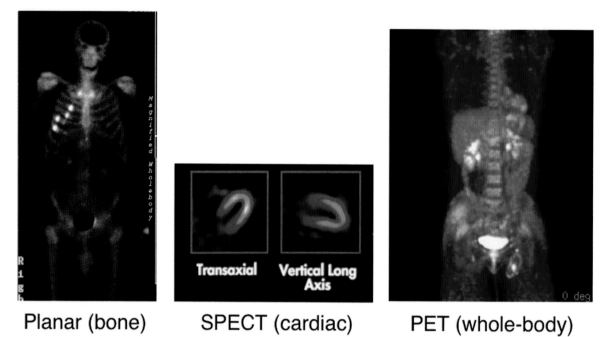

Planar (bone) | SPECT (cardiac) | PET (whole-body)

Figure 4.1. Examples of nuclear medicine images, including a planar bone scan with ^{99m}Tc-MDP, a cardiac SPECT scan with ^{99m}Tc-sestamibi, and a PET whole-body scan with ^{18}F-FDG.

(a)   (b)

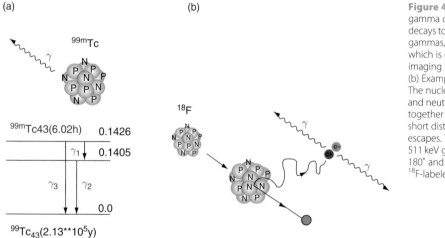

Figure 4.2. (a) Example of single photon gamma decay of ^{99m}Tc. The nucleus decays to a lower-energy state by emitting gammas, specifically the 140 keV gamma which is detected and used for imaging the ^{99m}Tc-labeled compound. (b) Example of positron decay of ^{18}F. The nucleus decays, emitting positron and neutrino, and the positron annihilates together with electron after traveling a short distance in tissue while the neutrino escapes. The annihilation produces two 511 keV gammas which are emitted at 180° and are used for imaging the ^{18}F-labeled compound.

The decay activity, A, of a radioactive nucleus is defined as the number of nuclei disintegrating or decaying (ΔN) per second (Δt). Mathematically:

$$A(t) = \frac{\Delta N}{\Delta t} \underset{\Delta t \to 0}{\longrightarrow} -\frac{dN}{dt} = \lambda N(t) \qquad (4.1)$$

where $A(t)$ is the activity at time t, λ is the probability for a single nucleus to decay (also known as the decay constant with units of 1/second), and $N(t)$ is the number of nuclei present at time t. The SI units for

activity are the becquerels (Bq) where 1 Bq = 1 decay per second. Another common unit for activity is the curie (Ci) where $1\,\text{Ci} = 3.7 \times 10^{10}$ Bq. With some mathematical calculation, Equation 4.1 is resolved into the Decay Law equation:

$$N(t) = N_0 e^{-\lambda t} \qquad (4.2)$$

where N_0 is the number of nuclei present at time $t = 0$, λ is the probability for a nucleus to decay, and the average life-time for a nucleus to decay is τ, defined as $\tau = 1/\lambda$. The amount of time it takes for N_o nuclei to decay into $N_o/2$ is called the half-life ($t_{1/2}$) of the nucleus and is defined as $t_{1/2} = \tau/1.44$. Commonly used isotopes in nuclear medicine are shown in Table 4.1, and examples of compounds are shown in Table 4.2.

Generally, SPECT isotopes are produced in nuclear reactors, and the half-life determines the manner in which they are delivered to the clinic. For example, ^{123}I is delivered by a radiopharmacy daily (depending

on need), whereas $^{99\,m}$Tc can be delivered as part of a "parent/daughter generator." The parent is ^{99}Mo, which decays ($t_{1/2} = 66\,h$) to the daughter $^{99\,m}$Tc, which can be eluted at any time, although a day is required between elutions in order to achieve a full dose of $^{99\,m}$Tc. After approximately one month, ^{99}Mo has decayed to a low level and the generator is replaced. In contrast, PET isotopes are usually produced in a cyclotron. Since ^{18}F has a half-life close to 2 hours, it can be produced and delivered by a commercial supplier, but a busy PET center may have a cyclotron on site, which enables the production of radiotracers for research investigations, labeled with either ^{18}F or short-lived isotopes such as ^{11}C. There are also parent/daughter generators for PET, notably ^{82}Sr/^{82}Rb; ^{82}Rb is used for cardiac imaging.

It is important to recognize that only a very small amount of radioactive material needs to be injected into the body in order to produce a signal of magnitude sufficient to produce a picture of the radiotracer distribution (see Chapter 10). For example, ^{18}F is used to label FDG (fluorodeoxyglucose), and we typically inject 10–15 mCi of activity in order to generate a picture of diagnostic quality in 10–20 minutes.

Table 4.1. Commonly used isotopes in nuclear medicine

SPECT	PET	$t_{1/2}$	Gamma energy (keV)
$^{99\,m}$Tc		6 h	141
^{201}Tl		3 d	~70
^{111}In		2.8 d	171, 245
^{123}I		13 h	159
	^{18}F	110 min	(2×) 511
	^{11}C	20 min	(2×) 511
	^{13}N	10 min	(2×) 511
	^{82}Rb	72 s	(2×) 511

Table 4.2. Examples of PET and SPECT radiolabeled tracers

	Tracer compound	Application
PET isotope		
^{11}C	Methionine	Protein synthesis, brain tumors
	Flumazenil	Benzodiazepine, epilepsy
	Raclopride	D_2 receptor agonist, movement disorders
^{13}N	Ammonia	Blood perfusion, myocardial perfusion
^{15}O	Carbon dioxide or water	Blood perfusion, brain activation studies
^{18}F	Fluoro-deoxyglucose	Glucose metabolism, oncology
	Fluoro-thymidine	Cell growth, oncology
	Fluoro-misonidazole	Hypoxia, response to radiotherapy
SPECT isotope		
$^{99\,m}$Tc	Sestamibi	Cardiac rest/stress
	MDP	Bone
	Neurolite	Brain blood flow
	DPTA	Renal imaging
	Sulphur colloid	Lymphoscintography
^{133}Xe	Gas	Lung ventilation
^{123}I	NaI	Thyroid
	MIBG	Neuroendocrine tumor
^{111}In	Prostascint	Prostate tumor
	Pentetreotide	Tumors

119

10 mCi corresponds to only 6 picomole or 1 nanogram of mass, which is only a trace amount and is inconsequential to the body's function. We therefore refer to the radioactive material as a radiotracer and, in fact, PET is often considered to be the most sensitive of imaging techniques.

Signal/sample interaction

In the energy range relevant to nuclear medicine imaging, gamma rays interact with matter by two main mechanisms, depending on the energy of the electromagnetic radiation. These are (1) the photoelectric and (2) the Compton interactions (Figure 4.3). Another type of interaction, known as pair production, takes place at energies greater than 1.022 MeV (twice the electron's rest mass), and therefore has little relevance in nuclear medicine.

Photoelectric effect

The photoelectric effect is an interaction of the gamma ray with orbital electrons in the inner shells of an atom. The photon transfers all of its energy to the electron, which overcomes the binding energy of the electron in the atom, leading to the ejection of the electron (photoelectron) from the atom with some residual kinetic energy. A more loosely bound outer orbital electron drops down to occupy the vacancy left in the ionized atom, emitting either a characteristic x-ray or

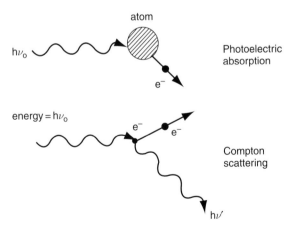

Figure 4.3. Gammas produced by nuclear medicine isotopes interact in tissue mainly by photoelectric absorption and Compton scattering. Photoelectric absorption results in complete absorption of the gamma by an inner-shell electron of the atom in the tissue, whereas Compton scattering results in scattering of the gamma by an outer-shell electron of the atom in the tissue, leading to a loss of energy and change of direction of the gamma.

an Auger electron in the process. The photoelectric effect dominates in human tissue at energies less than approximately 100 keV. It is of particular significance for x-ray imaging, and for imaging with low-energy radionuclides, but is a less frequent event at the energy of annihilation photons (511 keV) in PET, and therefore of less importance in that setting.

Compton scattering

Compton scattering is the interaction between a gamma ray and a loosely bound, outer-shell, orbital electron. After the interaction, the gamma ray undergoes a loss of energy and change in direction, and the electron is ejected from the atom with some resultant kinetic energy. The energy transferred to the electron does not depend on the properties of the material or its electron density. Compton scatter dominates in human tissue at energies above approximately 100 keV and less than ~2 MeV.

An important, though unwanted, contribution to the image background comes from the emitted gamma rays which undergo Compton scatter with an atomic electron inside the body. After a Compton scatter, the photon loses energy and changes direction, but might still be (falsely) detected as a true signal. The density of tissue in the human body is about the same as that of water, and so the mean free path is ~7 cm at 140 keV and ~10 cm at 511 keV. Since the cross-section of a human body is several multiples of 10 cm, many of the gamma rays originating from radiotracers injected into the human body are Compton-scattered before they are measured in the detector. In a PET or SPECT scanner some of these may be misinterpreted as a true signal, since the energy resolution of the detector is not precise enough to distinguish between the energy of the emitted gamma and a scattered gamma ray. The scattered gammas result in incorrect positioning, which fills in the background and, in turn, leads to a reduction of contrast of structure (or lesions) in the image.

Attenuation

Not all the photons emitted within the patient manage to exit the patient's body and reach the detectors. In some situations, the gamma rays are completely absorbed within the body or, more likely, scattered away from the detectors, since the scanner covers a limited solid angle around the body. This reduction in the number of detectable photons is referred to as attenuation. Although we take advantage of this property for x-ray and CT imaging, in PET as well as SPECT attenuation is an undesirable property, as the attenuation probability varies for different lines of response (LORs) and leads to severe modulations and loss of statistical quality in the collected data. In PET brain imaging as many as half the coincident events are lost due to attenuation, while in whole-body PET imaging, depending on the patient size and the region being imaged, as many as 90% of the coincident events are lost due to attenuation inside the patient. The transmission probability for a gamma ray through any material is characterized by its linear attenuation coefficient, μ, which depends on the photon energy, the atomic number of the material (tissue) through which it passes, and tissue density. For a collimated (i.e., narrow) beam of gammas passing through a material of thickness t, the transmission probability, $I(t)/I_o$ is given by:

$$\frac{I(t)}{I_o} = \exp\left(-\int_0^t \mu \, dt'\right) \quad (4.3)$$

where I_o is the incident number of photons, and $I(t)$ is the number of photons detected after passing through the material. For example, if we assume a patient's body is 30 cm thick, the number of gammas from the center of the body (15 cm depth) will be attenuated to 20% for 140 keV (SPECT) and to 25% for 511 keV. However, since in PET we need to detect two gammas in coincidence, the signal in this example is actually attenuated to 25% × 25% = 6%.

A mitigating property of attenuation in PET imaging comes from the two-gamma process. If we assume μ to be constant along a given LOR with a total length of intersection with the body of D, and the lengths of the two gamma segments are $d_1 + d_2 = D$, then the probability P that either of the photons is attenuated inside the body is given by:

$$P = e^{-\mu d_1} e^{-\mu d_2} = e^{-\mu(d_1+d_2)} = e^{-\mu D} \quad (4.4)$$

Thus the probability P is independent of the point of emission and it depends only on the object length along the LOR. Therefore, we can use an external radiation source such as in CT to correct for attenuation in PET. In SPECT imaging, however, only one photon is detected and so the attenuation probability P is a function of emission position within the patient, and correction with an external source is not as straightforward or accurate (Figure 4.4).

All contemporary commercial PET scanners are sold in combination with a CT scanner that is used both for attenuation correction and for co-registered anatomical information. An increasing proportion of SPECT scanners are sold as a combined unit as well. Since the attenuation coefficient μ is energy-dependent, the CT data need to be scaled to correspond to the energy of either the SPECT isotope or the PET isotope. The advantage of using CT for attenuation correction is that the data are acquired very quickly (< 1 minute for whole-body) and with very high statistical quality; however, there is the potential for bias if the data are not scaled accurately. In addition, there are some situations, such as patients who have metal prostheses, which make it more challenging to use the CT for this purpose.

Signal detection

Scintillation detectors are the most common and successful type of detectors for gamma-ray imaging in nuclear medicine, due to their high detection

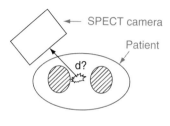

$I/I_0 = e^{-\mu d?}$

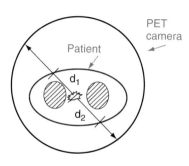

$I/I_0 = e^{-\mu d1} \, e^{-\mu d2} = e^{-\mu D}$

Figure 4.4. Attenuation in SPECT and PET. In SPECT we do not know the distance d the gamma must traverse to exit the patient's body, and therefore we can only approximate the correction factor for attenuation. In PET the attenuation depends on the total path length of the two gammas, $D = d_1 + d_2$, which can be measured, thereby allowing us to accurately correct for attenuation.

efficiency and good energy and timing resolution. They consist of a crystal or a scintillator which converts the gamma-ray energy into visible (blue) light, and a photodetector which converts the scintillation photons into a proportional electrical signal. The electrical signal gets converted into a digital value that can be stored in a computer and which is then used to generate an image of the radiotracer distribution.

As mentioned earlier, the electronic energy states of an isolated atom consist of discrete energy levels that are filled by the electrons, starting with the lowest energy level first. The last filled energy level is labeled the "valence" band, while the first unfilled energy level is called the "conduction" band. The energy gap, E_g, between these two levels is typically a few electronvolts. Electrons in the valence band can absorb energy by the interaction of the photoelectron or the Compton-scatter electron with an atom, and become excited to the conduction band level. Since this is not the ground state, the electron de-excites by releasing scintillation photons and returns to its ground state. Normally the value of E_g is such that the scintillation is in the ultraviolet region. By adding impurities to a pure crystal – adding, for example, a small amount (about 1%) of thallium to sodium iodide (NaI(Tl)) – we can modify the band structure to produce different energy levels between the valence band level and the conduction band level. Due to the reduced value of E_g, the scintillation process now results in an emission of blue light. Such a scintillation process is commonly known as luminescence. The scintillation photons produced by luminescence are emitted isotropically from the point of interaction.

The most common photodetector used in scintillation detectors is the photomultiplier tube (PMT), which is the oldest and most reliable technique to measure and detect low levels of scintillation light. The entrance window of a PMT consists of a photocathode that absorbs the energy deposited by the photons and transfers it into an electron in the photoemissive material. The quantum efficiency (QE) of the photocathode is a measure of the efficiency (typically 25%) with which electrons are emitted per incident photon and eventually produce a signal at the PMT anode. QE is a function of the incident wavelength and the photocathode material. The electrons released at the photocathode are then accelerated by an electric potential in the PMT and focused onto a dynode. Here we have a process of secondary emission of electrons similar to what takes place at the photocathode. However, due to the acceleration of the incident electron, a significantly larger number of secondary electrons are now emitted. A typical PMT has eight stages before the electrons reach the anode, and the resultant signal at the anode is, within statistical fluctuations, proportional to the energy of the incident photon.

In PET instrumentation, there are several techniques of arranging the scintillation crystals and coupling them to photodetectors for signal readout. The first is one-to-one coupling, where a single crystal is glued (with an optical coupling compound) to an individual photodetector. A closely packed array of small discrete detectors can then be used as a large detector, which is needed for PET imaging. The spatial resolution of such a detector is limited by the size of the discrete crystals making up the detector. In order to achieve good spatial resolution in one-to-one coupling, very small photodetectors are needed. Although early PET scanners used one-to-one coupling with PMTs, the smallest available PMT is about 10 mm in diameter and no longer sufficient for a high-resolution, state-of-the-art PET scanner. An alternative to using a standard PMT in the configuration is to use a multi-anode PMT, which consists of multiple anode structures in a single PMT housing with small anode pitch (about 5–6 mm in current versions available commercially) [1]. Another alternative is to use a semiconductor-based photodetector such as the avalanche photodiodes (APDs) instead of PMTs. The APDs are smaller in size relative to PMTs (available in 1–14 mm widths), can be implemented as an array instead of individual components, and are therefore ideal for use in such a detector design [2]. Large-size APDs can also be designed to be position-sensitive and can therefore accurately discriminate smaller crystals. APDs have higher QE than PMTs, but low gain and sensitivity to fluctuations in temperature and applied voltage makes their use in clinical PET scanners less practical than PMTs. Recent research has led to the development of a new semiconductor-based photodetector commonly known as the silicon photomultiplier or Geiger-mode APD that promises to produce much higher gains than APDs with less susceptibility to temperature and applied-voltage variations. While promising for use in detector designs such as one-to-one coupling, these solid-state photodetectors are currently very expensive. The cost and the inherent complexity (number of electronic

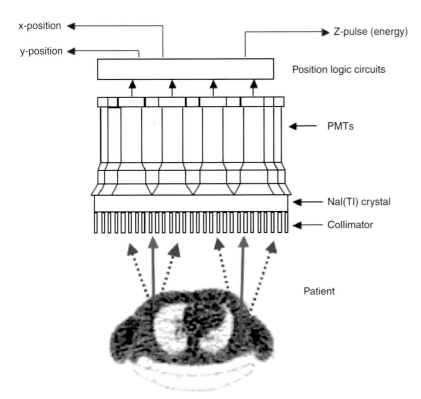

x-position

y-position

Z-pulse (energy)

Position logic circuits

PMTs

NaI(Tl) crystal

Collimator

Patient

Figure 4.5. Schematic of Anger camera used for single-photon imaging. The collimator restricts the number of gammas (green arrows) which pass through collimator, thereby defining their direction. The absorption of the gamma in the NaI(Tl) crystal leads to emission of scintillation light, which is detected and converted to an electronic signal by the photo-multiplier tubes and allows us to calculate energy and position using a weighted centroid algorithm.

channels) of a PET scanner based on solid-state detectors, or multi-anode, position-sensitive PMTs, limits their use to research tomographs, including small animal systems. For clinical PET and SPECT scanners, we currently rely on standard PMTs used in a light-sharing, Anger-logic configuration to achieve high spatial resolution.

The Anger detector [3], originally developed by Hal Anger in the 1950s, uses a large (e.g., 30–50 cm in diameter, ~9 mm thick) thallium doped sodium iodide (NaI(Tl)) crystal glued to an array of PMTs via a "lightguide." This camera is normally used with a collimator to detect low-energy single photons in SPECT imaging (Figure 4.5). A weighted centroid positioning algorithm is used for estimation of the interaction position within the detector. This algorithm calculates a weighted sum of the individual PMT signals and normalizes it with the total signal obtained from all the PMTs receiving light. The weights for the PMT signals depend on the PMT position within the array. Since the uncertainty of the weighted sum depends on the statistical uncertainty of the PMT signals, a high-light-output scintillator such as NaI(Tl) is needed to obtain good spatial resolution. The use of large PMTs in

the Anger detector leads to very good spatial resolution in a simple, cost-effective design. Also, using a large continuous scintillator leads to a very high packing fraction and high sensitivity for the detector.

The Anger detector has also been used in PET scanners by using thicker (2.5 cm) NaI(Tl) scintillation crystal plates [4], and without the collimator required for SPECT. Although this application was highly successful for many years, the limitations of this design became evident. The inherent disadvantage of this design, independent of the use of NaI(Tl) as a scintillator, is the link between the thickness of the detector and the spatial resolution. For PET, a thicker detector is needed to achieve high efficiency of detecting 511 keV gammas, but the spread of scintillation light within the crystal, combined with Compton scatter within the crystal, impacts spatial resolution and also leads to significant detector dead time at high count rates due to pulse pile-up. A more recent Anger-logic detector design uses small discrete crystals instead of a single large crystal coupled to an optically continuous lightguide [5]. The lightguide for this detector is optimized to restrict the light spread to within a seven-PMT cluster of a

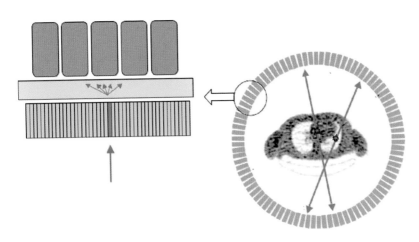

Figure 4.6. Schematic of PET camera based on Anger-logic detector consisting of many individual pixels whose cross-section determines the spatial resolution of the instrument. The energy and position of the gammas are calculated in a similar manner as for an Anger detector. Note that there is no need for a collimator, since the direction of the gammas is defined by the line between the two pixels which detect the gammas.

hexagonally close-packed PMT array (Figure 4.6). This leads to very good spatial resolution, determined by the width of the discrete crystals, as well as a significant reduction in dead time of the Anger-logic detector. Although this pixelated Anger-logic detector was originally developed for NaI(Tl), it has enabled the use of better scintillators for PET, resulting in higher stopping efficiency and faster decay time. This detector design was implemented in a dedicated brain scanner, G-PET, using gadolinium orthosilicate (GSO) at the University of Pennsylvania [6] and in the commercial Allegro and Gemini GXL whole-body PET scanners developed by Philips Medical Systems [7], as well as in the small-animal PET scanner A-PET (commercially available as Mosaic from Philips Medical Systems) based on another scintillator, lutetium yttrium orthosilicate (LYSO) [8].

A different Anger-logic detector design developed in 1985 is referred to as the block detector design, and was adopted by General Electric Healthcare and Siemens Medical Systems in their commercial PET scanners. The original design used an 8×4 array of bismuth germanate (BGO) crystals (each $6 \times 14 \times 30$ mm^3) glued to a slotted lightguide with signal readout performed by a 2×2 array of PMTs [9]. New block detector designs use different crystal sizes and types, as well as PMT size, in order to achieve the desired spatial resolution [10–15]. Compared to the pixelated Anger-logic detector, the block detector design has the benefit of reduced detector dead time, but this is achieved by increasing the number of detector channels (lower encoding ratio = number of crystals/number of PMTs), thus leading to increased cost. A modification of the block design, called the quadrant-sharing block design

[16], offset the crystal array with respect to the PMT array by one PMT – leading to either better spatial resolution with the same encoding ratio or the same spatial resolution with a higher encoding ratio, as in a standard block detector. This improvement, however, is achieved at the cost of increased dead time compared to the standard block detector.

The choice of scintillator in a PET detector is strongly tied to the detector and scanner design, and impacts the system spatial resolution, sensitivity, count-rate capability, and image contrast. The spatial resolution of a scanner is intrinsically related to the effective atomic number, Z_{eff}, which determines the proportion of photoelectric interactions within the scintillator or the photofraction. Z_{eff}, together with the density ρ of the scintillator, also determines the probability of an incident photon depositing most of its energy in the scintillator. Hence, a high-density scintillator helps to achieve a high-sensitivity scanner. For high count-rate imaging it is important to restrict the signal both spatially in terms of light spread (dependent on detector design) and temporally, which is determined by the scintillator signal decay time, τ. The light output of a scintillator is important for two reasons. First, high scintillator light output leads to good crystal discrimination in a block or pixelated Anger-logic detector and good spatial resolution in a conventional Anger detector. The second advantage of a high-light-output scintillator is the improved energy resolution achieved in the detector, which allows the use of a tight energy window around 511 keV to reject those events that scatter in the patient before reaching the detector. Table 4.3 contains a brief summary of properties for different scintillators which are currently (or were formerly) used in PET scanners.

Table 4.3. Comparison of properties of scintillators used in PET. The performance of the detector depends on these properties, whereby Z_{eff} and ρ determine the stopping power for gammas and impact on spatial resolution, τ determines the count-rate capability, and light output impacts energy and spatial resolution. LYSO typically has a ratio of 90/10 for lutetium/ytrium, and so the properties are similar to those of lutetium orthosilicate (LSO). LaBr$_3$ is the chemical formula for lanthanum bromide

Scintillator	NaI(Tl)	BGO	GSO	LSO, LYSO	LaBr$_3$
Z_{eff}	51	75	59	63	46
ρ	3.7	7.1	6.7	7.1–7.4	5.3
τ (ns)	230	300	60	40	27
Relative light output (%)	100	15	25	70	150

The performance of the detector depends on these properties, whereby Z_{eff} and ρ determine the stopping power for gammas and impact on spatial resolution, τ determines the count-rate capability, and light output impacts energy and spatial resolution. LYSO typically has a ratio of 90/10 for lutetium/yttrium, and the properties are similar to LSO.

The earliest PET detectors were composed of NaI(Tl), which continues to be the scintillator of choice in traditional nuclear medicine imaging such as SPECT. BGO became the more popular material beginning in the 1980s, since its very high Z_{eff} and high density leads to an increased sensitivity for detecting 511 keV photons. The block detectors were designed specifically to overcome the limitation of low light output (compared to NaI(Tl)) by using smaller PMTs and a tailored light distribution pattern to improve spatial resolution. The low light output, however, also leads to poor energy resolution, and so BGO scanners perform best as 2D imaging scanners where inter-plane septa are used to reduce the (out-of-plane) scatter rather than relying strictly on energy resolution, which allows one to raise the energy threshold. Scintillators with good energy resolution can operate in a fully-3D mode without inter-plane septa, which increases the sensitivity, while the high-energy threshold mitigates the increase of scatter. Both NaI(Tl) and BGO have the added disadvantage of slow decay (large τ), leading to higher dead time especially when using fully 3D PET designs. GSO, LSO, and LYSO have recently proven to be excellent PET scintillators for modern 3D scanners, due to the combination of high stopping power, short decay time, and good energy resolution. Lanthanum bromide, LaBr$_3$, represents a new generation of fast and very bright scintillators which have both excellent energy resolution and exciting potential for time-of-flight PET, which requires excellent timing resolution.

Image formation

Early efforts to achieve transverse-section images in nuclear medicine relied on iterative methods [17,18], but this changed rapidly with the introduction of x-ray, CT, and the filtered back-projection technique. Originally all PET scanners were used in a 2D mode, where slice-defining lead or tungsten septa placed at regular intervals along the axial length of the scanner divided it into multiple, thin 2D slices. Historically, the earliest PET scanners [19,20] were designed as single-slice scanners and sensitivity was increased by stacking multiple rings with inter-plane septa separating the rings. The width of each slice defines the axial resolution of such scanners, and oblique LORs (between different slices) are eliminated as the septa absorb the gamma rays along these lines (Figure 4.7). This reduces scanner sensitivity, and image reconstruction is performed on a slice-by-slice basis using a 2D algorithm. Today the scanners from GE Healthcare continue to use inter-plane septa, although they are short enough so that some oblique LORs are used, thereby improving sensitivity. In addition, these septa can be retracted so that the scanner can operate in a fully 3D mode, similar to scanners from Siemens and Philips, neither of which contain septa. In fact, some of the earliest efforts to develop PET used dual rotating detectors without septa, culminating in the development of a fully 3D acquisition [21] and reconstruction [22] in the late 1970s. The term "fully 3D" should not be confused with a three-dimensional or volumetric-image, as both 2D and fully 3D mode acquisitions produce volumetric images of tracer uptake. However, in the fully 3D mode, three-dimensional image reconstruction techniques are required.

There are two different classes of reconstruction algorithms, based either on analytic or on iterative methods. Filtered back-projection (FBP) is an analytic

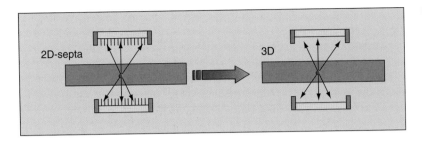

Figure 4.7. Comparison of PET scanners for 2D imaging with inter-plane septa and 3D imaging without septa. The inter-plane septa reject the out-of-plane gammas, thereby reducing the sensitivity of the instrument but simplifying the image reconstruction and data correction methods.

method and was the obvious initial choice to reconstruct PET images, since this was the standard method for CT and SPECT. Iterative algorithms have two major disadvantages: they are more computationally intensive, and the image changes both qualitatively and quantitatively as the number of iterations and the relaxation parameter(s) change. Since PET was largely if not exclusively used for research studies in its early years, quantitative accuracy was critical and more easily achieved with analytic approaches. This state of affairs did not change significantly until after attenuation correction through measured transmission scans became more generally available. This ultimately led to a significant image quality improvement, with iterative algorithms being used for both the emission and the transmission scans. Iterative algorithms have become the method of choice in attenuation-corrected clinical PET imaging, since the computing power is now sufficient to make iterative reconstruction practical.

Transform algorithms

These algorithms are based on the analytic techniques used to invert the projection data. They normally involve the back-projection of the data, which is expressed as the inverse Radon transform:

$$b(x, y) = \int_{\varphi=0}^{\varphi=\pi} p(x_r, \varphi)\partial\varphi \qquad (4.5)$$

where $p(x_r, \varphi)$ is the measured data as a function of linear position and angle (Figure 4.8). In SPECT, the detector or group of detectors (generally two or three) rotates around the body to collect data at all angles. In PET, the detector ring is stationary and collects data at all angles without motion. The projection data are actually a set of discrete points rather than a continuous curve, and so the integral in Equation 4.5 changes into a sum. Let us for simplicity consider

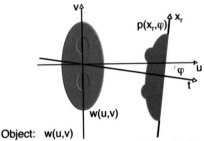

Object: w(u,v)
Projections: $p(x_r, \varphi) = \int x(u,v)dt$ = Radon transform $R \cdot w$

Figure 4.8. The process of image reconstruction used to estimate the activity distribution in the object is based on measurements of projections of the data sampled over both angular and linear directions.

a point source being imaged and ideal (perfect) spatial resolution for the detector. This means that the *point spread function* (PSF), which is the measured position spectrum of the source by the detector, is a delta function (i.e., PSF = $\delta(x)$). The Fourier transform of the PSF is called the *modulation transfer function* (MTF) of the detector, and in this ideal case it is equal to unity for all values of the spatial frequency v. However, the discrete sampling of the scanner results in a sampling MTF which is proportional to $\cos(\pi v d)/v$ (d is the sampling distance). As a result, the combined MTF of the point source in the scanner will also be proportional to $\cos(\pi v d)/v$. Since the inverse Fourier transform of this MTF is the image of the point source, this image will be blurred for high spatial frequencies v (smaller objects). Non-ideal detector behavior (PSF $\neq \delta(x)$) will only accentuate this blurring. Filtering techniques, where the MTF is multiplied by a function which helps boost the high-frequency components in the back-projection, are used to reduce this blurring, but must do so with consideration for noise amplification. This reconstruction technique is generally referred to as *linear superposition of filtered back-projection* (LSFBP).

In the 3D case for a PET scanner without septa, analytic solutions such as that of Colsher [22] are only valid if the scanner has a spatially invariant PSF. Unfortunately a practical scanner with a finite axial extent will have a spatial variant PSF due to incomplete projections for objects (patients) of finite size. Thus, either we do not use these incomplete projections, leading to a reduction in counts and increased image noise, or we estimate them by re-projecting (forward-projecting) through an initial estimate of the object. This re-projection approach has been implemented in both the spatial domain as 3D-RP [23] and the Fourier domain as 3D-FRP [24].

Alternatively, one can use an approximation method to sort the 3D oblique data into 2D parallel slices so that a 2D reconstruction method can be applied, either analytic or iterative. An early method was *single-slice rebinning* (SSRB) [25], which simply averaged the two axial (z) coordinates of the two gammas to determine the slice number. A more accurate method which operates in the Fourier domain is *Fourier rebinning* (FORE) [26], which is still in use in some commercial systems. In general, the approximation of these rebinning methods and resultant spatial resolution is best for systems with a small angular acceptance angle (for oblique rays), and for points in the object near the center of the transverse field of view.

Iterative or series expansion technique

In the cases of missing projection data or high levels of statistical noise, it is sometimes more efficient, and more accurate, to use iterative or series expansion techniques. These techniques attempt to optimize the reconstructed image so that its (forward) projection appears similar to the measured projection data. This normally involves minimizing a parameter such as an error term or maximizing a likelihood estimator through successive iterations until the solution reaches a steady state with very little change in further iterations. Since this technique involves solving several series of linear equations, it is computationally intensive as compared to the transform methods but, like the transform method, it is applicable to both 2D and 3D imaging. Examples are the *algebraic reconstruction technique* (ART), *expectation minimization* (EM), and the *row action maximum likelihood algorithm* (RAMLA). Although computers have greatly increased in speed, so too has the size of the data matrix, and it has become very important in practice to use acceleration techniques to decrease the reconstruction time. The *ordered subset expectation maximization* (OSEM) algorithm [27] uses ordered geometric subsets to accelerate the reconstruction, since fewer iterations are required to approach convergence. However, it is important to recognize that for OSEM, as with all iterative algorithms, convergence is not reached in practice and the stopping criterion (the number of iterations) is empirically determined, rather than mathematically derived.

An alternative to reconstructing from histograms (binned data) is to reconstruct from the list-mode data [28], which inherently preserves both the spatial and temporal information of the data. Although more computationally demanding than reconstructing from histograms, it is more easily extendable for incorporating time-of-flight (TOF) information, and more efficient in terms of data storage. The main advantage of iterative reconstruction algorithms is the ability to incorporate an accurate model of the physical process of the gammas which are detected and used to define the lines of response in the data matrix. For example, the statistical probability that gammas scatter or are attenuated in the body is accounted for in the update process of the iterative loop within the algorithm. Thus the system model typically includes scatter, attenuation, and detector efficiency, and for some state-of-the-art systems it also includes TOF and PSF modeling.

Scanner design

SPECT scanners

The fundamental detector unit in a SPECT camera is a large-area Anger detector functioning as a planar camera. To achieve a tomographic slice, one or more such planar detectors orbit in a trajectory around the patient to collect projection views at several angular positions in order to achieve a tomographic image with an image reconstruction algorithm. The direction of incident gamma rays in a SPECT detector is defined by the collimator which is attached to the Anger detector. A collimator consists of several small openings or holes in a base plate predominantly made of lead. These holes can be circular, square, or hexagonal in shape, and mainly allow only those gamma rays which hit the collimator surface parallel to the holes to hit the Anger detector, while absorbing the majority of the others. As the size of the hole increases, the spatial resolution of the SPECT scanner

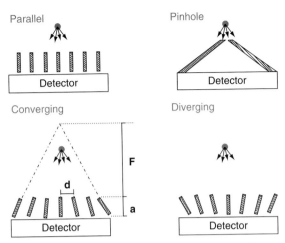

Figure 4.9. Comparison of different collimator types used in single-photon imaging.

degrades due to loss of gamma-ray direction information. The use of mechanical collimation with absorption represents a fairly inefficient process of signal detection in SPECT imaging, resulting in noisy images. There are four general collimator arrangements used in SPECT imaging (Figure 4.9): pinhole, parallel-hole, converging, and diverging collimators. In pinhole collimation a small hole cut in the collimator base plate leads to the magnification of a small imaging field of view (FOV) on the large detector surface. As a result, pinhole collimation can provide very high spatial resolution but limited imaging FOV. Parallel-hole collimation uses several larger holes placed normal to the detector surface, leading to a larger imaging FOV and higher sensitivity compared to a pinhole collimator, but at the cost of reduced spatial resolution. A refinement to the parallel-hole design is the converging collimation technique, which collects data from a limited FOV and uses some magnification to achieve improved spatial resolution. Finally, the diverging collimation technique is useful in situations where a large object is being imaged over a smaller detector surface, but the cost is reduced spatial resolution in the image.

Over the years SPECT cameras have been developed with one, two, three, or four detector heads, though in recent years almost all cameras available commercially from the major manufacturers are two-headed. In the last few years, interest in multimodality imaging has also led to the development of combined SPECT/CT systems, and the product list of the three major manufacturers (GE, Philips, and Siemens) is dominated by such systems as well. Besides adding anatomical information to the SPECT images, the CT data also allow more accurate attenuation correction of SPECT images, something which has been difficult to perform clinically in SPECT-only systems. A primary clinical application of SPECT over the years has been in cardiac imaging. Recent research into the development of high-performance detectors for cardiac SPECT imaging has seen the arrival of semiconductor-based detectors (cadmium zinc telluride, or CZT) in small-area cardiac SPECT cameras. However, the high cost and limited availability of high-uniformity CZT may still limit its uses in more general-purpose and large-area SPECT cameras.

PET scanners and system performance

A fundamental choice to make in whole-body PET imaging is whether to operate in the 2D versus fully 3D mode. As mentioned above, this impacts on the type of image reconstruction algorithm used, but also has a direct impact on the true sensitivity as well as the fraction of scatter and random coincidences. Scattered events, those in which at least one of the gammas undergoes Compton scatter, can be reduced either by energy rejection or by mechanical rejection through the use of inter-plane septa. Random events correspond to the detection of two gammas from two separate positron annihilations, but which happen to fall within the coincidence timing window (Figure 4.10). The number of randoms increases quadratically as the amount of activity increases and can quickly dominate the number of true events if not controlled through the use of a narrow coincidence timing window. Random events, as well as scatter events, lead to a reduction of image contrast if not compensated for. Thus it is critical to estimate the rate at which scatter events and random events are collected, so that the final image represents only true events after subtraction of scatter and randoms. Accurate compensation of both scatter and randoms is necessary not only to achieve good image contrast, but also to derive quantitative information from PET. Figure 4.11 shows a comparison of a PET image without any corrections, and with corrections for attenuation, scatter, and randoms. Note that with data corrections it is possible to make a quantitative comparison of the activity uptake in the lesions, particularly between deep and superficial lesions such as those in the mediastinum and the axilla.

However, even after subtraction, the presence of scatter and random events in the data collection increases the noise in the image. The amount of noise is characterized by a value referred to as the *noise-equivalent count-rate*, NEC, as shown in Equation 4.6 [29]:

$$\text{NEC} = T/(1 + S/T + R/T) \qquad (4.6)$$

where T is the trues rate, S is the scatter rate, and R is the randoms rate. Figure 4.12 shows the behavior of the NEC with activity as an illustration of how it

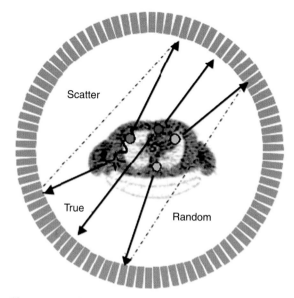

Figure 4.10. A PET scanner measures true coincidences, scatter coincidences in which at least one of the gammas undergoes Compton scatter, and random coincidences which result from two unrelated annihilations. As seen, the scatter and random coincidences are improperly positioned.

depends on scatter and randoms. The impact of scatter and randoms is even more significant for the new generation of PET/CT scanners, where the patient port diameter of the PET scanner is as large as 70–85 cm with reduced end shielding leading to even higher singles count-rates and random coincidences from activity outside the field of view. Since the overall image signal-to-noise is related to the NEC [29], an instrument is generally designed to produce a high NEC over a wide range of activity levels. It is important, though, to focus on the applications for which the instrument will be used most often, so, if the emphasis is on clinical imaging with FDG, then one should pay particular attention to the NEC that corresponds to an activity dose of 10–15 mCi, or ~0.1 μCi/cc for an average-sized patient of 70 kg.

Table 4.4 gives a summary list of commercially available whole-body PET/CT scanners currently being sold by the three major manufacturers. The scanners span a range of scintillators and detector designs in which a particular scintillator and detector combination is expected to provide the best possible scanner performance.

Time-of-flight PET scanners

In conventional PET imaging (both 2D and fully 3D) the location of the annihilation point along the line of response (LOR) is not precisely known, and the reconstruction algorithm assumes a uniform probability for its location along the length of LOR lying within the object boundary. In time-of-flight (TOF) PET, the detectors measure the difference in arrival times of the two coincident photons (t_1 and t_2)

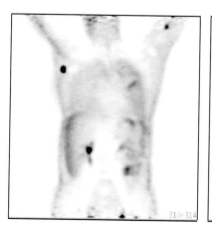
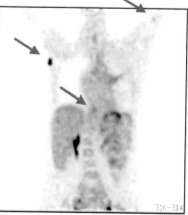

Figure 4.11. Comparison of PET image without any data corrections (left), and with attenuation, scatter, and randoms correction (right).

Table 4.4. Design specifications for several commercially available whole-body PET scanners

Manufacturer	Philips		Siemens	General Electric		
Product	Gemini GXL	Gemini TF	Biograph TruePoint	LS	ST	STE/VCT
Imaging mode	Fully 3D	Fully 3D with TOF	Fully 3D	2D and fully 3D		
Scintillator	GSO	LYSO	LSO	BGO		
Detector type	Pixelated Anger		Block	Block		
Individual crystal size (mm)	$4 \times 6 \times 30$	$4 \times 4 \times 22$	$4 \times 4 \times 20$	$4 \times 8 \times 30$	$6.3 \times 6.3 \times 30$	$4.7 \times 6.3 \times 30$
Axial FOV (cm)	18.3	18.0	16.2/21.6	15.2	15.7	15.7

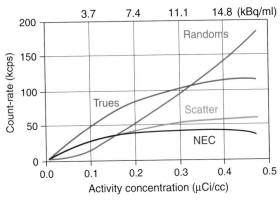

Figure 4.12. Example of a noise-equivalent count-rate (NEC) curve to illustrate the relationship between trues, scatter, and randoms as a function of activity. The typical range of activity concentration for a clinical FDG oncology study is 0.1–0.2 mCi/cm³. These data are courtesy of the University of Pennsylvania PET facility and were acquired on a Philips Allegro scanner.

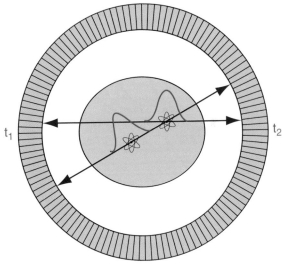

Figure 4.13. For a time-of-flight (TOF) scanner the time difference between the two gammas is measured precisely. The TOF information is used in the image reconstruction algorithm so that the data are back- and forward-projected over a limited distance corresponding to uncertainty of the measurement, thereby leading to improved signal-to-noise in the image.

precisely enough so that the emission point can be localized along the LOR within a region smaller than the object size (Figure 4.13). The error in this localization is determined by the coincidence timing resolution, Δt (full width at half maximum, FWHM), of the scanner. The FWHM of the spatial localization along the LOR is then calculated as $\Delta x = c\Delta t/2$, where c is the speed of light. Based upon this reasoning and its implementation in a back-projection reconstruction algorithm, it has been estimated that the TOF measurement is proportional to a sensitivity gain in the image given by $D/\Delta x$, where D is the size of the object being imaged [30,31]. The early TOF-PET systems were developed in the 1980s using scintillators such as cesium fluoride (CsF) and barium fluoride (BaF_2); however, the low stopping power and low light output of these scintillators led to reduced system sensitivity and spatial resolution compared to

conventional PET scanners of the day [32]. The recent development of crystals such as LSO, LYSO, and $LaBr_3$ has led even further to the reintroduction of TOF-PET imaging in modern scanner designs. Besides having good characteristics such as high stopping power, short decay time, high light output, and good energy resolution, it has also been demonstrated that these scintillators achieve very good timing resolution, which enables precise TOF measurement. As a result, it is possible to develop very high-performance fully 3D PET scanners with TOF capability without any of the drawbacks of the earlier TOF-PET scintillators. Commercially, a TOF-PET system using LYSO crystals with a timing resolution of <600 ps is currently

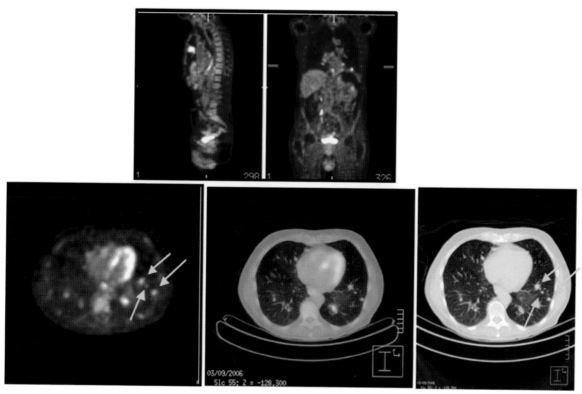

Figure 4.14. A patient with tongue cancer with lung metastases. The PET study was acquired one hour post-injection of 10 mCi, requiring 18 minutes of data collection. Note the correlation of the lung metastasis in the PET and CT images.

available from one manufacturer (Philips Medical Systems) [33]. An example of a study with this scanner is shown in Figure 4.14. A research system using LSO crystals (Siemens Medical Systems) has also been developed with similar timing performance [34], while at the University of Pennsylvania a research PET scanner using LaBr$_3$ crystals is under development with timing resolution of 360 ps [35].

In overview, while SPECT and PET have been in use for over 30 years, the performance and utility of these instruments have dramatically improved in the last decade and have expanded applications for both research and clinical studies. We can expect new technology to continue to be developed and implemented for nuclear medicine imaging, and to allow PET (or SPECT) to be acquired simultaneously with complementary imaging modalities, such as MRI.

References

1. Cherry SR, Shao Y, Silverman RW, *et al.* MicroPET: a high resolution PET scanner for imaging small animals. *IEEE Trans Nucl Sci* 1997; **44**: 1161–6.

2. Ziegler SI, Pichler BJ, Boening G, *et al.* A prototype high-resolution animal positron tomograph with avalanche photodiode arrays and LSO crystals. *Eur J Nucl Med* 2001; **28**: 136–43.

3. Anger HO. Gamma ray and positron scintillation camera. *Nucleonics* 1963; **21**: 10–56.

4. Adam LE, Karp JS, Daube-Witherspoon ME, Smith RJ. Performance of a whole-body PET scanner using curve-plate NaI(Tl) detectors. *J Nucl Med* 2001; **42**: 1821–30.

5. Surti S, Karp JS, Freifelder R, Liu F. Optimizing the performance of a PET detector using discrete GSO crystals on a continuous lightguide. *IEEE Trans Nucl Sci* 2000; **47**: 1030–6.

6. Karp JS, Surti S, Daube-Witherspoon ME, *et al.* Performance of a brain PET camera based on Anger-logic gadolinium oxylorthosilicate detectors. *J Nucl Med* 2003; **44**: 1340–9.

7. Surti S, Karp JS. Imaging characteristics of a 3-dimensional GSO whole-body PET camera. *J Nucl Med* 2004; **45**: 1040–9.

8. Surti S, Karp JS, Perkins AE, *et al.* Imaging performance of A-PET: a small animal PET camera. *IEEE Trans Med Imag* 2005; **24**: 844–52.

9. Casey ME, Nutt R. A multicrystal two dimensional BGO detector system for positron emission tomography. *IEEE Trans Nucl Sci* 1986; **33**: 460–3.

10. Wienhard K, Eriksson L, Grootoonk S, *et al.* Performance evaluation of the positron scanner ECAT EXACT. *J Comput Assist Tomog* 1992; **16**: 804–13.

11. Wienhard K, Dahlbom M, Eriksson L, *et al.* The ECAT EXACT HR: performance of a new high resolution positron scanner. *J Comput Assist Tomogr* 1994; **18**: 110–18.

12. Brix G, Zaers J, Adam LE, *et al.* Performance evaluation of a whole-body PET scanner using the NEMA protocol. *J Nucl Med* 1997; **38**: 1614–23.

13. DeGrado TR, Turkington T, Williams JJ, *et al.* Performance characteristics of a whole-body PET scanner. *J Nucl Med* 1994; **35**: 1398–406.

14. Brambilla M, Secco C, Dominietto M, *et al.* Performance characteristics obtained for a new 3-dimensional lutetium oxylorthosilicate-based whole-body PET/CT scanner with the National Electrical Manufacturers Association NU 2-2001 standard. *J Nucl Med* 2005; **46**: 2083–91.

15. Kemp BJ, Kim C, Williams JJ, Ganin A, Lowe VJ. NEMA NU 2-2001 performance measurements of an LYSO-based PET/CT system in 2D and 3D acquisition modes. *J Nucl Med* 2006; **47**: 1960–7.

16. Wong WH, Uribe J, Hicks K, Hu G. An analog decoding BGO block detector using circular photomultipliers. *IEEE Trans Nucl Sci* 1995; **42**: 1095–101.

17. Muehllehner G, Wetzel RA. Section imaging by computer calculation. *J Nucl Med* 1971; **12**: 76–84.

18. Kuhl DE, Edwards RQ, Ricci AR, Reivich M. Quantitative section scanning using orthogonal tangent correction. *J Nucl Med* 1973; **14**: 196–200.

19. Phelps ME, Hoffman EJ, Mullani NA, Higgins CS, Terpogossian MM. Design considerations for a positron emission transaxial tomograph (PETT III). *IEEE Trans Nucl Sci* 1976; **23**: 516–22.

20. Terpogossian MM, Mullani NA, Hood J, Higgins CS, Currie CM. A multislice positron emission computed tomograph (PETT IV) yielding transverse and longitudinal images. *Radiology* 1978; **128**: 477–84.

21. Muehllehner G, Buchin MP, Dudek JH. Performance parameters of a positron imaging camera. *IEEE Trans Nucl Sci* 1976; **23**: 528–37.

22. Colsher JG. Fully three-dimensional positron emission tomography. *Phys Med Biol* 1980; **25**: 103–15.

23. Kinahan PE, Rogers JG. Analytic 3D image-reconstruction using all detected events. *IEEE Trans Nucl Sci* 1989; **36**: 964–8.

24. Matej S, Lewitt RM. 3D-FRP: direct Fourier reconstruction with Fourier reprojection for fully 3D PET. *IEEE Trans Nucl Sci* 2001; **48**: 1378–85.

25. Daube-Witherspoon ME, Muehllehner G. Treatment of axial data in three-dimensional PET. *J Nucl Med* 1987; **28**: 1717–24.

26. Defrise M, Kinahan PE, Townsend DW, *et al.* Exact and approximate rebinning algorithms for 3D PET data. *IEEE Trans Med Imag* 1997; **16**: 145–58.

27. Hudson HM, Larkin RS. Accelerated image reconstruction using ordered subsets of projection data. *IEEE Trans Med Imag* 1994; **13**: 601–9.

28. Reader AJ, Ally S, Bakatselos F, *et al.* One-pass list-mode EM algorithm for high resolution 3-D PET image reconstruction into large arrays. *IEEE Trans Nucl Sci* 2002; **49**: 693–9.

29. Strother SC, Casey ME, Hoffman EJ. Measuring PET scanner sensitivity: relating count rates to image signal-to-noise ratios using noise equivalent counts. *IEEE Trans Nucl Sci* 1990; **37**: 783–8.

30. Snyder DL, Thomas LJ, Terpogossian MM. A mathematical model for positron-emission tomography systems having time-of-flight measurements. *IEEE Trans Nucl Sci* 1981; **28**: 3575–83.

31. Budinger TF. Time-of-flight positron emission tomography: status relative to conventional PET. *J Nucl Med* 1983; **24**: 73–6.

32. Lewellen TK. Time-of-flight PET. *Semin Nucl Med* 1998; **28**: 268–75.

33. Surti S, Kuhn A, Werner ME, *et al.* Performance of Philips Gemini TF PET/CT scanner with special consideration for its time-of-flight imaging capabilities. *J Nucl Med* 2007; **48**: 471–80.

34. Conti M, Bendriem B, Casey M, *et al.* First experimental results of time-of-flight reconstruction on an LSO PET scanner. *Phys Med Biol* 2005; **50**: 4507–26.

35. Daube-Witherspoon ME, Surti S, Perkins AE, *et al.* Imaging performance of a LaBr$_3$-based TOF-PET scanner. Paper presented at 2008 IEEE Nuclear Science Symposium and Medical Imaging Conference, 2008; Dresden, Germany.

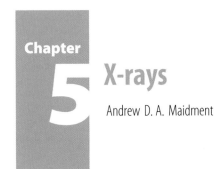

5 X-rays

Andrew D. A. Maidment

Signal

Electromagnetic radiation is utilized for much of medical imaging. Magnetic resonance imaging, optical and near-optical imaging, x-ray imaging, nuclear medicine, and radiation oncology portal imaging all use some form of electromagnetic radiation (Figure 5.1). Electromagnetic radiation consists of localized energy traveling at the speed of light. This energy can be characterized by a number of distinguishing properties, including energy (E), wavelength (λ), and frequency (v). These are related by two fundamental equations:

$$E = hv \qquad (5.1)$$

and

$$c = \lambda v \qquad (5.2)$$

where h is Planck's constant and c is the speed of light in the medium.

Electromagnetic radiation behaves differently depending upon the energy and mode of interaction. These two behaviors, the wave–particle duality, originally caused physicists great consternation. In the early days of physics, it was not clear how one entity (light) could sometimes behave like a wave (for example, diffracting) and at other times behave like a particle (for example, the photoelectric effect). It is now known that the mode of interaction of light determines its behavior; thus light will behave like a wave and diffract when passing through a slit, while light will typically behave like a particle when absorbed. For the purposes of x-ray imaging, we will concentrate almost exclusively on particulate behavior.

We can learn much about the behavior of x-rays by examining light. For example, light (and x-rays) travels in straight lines. This presents us with one of the fundamental principles of x-ray imaging – x-rays record information in straight lines from the x-ray source to the point of detection (Figure 5.2). Light refracts at the boundaries of materials because of the difference in refractive index of light between materials. The refractive index at x-ray energies is nearly identical for all materials, this effect is quite small and is typically ignored. X-rays also demonstrate two other properties of light – polarization and phase. Again, these are not commonly utilized in medical imaging because of the nature of the x-ray sources used; however, it is possible to produce both coherent and polarized x-ray sources using a synchrotron.

Signal source

In medical imaging, x-rays are most commonly produced with an x-ray tube (Figure 5.3). The x-ray tube is powered by an x-ray generator. The x-ray generator produces a high voltage to accelerate electrons from the cathode to the anode in the tube. The resulting high-energy electrons produce x-rays when they strike the anode.

There are two principal electron interactions that produce x-rays: bremsstrahlung and characteristic x-ray emission. The word bremsstrahlung, from the German *bremsen*, "to brake," and *strahlung*, "radiation," refers to electromagnetic radiation produced by the deceleration of a charged particle, such as an electron, when deflected by another charged particle such as an atomic nucleus. The efficiency of bremsstrahlung is proportional to the charge squared of the moving particle and inversely proportional to the mass. The efficiency of bremsstrahlung is also proportional to the atomic number (Z) squared of the interacting material. Thus bombarding high-atomic-number materials with high-energy electrons produces substantial bremsstrahlung.

Introduction to the Science of Medical Imaging, ed. R. Nick Bryan. Published by Cambridge University Press. © Cambridge University Press 2010.

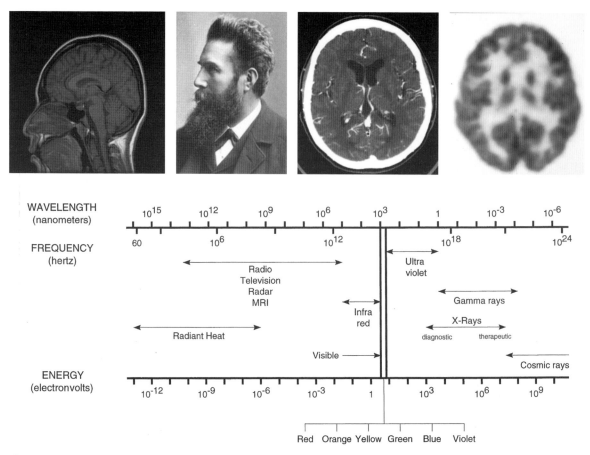

Figure 5.1. Medical imaging utilizes the full gamut of the electromagnetic spectrum (bottom) to produce images. Key examples are shown, including radio-frequency waves used in MRI (top left), visible light (middle left), x-rays used in computed tomography (middle right), and gamma rays used in positron emission tomography (top right).

Bremsstrahlung results in a continuous spectrum of x-ray energies. By comparison, characteristic radiation is, as suggested by the name, a characteristic of each material. While bremsstrahlung is predominantly an electron–nucleus interaction, characteristic radiation is an electron–electron interaction. In characteristic-radiation production, an incident electron interacts with a bound orbital electron, ejecting that electron from the atom. The empty orbital shell is subsequently filled by an outer-shell electron, resulting in the emission of a characteristic x-ray. This interaction is the electronic equivalent of the photoelectric effect described later in this chapter.

The efficiency of production of characteristic radiation is proportional to E^2 (where E is the energy of the incident electron) and increases rapidly with Z. A competing interaction results in the production of

Auger electrons. The fraction of characteristic x-rays that are produced is called the fluorescence yield. The yield scales non-linearly with atomic number, being very low for low-Z materials typical of tissue, and very high for high-Z materials; thus preference is again given to anodes of higher atomic number.

X-ray tubes are designed to take primary advantage of the K-shell electrons, resulting in K-characteristic radiation. Radiation from L-shell (and lower shell) electrons is detrimental, as the x-ray energy is too low to penetrate the body fully; as a result, spectral shaping with metallic filters is required before an x-ray beam interacts with the patient.

An x-ray tube consists of two main components, the insert containing the x-ray-producing elements and a housing which surrounds the insert with high-voltage oil (for thermal and electrical protection) in a

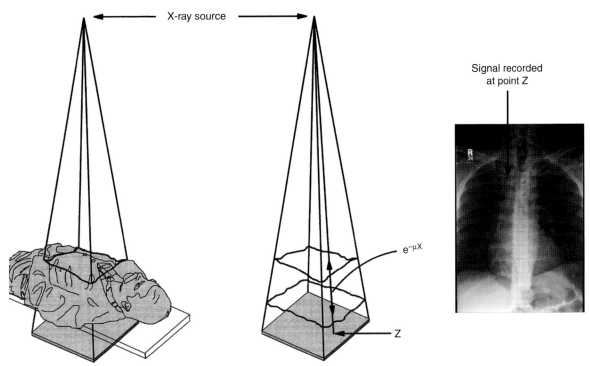

X-ray source

Signal recorded
at point Z

$e^{-\mu x}$

Z

Figure 5.2. X-rays travel in straight lines from the x-ray source through the patient to the detector. The signal at any point in the image is proportional to the number of x-rays that propagate through the patient.

lead-lined shell (for protection against unwanted radiation) (Figure 5.4). The insert consists of a sealed, evacuated vessel (either glass or metal) to allow free movement of energetic electrons from the cathode to the anode. The cathode consists of a tungsten filament wire which is heated until it glows red. This filament is the source of electrons. The filament is positioned within a focusing cup. The cup is designed to alter the electron trajectories from the cathode to the anode; as a result, virtually all of the accelerated electrons strike the anode within a small region called the focal spot. While typically achieved passively, the focusing cup can be biased with an applied voltage to alter the focus or even stop the flow of electrons to the anode to provide rapid switching of x-rays on and off (called grid control).

A by-product of the electrons striking the target is heat. In fact, only about 1% of the energy incident on the anode results in x-rays; more than 99% of the energy is transmuted into heat. Thus the single greatest design constraint of x-ray tubes is heat management. There are a number of innovations in this regard. The anode is constructed with an outer surface of tungsten (molybdenum or rhodium may be used in mammography

due to favorable characteristic radiation). This has two advantages: firstly, tungsten has one of the highest melting points of all materials (3422 °C); secondly, the high atomic number of tungsten ($Z = 74$) means that x-ray production is relatively efficient. Tungsten is often alloyed with trace elements to improve the life expectancy of the anode. The tungsten is frequently backed with a material that has high heat capacity and high thermal conductivity, such as copper or graphite, to better radiate the heat to the surrounding oil.

Two other innovations are used to increase x-ray production. The first is to angle the anode. As a result, the focal spot is viewed from the side, producing the appearance of a smaller focal spot. Thus, for the same apparent size, the actual focal-spot size can be increased with decreasing angle. This line focus allows for greater tube current, the current between the cathode and the anode, resulting in greater x-ray production. The second innovation is to rotate the anode. This is done in all but the simplest applications (e.g., dental radiography). The result is that the electron beam constantly strikes the anode on freshly cooled metal, allowing greater tube current, instantaneous heat loading, and x-ray production.

135

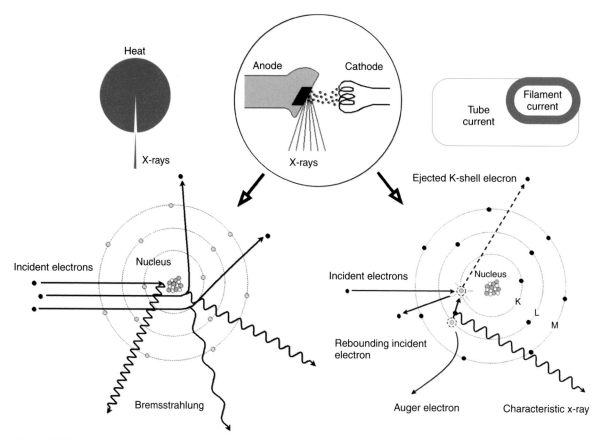

Figure 5.3. An x-ray tube is shown in schematic (top center). All modern x-ray tubes use a heated filament cathode, the tube current being 25 times smaller (or more) than the filament current. Electrons accelerated from the cathode to the anode produce x-rays. The high-energy electrons interact with atoms in the anode to produce bremsstrahlung (bottom left) or characteristic radiation (bottom right). In the latter case, either a characteristic x-ray or an Auger electron will be produced. Only 1% of the electron's energy is converted to x-rays, with the remainder converted to heat.

X-ray generators can be thought of as power supplies for x-ray tubes. X-ray generators control three factors: the applied voltage (kV), the tube current (mA), and the exposure time (ms). The applied voltage and the exposure time are controlled directly by the amplitude and duration of the high voltage. The tube current, however, is controlled indirectly by the filament current. The higher the filament current, the higher the filament temperature; hence, the greater the availability of unbound electrons on the filament. These unbound electrons are accelerated in the strong electric field that results from the applied voltage between the cathode and the anode; thus, the more electrons that are available, the greater the tube current and hence the more x-rays that are produced.

Signal/sample interaction

Sample effect on signal

X-rays interact with matter in accordance with Beer's law:

$$I = I_0 e^{-\mu t} \tag{5.3}$$

where I_0 is the number of x-rays entering an object, I is the number of x-rays exiting an object, t is the thickness of the object and μ is an intrinsic property of the material called the linear x-ray attenuation coefficient. This relationship is frequently termed exponential attenuation. More commonly, one normalizes by the density of the material to yield the mass attenuation coefficient (Table 5.1).

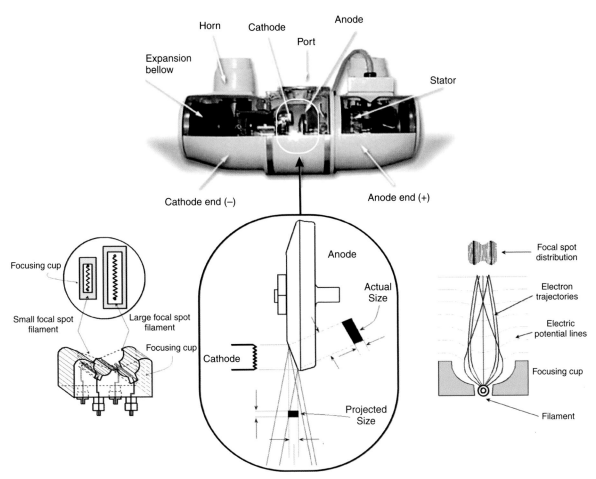

Figure 5.4. An x-ray tube is shown in cross-section. The glass insert forms an evacuated envelop containing the cathode and anode. The cathode consists of one or two filaments set within a focusing cup (lower left). Electrons accelerated from the cathode to the anode are focused so as to arrive on the anode within a well-defined focal spot (lower right). The actual size of the focal spot is larger than the projected size by virtue of the anode angulation (lower middle); this, combined with rotation by the stator, increase the heat loading. The glass insert is contained within a lead-lined vessel; the x-rays are emitted through a low Z port; the intermediate space is filled with oil for thermal protection; an expansion bellows is provided to allow for thermal expansion of the oil.

Attenuation occurs via two fundamental processes at diagnostic x-ray energies: the photoelectric effect and Compton scattering (Figure 5.5). The photoelectric effect is an interaction between an incident x-ray and a bound orbital electron. In the photoelectric effect, the x-ray is completely absorbed by an orbital electron. The x-ray energy is used to promote the electron from its orbit; the remaining energy is converted to kinetic energy for the electron. The photoelectric effect is proportional to the cube of the atomic number (Z^3) and inversely proportional to the cube of the x-ray energy (E^{-3}); thus it is predominantly a low-energy effect. The exception to this rule occurs at discrete energies related to the binding energy of the orbital electrons. At x-ray energies lower than the binding energy, such bound electrons cannot interact by the photoelectric effect. However, when the x-ray energy is increased above the binding energy, the previously prohibited electrons become the preferred electrons in x-ray interactions. For example, iodine has 53 electrons. At the K-shell binding energy (33.2 keV), the two K-shell electrons are six times more likely to interact with x-rays than the remaining 51 electrons combined. For this reason, the photoelectric effect is the primary determinant of contrast in x-ray imaging, displaying compositional differences with substantial contrast (Figure 5.6).

Compton scattering is a form of incoherent scattering. In incoherent scattering, the x-ray interacts

Table 5.1. X-ray mass attenuation coefficients for three energies [4], representative of mammography (20 keV), musckuloskeletal and interventional radiography (40 keV), and chest radiography (60 keV)

| | Density (g/cm^3) | Mass attenuation coefficient (cm^2/g) | | |
		20 keV	40 keV	60 keV
Water	1.000	0.7613	0.2629	0.2046
Air	0.0012	0.7334	0.2429	0.1861
Muscle	1.040	0.7777	0.2635	0.2036
Bone	1.650	2.753	0.5089	0.2727
Fat	0.916	0.5332	0.2353	0.1961
Iodine		25.43	22.10	7.579
Barium		29.38	24.57	8.511
Aluminum	2.699	3.441	0.5685	0.2778
Copper	8.960	33.79	4.862	1.593

with an electron, converting a fraction of the x-ray energy into kinetic energy of the electron, setting the electron into motion. The x-ray and the electron interact in compliance with two fundamental laws of physics: conservation of energy and conservation of momentum. In the most idealized description of incoherent scatter it is presumed that the interaction occurs between an x-ray and a free (or unbound) electron. Compton scattering differs from the conceptual ideal of incoherent scatter, in that one must account for the binding of electrons (no electron in matter is unbound at room temperature). A relativistic correction is also needed, since electrons can travel near the speed of light (a 100 keV electron will travel at 55% the speed of light).

Compton scattering is virtually independent of both x-ray energy and atomic number. Compton scatter is, instead, almost solely dependent upon electron density. For the materials found in the body, electron density is essentially a constant. The primary determinant of electron density is, in fact, the physical density. Thus, images produced at an energy dominated by Compton scattering almost solely reflect the physical density of materials in the body.

Note that the energetic electrons created in the photoelectric interaction and Compton scattering will travel some distance through the surrounding tissue before stopping. Also note that the vacancy in the orbital shell in the photoelectric effect will be filled by an outer-shell electron, resulting in the production of a characteristic x-ray or more commonly

an Auger electron. These energetic electrons will continue to interact in the tissue through multiple interactions until they are captured.

The signal in x-ray imaging is quantified as the number of x-rays incident on a small area of the detector. This area can be defined by the individual detector elements or the size of the object. Although we rarely care about the actual signal, we do care about the difference in signals between the object and the background, or the relative signal difference (i.e., contrast). To a first approximation, the number of x-rays incident on a patient is a constant. The recorded signal is modulated (reduced) by the intervening tissues. It is for this reason that signal difference is preferred as a performance metric; the signal difference is a record of the difference in materials along various paths through the patient.

According to this definition, the contrast (C) is the relative difference in the x-ray signal between an object and the background. Thus:

$$C = 1 - e^{-\Delta\mu\Delta t} \tag{5.4}$$

where $\Delta\mu$ is the difference in attenuation between an object and the background and Δt is the thickness of the object (Figure 5.6).

We began this discussion by assuming that the number of x-rays incident across a patient is a constant. In fact, the formation of x-rays occurs randomly in both space and time. As a result, a measurement of the number of x-rays that pass through a small region (for example, an object of interest or a detector element) is a random variable. By making repeated measurements, one can estimate the average (mean) and variance (standard deviation squared). The underlying statistical process of x-ray generation is Poisson-distributed. As a result, the variance is equal to the mean. Defining the signal as the mean number of x-rays (N) and the noise as the standard deviation of that number ($\sqrt{N}$) results in a definition of the signal-to-noise ratio (SNR) that is equal to the standard deviation; thus:

$$\text{SNR} = N/\sqrt{N} = \sqrt{N} \tag{5.5}$$

As a result, the greater the number of x-rays, the greater the signal-to-noise ratio (Figure 5.6).

Since we typically are more interested in the contrast than the signal, we can equally define a contrast-to-noise ratio (CNR). The CNR is dependent on the number of x-rays incident on the patient, the difference in the attenuation of the object to the background, and the thickness of the object. It has been

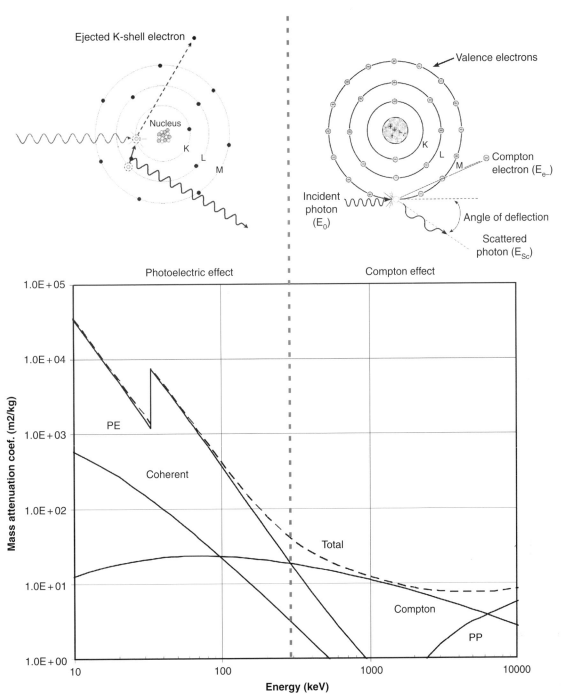

Figure 5.5. The two primary x-ray interactions with matter are the photoelectric effect (PE) and the Compton effect. The mass attenuation coefficient of each interaction is plotted as a function of energy. In addition, the attenuation coefficient for coherent scatter and pair production (PP) is shown. The total attenuation is the sum of the individual components. The vertical dashed line at 290 keV marks the boundary between where the PE is dominant and the Compton effect is dominant.

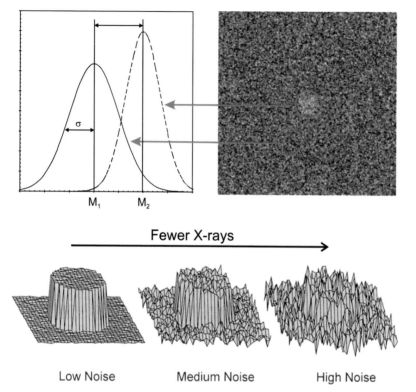

Figure 5.6. Image of a lesion in a uniform background (upper right). Although the lesion is clearly brighter than the background, both the lesion and the background have a distribution of pixel values. The histogram of pixel values (upper left) shows that the distributions, while having unique mean values, do overlap. The extent of the overlap is determined by the difference in the mean and the breadth of the distributions. In the lower half, images of the lesion are simulated with various x-ray intensities; as the number of x-rays is reduced, the noise increases relative to the signal difference. This is further illustrated by the associated histograms.

found experimentally that CNR = 5 is the lower limit for which an observer can reliably detect an object. In clinical radiography, the quantity of radiation used to produce an image is determined by the CNR of the clinically relevant structures.

Signal effect on sample

Both the photoelectric effect and Compton scatter result in the creation of high-energy electrons in the body. These electrons will travel some distance in the tissue before stopping. The distance traveled is dependent upon the tissue composition and the electron energy. However, unlike x-rays, this distance has an upper limit, defined as the electron range. The moving electrons will interact continuously with intervening atoms in a series of electron–nucleus and electron–electron interactions. These interactions are analogous to those that occur when an energetic electron is incident on the x-ray tube anode, with the proviso that the electron energies are typically much lower and tissue generally has a low atomic number, resulting in more Auger electrons.

Electron–electron interactions which result in an energy transfer of more than approximately 10 eV are said to be *ionizing* (the exact value is dependent upon the material). Such interactions have the potential to ionize the atom involved in the interaction. As a result, either an atomic bond may be broken, resulting in a chemical alteration in the body, or the ionized atom may become chemically reactive, resulting in the potential to alter surrounding molecules. In either case, the resultant chemical change can in turn produce a biological change that can deleteriously affect the organism.

The primary agent of such change is water. Water is the most common constituent of the body and one

Table 5.2. Effective doses for various adult diagnostic radiology procedures. The data were obtained from an extensive literature survey [5], in which both the average values and the range of values were reported; the former account for trends and statistical outliers

Examination	Average effective examination dose (mSv)	Values reported in literature (mSv)
Skull	0.1	0.03–0.22
Cervical spine	0.2	0.07–0.3
Thoracic spine	1.0	0.6–1.4
Lumbar spine	1.5	0.5–1.8
PA and lateral chest	0.1	0.05–0.24
Mammography	0.4	0.10–0.60
Abdomen	0.7	0.04–1.1
Pelvis	0.6	0.2–1.2
Shoulder	0.01	–
Upper gastrointestinal series	6	1.5–12
Small-bowel series	5	3.0–7.8
Barium enema	8	2.0–18.0
Head CT	2	0.9–4.0
Chest CT	7	4.0–18.0
Abdomen CT	8	3.5–25
Pelvis CT	6	3.3–10
Intraoral radiography	0.005	0.0002–0.010

of the easiest to ionize. Water can form a variety of free radicals that are highly reactive. The primary target of concern for these and other reactive species is DNA. The double-helix structure of DNA is relatively robust to radiation injury. However, if DNA undergoes an unrepaired double-bond break, then the resulting genetic changes can either result in cell death (the most common outcome and a feature capitalized for radiation therapy), or can transform the cell (potentially resulting in the future formation of a malignancy).

The potential for injury is quantified by the radiation dose. Dose is defined as the energy absorbed in the medium per unit mass. Radiation dose has a special SI unit, the gray, where 1 Gy is equal to 1 J/kg. Formerly, the rad was used; 1 Gy = 100 rad. It is important to note, however, that not all tissues are equally sensitive to radiation, nor are all radiations equally damaging (e.g., neutrons are more damaging than x-rays). The likelihood that irradiation of a specific tissue type will result in an organism's death can be estimated from experiments on similar organisms. This relative tissue sensitivity is denoted by the tissue weighting factor (w_T), while the relative sensitivity to different radiations is given by the radiation weighting factor (w_R) [1]. Thus the *effective dose* is calculated as the weighted sum of the dose to each organ by each radiation type [1]. The effective dose is specified in sieverts (Sv); the former unit was the rem, where 1 Sv = 100 rem. The effective dose is a measure of the total risk to an organism. In humans, a whole-body irradiation of 3.2–3.6 Sv will result in the death of 50% of the irradiated population in 60 days without medical intervention [2].

The likelihood of an adverse biological effect is dependent upon the radiation dose. The effects are typically divided into deterministic and stochastic effects. Deterministic effects include cataracts, skin injury, denudement of the hematopoietic stem cells, and other effects. Such effects are extremely rare in diagnostic imaging, with only the first two occurring sporadically when a threshold dose to the specific tissue is exceeded. Stochastic injury refers to the likelihood that the organism has incurred a fatal alteration to the genotype based on the x-ray exposure. Today, international standards organizations prefer a linear, non-threshold risk model for stochastic injury; that is, the risk of injury scales linearly with the radiation dose [3], and even small amounts of radiation can result in small but potentially measurable risks. The current estimate of a stochastic injury, namely a fatal cancer, is about 0.04 Sv^{-1} (4% incidence per Sv). In current medical practice, typical radiation doses from diagnostic radiology are on the order of μSv to mSv (Table 5.2). Thus the risk of carcinogenesis in diagnostic imaging is extremely low, though of increasing concern with the increased use of newer CT scanners.

Signal detection

Radiography

X-ray detectors used in medical imaging consist of an x-ray attenuator that transduces the x-ray signal into either an optical signal (typically by a phosphor) or an electronic signal (typically by a semiconductor), and a device for recording the light or electrons. While historically the optical signal (light) was recorded by film, this has largely fallen out of practice. Today, two broad classes of digital detectors are most

141

Computed Radiography

x-rays

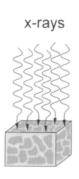

laser light

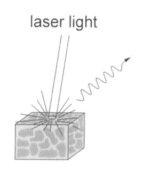

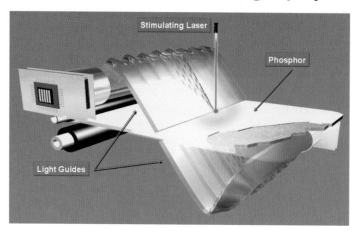

Digital Radiography

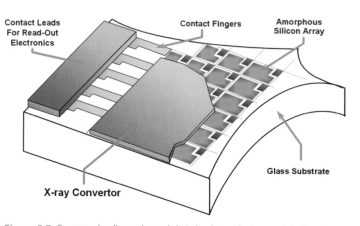

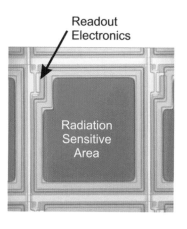

Figure 5.7. Computed radiography and digital radiography image detectors. In computed radiography (CR), x-rays excite a phosphor which traps the liberated charge (top left). The phosphor plate is then raster-scanned by translating a plate past a scanning laser. The laser stimulates the emission of light (top right). The stimulated light is collected by lightguides and recorded to produce the radiograph. In digital radiography (DR), a flat-panel detector consists of an array of photodetectors coupled to an x-ray converter (bottom left). Each photodector consists of a radiation-sensitive area and readout electronics made up of thin-film transistors. The array of detector elements is read in a raster fashion to produce an image.

commonly used; these go by the rather confusing names of computed radiography (CR) and digital radiography (DR) (Figure 5.7).

CR systems consist of two elements: a photostimulable phosphor (PSP) plate stored in a light-tight cassette, and a PSP reader. The PSP plate is prepared by exposure to an intense light source to erase any residual signal on the plate. The plate is then placed behind the patient and irradiated. The PSP is designed to trap energetic electrons produced by the incident x-rays in the crystalline lattice of the PSP. This stored charge (PSPs are also called storage phosphors) is liberated in the form of blue/ultraviolet light in the reader by way of a stimulating infrared light. The reader consists of a scanning laser assembly which irradiates the plate point-by-point. The stimulated blue light is separated from the stimulating red light by an optical filter. The blue light is then recorded; the intensity of the recorded signal at each point is linearly proportional to the intensity of the x-ray signal at that point.

DR detectors consist of either a phosphor or a photoconductor coupled to a thin-film transistor

of a large num-
rranged in rows
or element con-
capacitor) and a
rational mode of
to remove any
r; the configura-
rage of any inci-
reate either light
to an electronic
rons which are
he configuration
ation and begin
-by-row, reading
v sequentially. In

s are used exclu-
can be used for
The rapid (up to
DR fluoroscopy
itable for certain
al tomosynthesis.

Γ) revolutionized
irst non-invasive
high-quality cross-sectional images of the body. CT
scanners do not intrinsically acquire image data that
are human-readable; rather, data are acquired in a
manner to facilitate subsequent reconstruction of an
interpretable image. CT scanners consist of an x-ray
tube and an opposing x-ray detector mounted on a
circular ring. In most CT scanners, the x-ray generator
and data processing system are also mounted on the
ring. These elements rotate about the patient to
acquire projections through the patient at various
angles. The rotating ring is most commonly arranged
in a vertical plane, while the patient is prone or supine
on a horizontal bed. The bed is advanced through the
center of the ring as the acquisition system is rotated
about the patient (Figure 5.8).

The x-ray tube and generator for CT are designed to
allow substantially longer exposure times than conventional radiographic systems. The CT detectors typically
consist of discrete arrays of photodetectors coupled to
phosphors with very high light output and fast temporal
response; the latter is necessary to allow rapid readout
of the image data. While early CT scanners acquired a
single plane of projection through the patient at one
time, i.e., a slice (moving the patient between

acquisitions to produce a 3D image), all modern CT
scanners simultaneously acquire multiple projection
planes while moving the patient continuously. These
so-called multislice helical CT scanners are capable of
acquiring an isotropic 3D image of the entire body in
less than 30 seconds. Prior to display, the "raw" data
must be reconstructed, as detailed below.

Spatial encoding

Projection

X-ray images are acquired in a projective geometry.
X-rays emanate from the point-like x-ray source and
travel in straight lines to the detector (Figure 5.2). The
x-rays are attenuated as they traverse a path through
the tissue; the exact attenuation in each path is dependent upon the various tissues traversed.

The recorded attenuation is energy-dependent; the
x-ray energy spectrum is chosen based on the anatomy
of interest. For example, when imaging the thorax, one
may be interested in the bony anatomy or the lung
parenchyma; the former is imaged at low energy to
emphasize the photoelectric effect, which is strongly
dependent upon composition, allowing one to easily
distinguish bone from soft tissue; the latter is imaged
at high energy, emphasizing the Compton effect,
which is dependent upon density, thus allowing one
to more readily visualize soft tissue from air. This is
illustrated in Figure 5.9.

The secondary x-rays created in Compton scatter
are emitted essentially isotropically. These eponymous
scattered x-rays reduce the contrast of images. The
contrast is proportional to $1/(1 + S/P)$, where S/P is
the ratio of scatter to primary. S/P ranges from 1 to 5
in medical imaging, increasing with x-ray energy; thus,
contrast can be severely reduced by scatter. As a result,
most radiographs are acquired with a radiographic
grid interposed between the patient and the detector.
Grids are composed of alternating lamina of lead and
a minimally attenuating material. Grids preferentially
attenuate x-rays incident at an acute angle; as a result,
scattered x-rays are up to 10 times more likely to be
attenuated than primary (non-scattered) x-rays,
restoring contrast, although at a cost of increased dose.

The projective geometry results in images of objects
which are magnified relative to the size of the actual
object. The magnification is dependent upon the position of the object. Objects closer to the detector are less
magnified; objects closer to the x-ray source are more
magnified. This effect has both benefit and detriment.

143

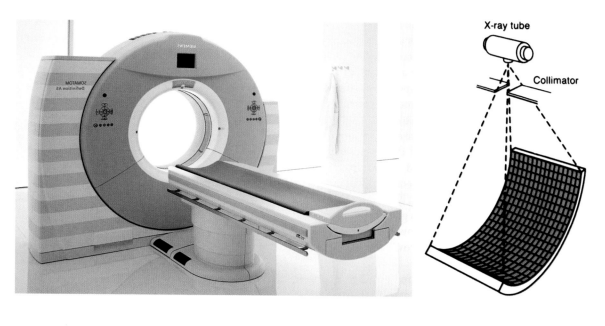

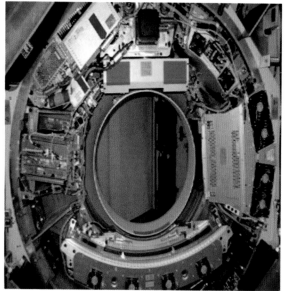

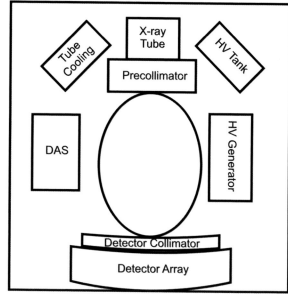

Figure 5.8. A modern CT scanner. The two main elements are an x-ray source and an opposing detector array; these rotate about the patient, as the patient is advanced through the scanner. The actual scan is complex, consisting of multiple elements mounted on a rotating stage. The stage is powered through a slip-ring. Mounted on the stage are an x-ray and pre-collimator, the x-ray generator and high-voltage (HV) tank, the detector array and collimator, and the data acquisition system (DAS).

Magnification can be used to enlarge the image of small objects to aid in diagnosis; however, excessive magnification results in the blurring of an object's edges. This latter effect, called the penumbra effect, is the result of the finite size of the x-ray focal spot; the larger the focal spot, the greater the blurring. X-ray geometry is the subject of extensive work in procedural optimization; for example, smaller focal spots result in less blurring from penumbra, but result in greater blurring from patient motion, since smaller focal spots are operated with lower tube current.

Tomography

Unlike projection radiography, CT images are acquired in a non-Cartesian coordinate system. CT

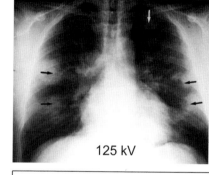

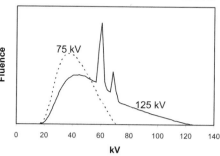

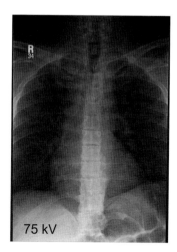

Figure 5.9. Two thoracic radiographs. The first (upper left) is acquired at 125 kV; an x-ray spectrum which is dominated by the Compton effect. The result is a radiograph that emphasizes physical density differences, providing high contrast to the lung parenchyma and low contrast to the bony structures. The second radiography (right) is acquired at 70 kV; an x-ray spectrum that is dominated by the photoelectric effect. The result is an image that emphasizes atomic number differences, providing high contrast to the bony structures.

image data are, instead, acquired in a rotational-projective coordinate system. In this coordinate system, the location of any object in space is recorded as a sinusoidal wave, in which location is denoted by the amplitude and phase of the sine wave, comparable to the Radon transform of the object. While these data can be visualized graphically in a sinogram (Figure 5.10), such displays are not readily interpretable by human observers for any but the simplest scenes. Fortunately, the CT rotation-projection space can be transformed to a Cartesian space by application of the inverse Radon transform.

The Radon transform was developed in 1917 by the mathematician Johann Radon. While the forward transform is mathematically tractable, the inverse transform is not. As a result, numerous approximate solutions have been developed. The method most commonly used in CT imaging is an analytical technique called filtered back-projection (FBP); iterative techniques are more commonly used in tomographic imaging in nuclear medicine (see Chapter 4). The resulting CT image is a spatial map of x-ray attenuation coefficients.

FBP consists of two steps. First, each projection is filtered; most commonly with a ramp filter and a band-limiting filter. This filtering operation is usually performed in the Fourier domain for computational expediency. The filtered projection is then back-projected in a fashion that accounts for the geometry of image acquisition. Computation efficiency is achieved by sorting the projection data (prior to filtering) so that parallel back-projections can be computed.

The image data created by CT imaging systems have numerous deficiencies which must be addressed either prior to or after back-projection; the order depends upon the nature of the artifact. Failure to address these concerns will result in unacceptable image artifacts. For example, imaging with a poly-energetic x-ray spectrum results in beam-hardening – low-energy x-rays are more readily attenuated than high-energy x-rays – and, as a result, the mean energy of the x-ray beam increases as more tissue is traversed. This effect causes a cupping artifact in FBP images, which is corrected through image processing.

The final step in CT reconstruction is normalization of the image data. As stated, the CT image data are proportional to the x-ray attenuation coefficients. Such values are not easily interpretable, as they depend upon the energy of the x-ray spectrum and other factors. As a result, CT data are normalized to the attenuation coefficient of water. The normalized data are then multiplied by a constant (typically 1000) to generate integer values called Hounsfield units (HU) in honor of Sir Godfrey Hounsfield, one of two scientists awarded the Nobel Prize in Physiology or Medicine in 1979 for the invention of CT. Hence, CT signal intensity is reported using a ratio numeric system. In this scheme, water has a value of 0 HU, air

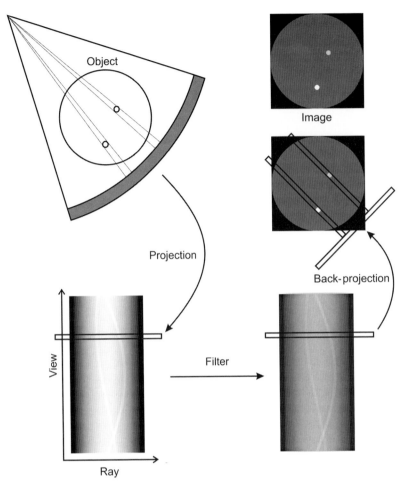

Figure 5.10. CT acquisition and image reconstruction is illustrated for a simple object consisting of two rods in a large cylinder. Multiple projections are obtained at specific view angles, each view containing multiple divergent rays, as shown. In this way, the CT scanner acquires an image (the sinogram) that is the Radon transform of the object. The inverse Radon transform is approximated through filtered back-projection, where first the sinogram is filtered and then back-projected. Computation efficiency is obtained by reordering the data prior to back-projection (not shown), so that parallel-ray back-projection can be used. The result is an image of the object in cross-section.

has a value of −1000 HU, and fat, blood, and bone have values of approximately −100, 50, and 1200 HU, respectively.

References

1. International Commission on Radiological Protection. 1990 Recommendations of the International Commission on Radiological Protection. *Ann ICRP* 1990; **21** (1–3): 1–201.

2. National Council on Radiation Protection. *Guidance on Radiation Received in Space Activities*. NCRP Report 98. Bethesda, MD: NCRP, 1989.

3. BEIR VII: *Health Risks from Exposure to Low Levels of Ionizing Radiation*. Washington, DC: National Academies Press, 2005.

4. Johns HE, Cunningham JR. *The Physics of Radiology*, 4th edn. Springfield, IL: Charles C. Thomas, 1983.

5. Mettler FA, Huda W, Yoshizumi TT, Mahesh M. Effective doses in radiology and diagnostic nuclear medicine: a catalog. *Radiology* 2008; **248**: 254–63.

General reading

Bushberg JT, Seibert JA, Leidholdt EM, Boone JM. *The Essential Physics of Medical Imaging*, 2nd edn. Philadelphia, PA: Lippincott, Williams & Wilkins, 2002.

Buzog TM. *Computed Tomography: from Photon Statistics to Modern Cone-Beam CT*. Berlin: Springer-Verlag, 2008.

Curry TS, Dowdey JE, Murry RC. *Christensen's Physics of Diagnostic Radiology*, 4th edn. Philadelphia, PA: Lea & Febiger, 1990.

Chapter 6

Non-ionizing radiation
Ultrasound imaging

Peter H. Arger and Chandra M. Sehgal

Ultrasound (US) consists of high-frequency sound waves that are above the range of human hearing, at frequencies higher than 20 kHz. Medical ultrasound imaging is performed at much higher frequencies, typically in the MHz range. Ultrasound differs from other conventional imaging methods in important ways. First, unlike electromagnetic radiation, ultrasound waves are non-ionizing pressure waves. Second, the ultrasound signal is recorded in the reflection mode rather than the transmission mode used for x-ray and CT imaging. In ultrasound imaging, the imaged structures are not the sources that emit radiation. Instead, the sample is imaged by applying external acoustic energy to it. A "pulse echo" technique is used to create an image from longitudinal mechanical waves that interact with tissues of the body. The applied energy is reflected to the source by tissue inhomogeneities. The resulting signals carry information about their source as well as about the sample. Decoding these signals into an image requires separating the detected signal components due to the external source from those due to the sample.

Medical ultrasound imaging systems typically incorporate a piezoelectric crystal as the external signal source. This crystal vibrates in response to an oscillating electric current, producing longitudinal mechanical waves. The ultrasound signal propagates linearly through various media, including water and soft tissue, at an average speed of 1540 m/s, but does not propagate satisfactorily through bone or air. As a result, ultrasound is most suited for imaging soft tissues. The ultrasound signal is absorbed and reflected differently by different tissue types, allowing precise delineation of organs and individual tissue structures in the images. Figure 6.1 shows an example of an intrauterine fetus with a large facial teratoma, demonstrating the exquisite detail possible using diagnostic ultrasound today.

In this chapter we describe the basics of biomedical ultrasound imaging. The imaging path is traced from the signal source through signal/tissue interactions, detection, signal processing, and image display. Topics to be covered include instrumentation, modes of ultrasound interaction and display, Doppler flow imaging, contrast agents, and bioeffects. At the conclusion, future applications of ultrasound imaging are discussed.

Ultrasound signal and source

Depending on the application, US imaging is performed using 2–50 MHz ultrasound signals. Medical ultrasound typically uses ultrasound waves between 2 and 20 MHz, although ultrasound systems that operate at frequencies up to 50 MHz are also available. However, at these high frequencies ultrasound penetration is limited to a few mm (10–12 mm) on research scanners principally used for imaging small animals.

Ultrasound signals are produced when an electric current stimulates a piezoelectric crystal, usually constructed from lead zirconate titanate. Figure 6.2 illustrates the concept for a single-element piezoelectric crystal composed of diagonally aligned molecular dipoles [1]. When an oscillating external voltage is applied, the crystal expands and compresses alternately due to the realignment of the molecular dipoles between horizontal and vertical (Figure 6.2a). The compressions and expansions of the crystal are transmitted as mechanical sound waves to the medium coupled to the piezoelectric element. Conversely, when the same crystal is exposed to sound waves, it expands and contracts to generate electrical voltage as a function of time (Figure 6.2b). That is, the same crystal can be used to transmit and receive ultrasound.

Introduction to the Science of Medical Imaging, ed. R. Nick Bryan. Published by Cambridge University Press. © Cambridge University Press 2010.

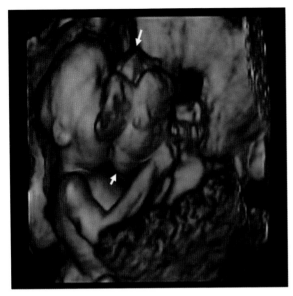

Figure 6.1. A large teratoma seen during the intrauterine ultrasound examination. Note the large lobulated mass which extends from the face of the fetus (arrows).

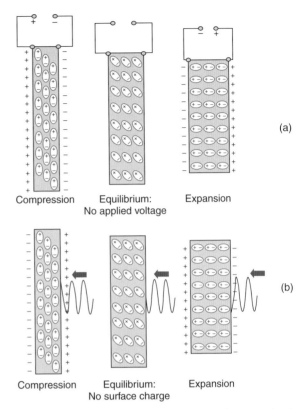

Figure 6.2. Ultrasound generation and reception by a piezoelectric element consisting of molecular dipoles: (a) generation of ultrasound by the piezoelectric element in response to external oscillating voltage; (b) generation of electrical signal by the ultrasound incident on the piezoelectric element. (Reproduced from Bushberg *et al.*, 2002 [1], with the permission of Lippincott Williams and Wilkins.)

Ultrasound waves are pressure waves that propagate through matter via compression and expansion of the medium. The particles in the medium move closer and further apart during the propagation, but their mean positions remain unchanged. An ultrasound wave with pressure (p) varying in spatial direction (x) and time (t) is called a plane wave. Its physical behavior is described by the one-dimensional wave equation:

$$\frac{\partial^2 p}{\partial x^2} = \frac{1}{c^2}\frac{\partial^2 p}{\partial^2 t} \tag{6.1}$$

whose general solution can be represented by a sinusoidal function:

$$p(x, t) = \cos\left(\frac{2\pi f}{c}\right)(x - ct) \tag{6.2}$$

In Equations 6.1 and 6.2, c is the speed of sound and represents the distance traveled by the wave per unit time; f is the frequency and represents the number of times the wave oscillates per unit time; and λ is the wavelength and represents the distance between two consecutive compressions or refractions. The sound speed, frequency, and wavelength are interrelated by the equation:

$$c = \lambda f \tag{6.3}$$

Equation 6.2 is for a continuous wave in infinite space and infinite time. Ultrasound images are constructed using pulsed ultrasound, and the wave form is approximately sinusoidal, when viewed locally over a short period of time.

Different interactions occur between the ultrasound waves and various body tissues. The interactions depend on the acoustic properties of the tissues being examined, and include absorption, scattering or dispersion, refraction, and reflection.

Signal/sample interactions

Tissue absorption and scattering of the ultrasound beam cause signal *attenuation*, a loss of acoustic energy as the distance that the sound wave travels increases. The strength (pressure amplitude) of an ultrasound wave decreases exponentially with the propagation distance and follows the Beer–Lambert law of attenuation. A thorough understanding of attenuation effects is critical in biomedical ultrasound imaging because the reduced signal strength from attenuation must be compensated for during image construction. Also, the absorption of acoustic energy heats the tissue and can be potentially hazardous, especially in obstetrical ultrasound.

The interactions of the ultrasound beam with tissue depend upon differences in acoustic impedance at the tissue interfaces. Adjacent tissue interfaces larger than the wavelength are called specular reflectors. Ultrasound incident on these interfaces undergoes reflection and refraction. *Scattering* occurs at rough or non-specular reflector surfaces where the tissue interface size is comparable to or smaller than the wavelength.

Reflection occurs when the ultrasound beam is incident on an interface with a significant difference in acoustic impedance (Z). Acoustic impedance is a material property that measures resistance to the propagation of acoustic energy. It is the product of density of the medium (ρ) and the sound speed (c). When an ultrasound wave is incident on an interface of two layers with different acoustic impedance, a portion of the energy is reflected back to the transducer. For a perpendicular incident ultrasound wave, the fraction $R_{intensity}$ of the incident energy reflected back is related to the difference in the impedances of the two layers 1 and 2:

$$R_{intensity} = \left[\frac{Z_2 - Z_1}{Z_2 + Z_1}\right]^2 = \left[\frac{\rho_2 c_2 - \rho_1 c_1}{\rho_2 c_2 + \rho_1 c_1}\right]^2 \quad (6.4)$$

The remaining energy ($1 - R_{intensity}$) is transmitted to layer 2 and continues to propagate until it arrives at another tissue interface, where it undergoes similar reflection and transmission. Because ultrasound can transmit through multiple layers, it is possible to image structures that are located behind one another at different depths along the direction of the beam.

As the sound beams progress through tissue, each layer may cause reflection, refraction, scattering, or absorption, and only a small portion of the initial ultrasound energy from the transducer returns for constructing images. The transformation of this reduced beam signal into an ultrasound image is discussed below.

Refraction is a change in the direction of the transmitted ultrasound energy beam at a tissue interface that is not perpendicular to the transmitted energy. The bending of the incident beam follows Snell's law, where the angle of refraction (θ_t) depends on the angle of incidence (θ_i) and the sound speed of the two layers at the interface:

$$\frac{\sin(\theta_t)}{\sin(\theta_i)} = \frac{c_2}{c_1} \quad (6.5)$$

The echo amplitude from the various interfaces determines the tissue's appearance on the actual ultrasound image. Differences in scattering amplitude in different areas of the same organ, for example, cause brightness changes on the final ultrasound image. Image appearance depends on a number of factors in addition to acoustic impedance differences, including the number of scatterers per unit volume, the size of the scatterers, and the frequency of the ultrasound beam. *Hyperechoic* areas have higher scatterer amplitude relative to the background, and appear bright in an image. *Hypoechoic* areas, on the other hand, have lower scatterer amplitude compared to the background and appear as dark regions in an image. In essence, hyper- and hypoechogenicity create contrast in an image, as discussed in more detail later. Figure 6.3 shows examples of hypoechoic breast mass and hyperechoic gallstone.

Signal detection

A unique feature of ultrasound imaging is that the same piezoelectric crystal is used for generating the source signal and for detecting echo signals from the tissues. The *transducer* used for signal detection is more complex than suggested previously. In addition to the piezoelectric element, the transducer parts include an insulating cover, a matching layer in front of the piezoelectric element, a damping layer at the back of the element, and electrodes. The matching layer facilitates the exchange of acoustic energy between the transducer and a patient. The backing material absorbs acoustic vibrations and reduces the ultrasound pulse length. Short pulses are necessary for resolving tissue structures along the beam axis. The shortening of ultrasound pulses by damping or ring-down of vibrations introduces a band of frequencies above and below the center frequency. That is, the short pulse of ultrasound emanating from the transducer source has a bandwidth characterized by Q factor. High spatial resolution requires a low-Q broadband transducer.

The imaging transducers used in modern scanners consist of multiple individual piezoelectric elements arranged in curvilinear or linear arrays, depending on the application. Some transducers have a phased array configuration. A *linear* or *curvilinear array* typically consists of 128–512 elements. The ultrasound beam is formed by activating only a small group of adjacent transducer elements at a time. The beam is steered

(a)   (b)

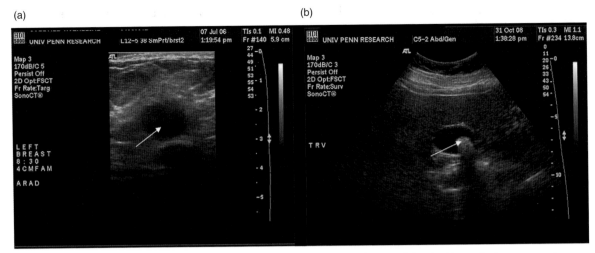

Figure 6.3. Examples of hypoechoic and hyperechoic areas. (a) Moderate-size breast lesion with low-level internal echoes represents a hypoechoic mass (arrow). (b) A large hyperechoic gallstone (arrow) located within the fluid-filled lumen of the gallbladder. Note the posterior shadowing behind the gallstone caused by the attenuation of ultrasound.

electronically by shifting the transducer elements that participate in beam forming. A *phased array* typically consists of 64–128 elements. Unlike linear and curvilinear arrays, the phased array simultaneously activates all the elements to produce an ultrasound beam. The beam is steered by using a small time delay in the electrical activation of the individual elements. It is important to note that with either the phased-array or linear-array transducer, the beam is steered electronically without moving the transducer.

Spatial encoding of the signal for image formation

Ultrasound images are constructed by a pulse–echo technique that involves transmitting a burst of ultrasound energy along a narrow beam (A-line/scan line) and listening to the echoes (reflected and backscattered ultrasound) from the tissue along the path of the beam. The transmit–receive process is repeated by steering the ultrasound beam along several A-lines to scan the tissue of interest. The resulting echoes are received by the piezoelectric element of the imaging transducer and transformed into electric signals. These signals are displayed as gray-scale images, where brightness represents echo amplitude and depth represents distance of the tissue interface from the transducer. Depth is computed from the time it takes for the ultrasound pulse to travel to

the tissue interface and then return to the transducer. If the time taken by the ultrasound pulse to travel to the interface is T, the depth d of the tissue interface relative to the transducer is described by the equation:

$$d = \tfrac{1}{2}cT = \tfrac{1}{2} * 1540 * T \qquad (6.6)$$

where sound speed c is assumed to be 1540 m/s. During imaging, an ultrasound pulse can only be transmitted after the echo from the previous transmission has been completed. If the maximum depth to be imaged is d_m and there are n scan lines per image, then the frame rate F for imaging is:

$$F = \frac{c}{2nd_m} \qquad (6.7)$$

For example, using 256 scan lines per image, a 10 cm depth can be imaged at the video-frame rate of 30 frames/second. Thus, ultrasound allows real-time imaging.

The *spatial resolution* of ultrasound images is defined along the axial and lateral directions in the image plane. Ultrasound pulses with shorter spatial lengths yield higher axial resolution along the axis of the beam. Higher frequency combined with strong damping of the transducer element leads to shorter pulses and higher resolution. At 5 MHz, axial resolution is on the order of 0.5 mm. Lateral resolution is determined by the beam size in the image plane.

Because the beam size changes with depth (due to focusing) lateral resolution is strongly dependent on depth. Typically, lateral resolution is of an order of magnitude lower than axial resolution, on the order of 2–5 mm.

Image contrast

Tissue contrast in the images results from the difference in acoustic impedance and compressibility between tissue structures and the surrounding tissue. Larger differences result in stronger image contrast. Other factors also contribute to image contrast. The displayed ultrasound images are a result of considerable processing of the raw pulse–echo signals, including the following: time-gain compensation to offset the signal loss due to attenuation; logarithmic compression of the pulse–echo signals to match the broad dynamic range of the acoustic signal to the limited dynamic range of the display monitor; non-linear display of the signals to accentuate or suppress certain gray levels; and spatial and temporal averaging to reduce noise. Each signal-processing step influences the histogram and the contrast of the displayed images in a complex fashion specific to the processing algorithm.

Contrast is also influenced by the texture or speckle in the images. Speckle is a consequence of wave interference between the echoes from the pulse volume. It is related to the microstructure of the tissue as well as to the characteristics of the imaging device, such as transducer frequency and bandwidth. Since the presence of speckle may obscure small structures and margins, image-compounding techniques using incoherent averaging of the images have been proposed to reduce speckle. Although either frequency compounding or spatial compounding can be used to reduce speckle, spatial compounding is more common on commercial scanners. It involves acquiring multiple images (five to nine) of the same region from different view angles by reorienting the ultrasound beam. The images from different angles have slightly different speckle patterns, and when averaged they produce a *compound* image with reduced speckle and clearer margins and structures. Since the view angles are changed rapidly by electronically updating the direction of the ultrasound beam, compound imaging is performed in real time. Although compound imaging reduces speckle effectively, it is prone to motion-blurring when there is rapid tissue movement.

The final image is modified by parameters such as acoustic power (*gain*) and *time-gain compensation* (TGC), a depth parameter that is programmed into the machine to compensate for the attenuation of sound at different depths as the beam progresses through and reflects from the scanned object. This compensation makes it appear as if the amount of sound from each tissue interface depth is the same, resulting in consistent image brightness for either clinical or investigational purposes. TGC can be manipulated manually by the scanner operator, as can the near field, the slope, and the far gain of the echo signals. The final image also depends on the physical characteristics of the near field, the focused area, and the far field, as mentioned above and described below.

The *near field* is called the Fresnel zone. There is both constructive and destructive sound-wave interference in this area nearest to the transducer. The interference may cause the resulting near-field image to be more poorly defined than the rest of the image.

In the *far field*, known as the Fraunhofer zone, the beam diverges, resulting in progressively less definition as the beam travels further from the transducer.

The *focus area* occurs where re-phasing of the individual signals synthesizes them into an image that has the highest definition. Phase-array transducers with dynamic depth function, electronic delays, or just time delays, have adjustable focus areas.

Ultrasound transducers detect a wide range of ultrasound energy, up to 120 dB. This is called the *dynamic range*. Due to the limitations of the display system, the signals are non-linearly compressed. The human eye can only perceive a small range of intensities. To emphasize specific tissue structures, the echo signals are mapped non-linearly in gray scale. The non-linear mapping of echo signals and freedom to choose different scanner settings to construct optimal images make ultrasound imaging operator-dependent. Figure 6.4 shows an example of an image that was constructed using different scanner settings, showing marked differences in image quality. For example, improper TGC and overall gain result in inferior-quality images. An excellent example of a transvaginal coronal image of the bicornuate uterus acquired under optimal scanner settings is shown in Figure 6.5 (a–c). The 3D reconstruction from 2D images acquired at

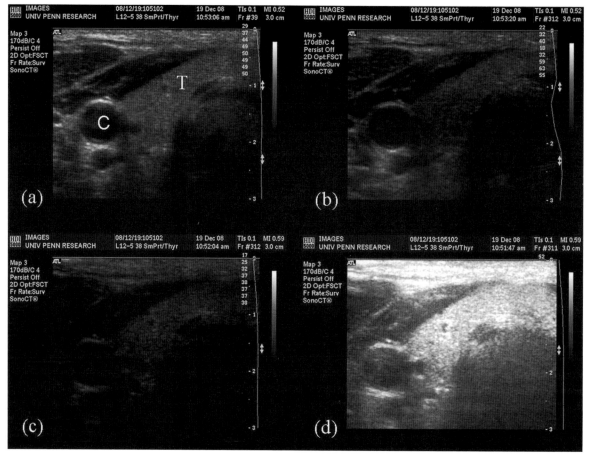

Figure 6.4. (a) A transverse image of the right thyroid (T) with common carotid artery (C) acquired at appropriate scanner settings; (b) the image acquired with improper time-gain compensation; (c) the image acquired with low overall gain; (d) the image acquired with high overall gain.

multiple parallel planes reveals a polyp (arrow) within the endometrial canal that renders the patient infertile (Figure 6.5d).

Doppler ultrasonography

A moving ultrasound reflector causes a shift in the frequency of an ultrasound wave in proportion to its velocity. In *Doppler ultrasound* the shift in frequency is used to trace the velocity of the reflector (blood) as a function of time (spectral Doppler) or to construct color images where Doppler information is superimposed in color on the gray-scale images. As illustrated in Figure 6.6, Doppler shift is measured by comparing the incident ultrasound frequencies with the reflected ultrasound frequency from the blood [2]. If f_0 and f_r are the frequencies of the transmitted and

reflected ultrasound, the shift in frequency, Δf, is the velocity v of the moving scatterer as described by the Doppler equation:

$$f_0 - f_r = \Delta f = \left(\frac{2f_0 \cos\theta}{c}\right) v, \qquad (6.8)$$

where θ is the angle between the direction of flow and the incident ultrasound beam measured on the ultrasound image. The angle at which the Doppler study is performed is important, as slight changes in angle may cause significant changes in velocity. The Doppler shift can be either positive or negative, depending on the direction of flow. Since all the parameters in Equation 6.8 are known, measuring Δf every few milliseconds gives flow velocity v as a function of time. The changing flow velocities during cardiac cycles are

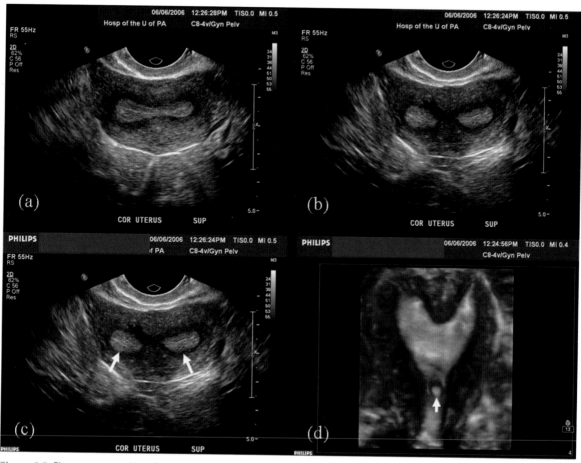

Figure 6.5. Bicornuate uterus. Note that as the examination progresses inferiorly to superiorly, as shown in the gray-scale images, the endometrial stripe divides (arrows). The coronal view (d) shows a polyp which is the cause of the patient's infertility (arrow).

displayed as a velocity–time tracing on the monitor. Because the Doppler shifts occur in the audible kHz range at physiological flow velocities, the Doppler signals are also played through loudspeakers for audible monitoring.

In principle, both continuous and pulsed ultrasound can be used for measuring Doppler shifts, but it is the latter that is often chosen for clinical studies because it allows range discrimination. Echo from a single transmitted ultrasound pulse, however, does not contain sufficient information to determine Doppler shift. Therefore, an ensemble of pulses at a pulse repetition frequency (PRF) is targeted to the site of measurement, and the phase of echo from each transmitted pulse is analyzed to determine frequency shift. Although this approach measures Doppler shifts accurately, it is limited by aliasing. To

determine Doppler frequency shift unambiguously, the Nyquist sampling condition must be satisfied: the sampling rate (pulse repetition frequency) should be at least equal to Doppler frequency shift. At a pulse repetition frequency (PRF), the maximum Doppler shift Δf_{max} that is unambiguously determined is:

$$\mathrm{PRF} = 2\Delta f_{max} = \frac{4 f_0 v_{max} \cos\theta}{c} \qquad (6.9)$$

or the maximum velocity v_{max} that can be measured without aliasing is:

$$v_{max} = \frac{c\mathrm{PRF}}{4 f_0 \cos\theta} \qquad (6.10)$$

Unlike spectral Doppler, which shows change of flow velocity with time, Doppler imaging provides

153

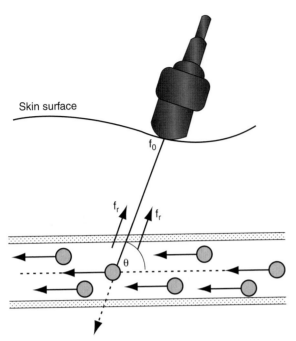

Figure 6.6. Configuration of ultrasound transducer and ultrasound beam in relation to blood flow and Doppler flow measurement. (Reproduced from Sehgal, 1996 [2], with the permission of Blackwell Science.)

a two-dimensional display of the moving blood in the vasculature. The Doppler signal is detected for each pixel within a region selected by the user on the gray-scale image. Due to the constraints imposed by real-time imaging, autocorrelation techniques are used to detect only the mean frequency and the mean amplitude of the Doppler signal. The pixels with Doppler signal exceeding a threshold are coded in color and superimposed on the gray-scale image. In color Doppler images, mean Doppler shift frequency is displayed in two colors: red and blue. The colors represent direction of flow. The brightness of the color represents the magnitude of the frequency shift or the mean velocity of flow. In power Doppler images, the strength of Doppler signal (amplitude) related to blood volume is displayed in color. Since the amplitude lacks direction, only a single color is used to display the Doppler information. The power Doppler images do not have aliasing problems and are highly sensitive to motion. Power Doppler allows detection of slow flow regions but also suffers from significant flash artifacts from tissue and patient motion. Figure 6.7 shows an ultrasound comparing a normal and an abnormal carotid artery for both duplex Doppler and color Doppler imaging.

Biological effects

So far we have covered how tissues change ultrasound signal and how the changed signal can be used to construct an image. It is important to recognize that under appropriate conditions of sonication, the ultrasound signal can change tissues and produce biological effects. The acoustic power output of the scanner, which determines the exposure of the patient to ultrasound, is regulated in the USA by the Food and Drug Administration (FDA). Acoustic power at the diagnostic ultrasound level is low enough so that no definite side effects have been shown to date. However, at high acoustic power, ultrasound has several measurable thermal and non-thermal effects, including tissue heating, blood vessel damage, tissue cavitation, and cell destruction.

Ultrasound energy is absorbed by biological tissues and converted into heat. All areas scanned are heated by the ultrasound beam. Whether the tissue exhibits any thermal effect from this heat depends on how much heat is deposited by the ultrasound beam and on how fast the heat can be removed by blood flow or other means. Tissue absorption coefficients and the intensity of the ultrasound beam determine how much heating occurs within the scanned tissue. Higher-frequency ultrasound is absorbed more than lower frequencies, but heating also depends upon tissue type. Diagnostic ultrasound generates tissue temperature rises of 1–2 °C [1], well below the temperatures likely to cause any damage. However, Doppler ultrasound can produce greater tissue heating.

In addition to thermal effects, there are secondary mechanical effects from the ultrasound beam. At very high outputs of ultrasound power, tissue damage and cell disruption can be seen with a microscope. The mechanical movement of tissue particles subjected to the ultrasound beam creates a steady circulatory flow, since radiation pressure produces tissue torque and acoustic streaming. When gas and vapor are present in the tissues, cavitation can occur. Cavitation may be subtle or obvious, so predicting whether it will occur is difficult. Ultrasound intensities used clinically may actually produce some persistent bubbles in the tissues. For this reason, ultrasound machines must display a mechanical index (described below) to indicate cavitation likelihood. At higher ultrasound intensities, the bubbles can collapse or dissolve and change water into free radicals that can damage DNA. However, in clinical diagnostic imaging, the intensity of the beam is below the level for transient cavitation.

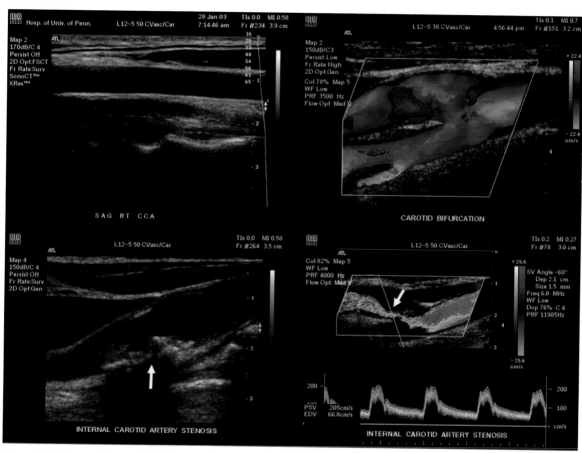

Figure 6.7. Ultrasound images of carotid artery. The two top figures show a normal gray-scale on the left and a normal color Doppler of the carotid bifurcation. The lower left gray-scale image shows arteriosclerotic plaque and debris. The color Doppler on the right indicates the marked degree of stenosis (arrows).

The peak pulse power needed for transient cavitation is on the order of $1\,kW/cm^2$.

The *thermal index* (TI) is the ratio of the acoustic power produced by the transducer to the power required to raise the tissue in the ultrasound beam by $1\,°C$. The acoustic output power of the transducer, the ultrasound frequency, and the areas scanned are used to estimate this index. Assumptions are made for exposure time, the thermal properties of the tissues related to exposure time, and the attenuation of the ultrasound beam

The *mechanical index* (MI) estimates the potential for mechanical effects such as cavitation associated with ultrasound. Cavitation occurs when the negative pressure of the ultrasound wave extracts gases from the tissue and forms microbubbles. When these microbubbles oscillate and collapse, the mechanical effects associated with them can often cause tissue

damage. The mechanical index estimates whether the ultrasound beam is likely to cause cavitation. It depends on two ultrasound wave parameters, the peak rarefaction pressure and the ultrasound frequency. As ultrasound power output increases, the mechanical index increases linearly. However, increasing the transducer frequency decreases the mechanical index inversely.

Diagnostic ultrasound has an excellent safety record, with no history of serious bioeffects. Even so, it is important to take precautions to ensure maximum benefit with minimal risk. The official policies of the ultrasound professional organizations recommend ALARA principles [3]. ALARA (as low as reasonably achievable) calls for prudent use of diagnostic ultrasound to ensure that total exposure is minimized while diagnostic information is preserved. The FDA requires ultrasound equipment to display TI and MI on the

155

screen, so that operators can assess the possible risks due to heating and cavitation during imaging.

Contrast agents

Red blood cells are weak scatterers of ultrasound and significantly less echogenic than soft tissues, making the detection of small blood vessels difficult. This limitation has prompted the development of highly echogenic contrast agents which, when injected intravenously, increase the intensity of the signal from the vessel lumen to facilitate vessel visualization [4]. These agents typically consist of microbubbles of insoluble gases encapsulated in thin shells of phospholipids or denatured albumin. The microbubbles are highly compressible and undergo resonance oscillations when exposed to ultrasound. As a consequence, they are very effective scatterers, even though their diameters are small (< 10 μm), comparable to the diameters of red blood cells (~ 5 μm). Even low concentrations of contrast agent after systemic dilution enhance echoes from blood by 20 dB or more. Unlike x-ray and MRI contrast agents, which diffuse into interstitial space, ultrasound contrast agents are vascular agents and the microbubbles do not cross the endothelium. The vascular enhancement typically lasts 3–4 minutes, and the gases from the microbubbles are primarily exhaled through the lungs, although there is some evidence that some microbubbles may be taken up by phagocytosis in the liver and spleen.

At low ultrasound amplitudes, the microbubbles behave as harmonic oscillators and emit ultrasound of frequency equal to the imaging frequency. When the microbubbles are driven at higher amplitudes, they oscillate non-linearly, expand easily, but compress with difficulty. The asymmetric or anharmonic vibrations of the bubbles emit a spectrum of *harmonic* overtones at two, three, or more times the ultrasound frequency. They also emit subharmonic signals at one-half or one-third of the ultrasound frequencies. The pulse–echo ultrasound scanners described above are modified to use the harmonic (or subharmonic) signals to construct ultrasound images. Since the harmonic signal is generated by bubble oscillations, the signals from the tissues are suppressed and clearer images of the vasculature are produced.

The thin encapsulating shells of the microbubbles are relatively fragile, so the microbubbles are readily destroyed during ultrasound imaging. This has led to new forms of contrast-enhanced imaging that use low MI as well as intermittent and multigating schemes to preserve microbubbles for improved visualization. Techniques using different imaging strategies for selectively destroying microbubbles and monitoring their replenishment have been proposed to estimate microvascular flow.

Recent advances in ultrasound contrast agents are in *molecular imaging* and *therapeutics*. The microbubble surfaces are labeled with disease-specific ligands or antibodies (Figure 6.8). When these conjugated microbubble–ligand or microbubble–antibody assemblies are injected into the blood stream, they bind to the disease markers at the site of the disease within the vasculature. The ligands or antibodies provide specificity, whereas the microbubbles act as beacons which scatter ultrasound and can be visualized by ultrasound imaging. Targeted ultrasound contrast agents have been used for imaging inflammation, angiogenesis, and thrombus.

The oscillations and collapse of microbubbles under suitable conditions of sonication can release high energy, resulting in bioeffects. Microbubble bioeffects are being studied for therapeutic applications. Microbubbles have been shown to accelerate thrombolysis and enhance drug delivery by temporarily permeating the blood–brain barrier and cell membrane.

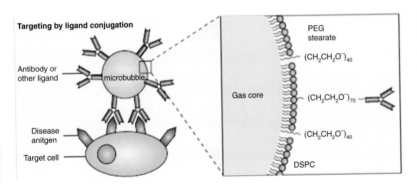

Figure 6.8. Molecular imaging by microbubble targeted contrast agent. The conjugated assemblies of microbubbles and ligands or antibodies attached to disease-specific antigens can be visualized by ultrasound imaging. (Adapted from Lindner, *Nat Rev Drug Discov* 2004; **3**: 527–32 [4].)

The temporary permeabilization of cell membranes to increase the uptake of DNA and drugs is often referred to as *sonoporation*.

Our own research has shown that the fragile blood vessels of tumors are disrupted by contrast agents in the presence of continuous ultrasound [5]. There is currently significant interest in developing vascular disrupting drugs to treat tumors, and the use of contrast agents with ultrasound could be an option for treating such tumors. Even though the therapeutic applications of microbubbles are promising, there are substantial obstacles to overcome for clinical application.

Applications

The diagnostic clinical and research applications of ultrasound are diverse. The clinical applications include brain evaluations, both in the adult and in the neonatal head. Vascular diagnosis of both arteries and veins can be made from scans anywhere on the body, from carotid arteries to arterial and venous analysis of legs and arms. Echocardiography is routinely used for imaging the heart in the clinical management of cardiac patients. Nearly all abdominal organs can be evaluated by diagnostic ultrasound unless obscured by bowel gas. As described previously, ultrasound is poorly transmitted in air and is reflected back from bone, so pulmonary and bone US imaging are restricted. Obstetrics and gynecology are being revolutionized by the technological advances in ultrasound.

Ultrasound has extensive applications not only in human research, but also in animal research and basic science. Clinical trials both in humans and in animals illustrate how ultrasound techniques continue to advance. Instructive examples of current ultrasound human clinical trials can be obtained from ACRIN (American College of Radiology Imaging Network). This organization is devoted to research using various imaging modalities, including ultrasound. An example of one of their clinical trials of breast ultrasound is described in references [6] and [7].

In pre-clinical research using small animals such as mice, the increasingly common use of new high-frequency, high-spatial-resolution scanners illustrates the state of ultrasound technology today. Because the mouse is a preferred model for phenotypic study, genetic research, and drug applications, the high-frequency VisualSonics Vevo 770 has been developed, offering spatial resolution down to 30 μm, the highest resolution available in real time. Figure 6.9 shows an

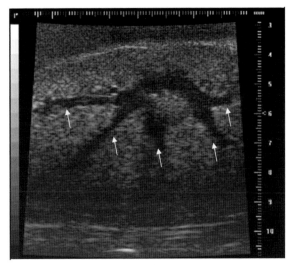

Figure 6.9. A high-frequency (40 MHz) ultrasound image of a mouse kidney in the sagittal plane demonstrating renal blood vessels (arrows) at the level of the hilum. This kidney measured approximately 12 mm in length and 6 mm in depth.

image of a mouse kidney acquired at 40 MHz. The submillimeter blood vessels within the kidney can be easily seen at the high frequencies. Since the system is not invasive, it is ideal for longitudinal studies and reduces the number of animals required. The equipment and technology are readily transferable and adaptable to other small-animal models such as the rat, chick, and zebrafish [8]. Pre-clinical trials using this equipment have been described by various researchers [9,10].

Future developments

Current and future research, both clinical and non-clinical, will lead to technological advances that expand the role of diagnostic ultrasound. For example, ongoing research cited in the medical press suggests that whole milk is as effective a US oral contrast agent for bowel imaging as diluted 0.1 percent barium suspension, the standard oral contrast agent for body CT. In other developments:

- The agent dutasteride has been found to decrease blood flow in benign prostate tissue, helping reduce unnecessary prostate biopsies, since the remaining areas of increased blood flow in the prostate are twice as likely to be positive for cancer. Since ultrasound color and power Doppler both with or without ultrasound contrast agents show prostate vascularity extremely well, this could help increase the percentage of positive prostate biopsies by helping to focus on the areas which are hypervascular.

- Ultrasound is being used to assess surgical margins in patients with breast cancer, minimizing the need for re-excision.

- Investigators are evaluating whether ultrasound should be the preferred imaging modality for preliminary diagnosis of acute appendicitis, instead of CT.

- Ultrasound may also be more sensitive than CT for chest-wall invasion by lung tumors.

- Combined ultrasound and mammography screening improves breast-cancer diagnosis over mammography alone.

- Sonoelastography, depicting tissue motion and elasticity, is one of the newer areas of investigation in both clinical and basic research. It is known that as some tumors grow they cause inflammation and desmoplasia, a reaction in specific dense tumors such as breast cancers that leads to cross-linking of collagenous fibers and stiffening of tissues. Elasticity measurements quantify tissue viscoelasticity, and require imaging that resolves both spatial and temporal variations.

Among advances in ultrasound technology, the miniaturization of ultrasound equipment is being pursued by almost all equipment manufacturers. Small hand-held units are already in use. A 0.7 kg ultrasound unit is available that fits inside the top pocket of a lab coat and is useful in emergency medicine, obstetrics, radiology, and cardiology (Figure 6.10). The system is not expected to replace traditional, cart-based ultrasound soon, but as the equipment becomes more portable the technology approaches the goal of the "electronic stethoscope."

The combination of technological advances in ultrasound and the advent of ultrasound contrast agents has greatly expanded both clinical research and basic research applications. With the advent of compound imaging, native harmonic imaging, 3D imaging, and M-mode, this expansion has accelerated significantly in recent years. Ultrasound has both an anatomic and a physiologic role in research. Blood-flow evaluations with Doppler ultrasound are important clinically and in the laboratory. Ultrasound contrast agents can also be used to actively target therapies. Actively targeted contrast agents contain biologically active molecules that will localize or be

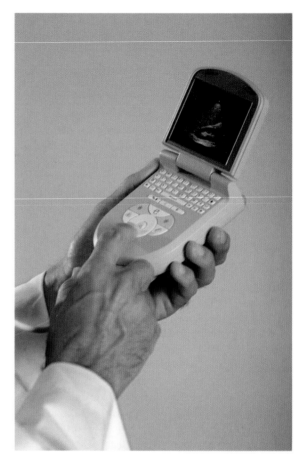

Figure 6.10. A handheld ultrasound unit, as featured on the Siemens Medical website (www.medical.siemens.com). (Reproduced with permission of Siemens Healthcare.)

trapped in a specific interest area. In other experimental ultrasound research, pathologic areas are being evaluated using disease-associated molecular signatures in order to produce a molecular delineation of disease mechanisms and even gene expression. A complementary receptor ligand can direct the contrast agents to the cellular areas of interest. This facilitates earlier detection of disease as well as better pathologic assessment and treatments commensurate with the pathology.

References

1. Bushberg JT, Seibert JA, Leidholdt EM, Boone JM. Ultrasound. In: *The Essential Physics of Medical Imaging*, 2nd edn. Philadelphia, PA: Lippincott Williams and Wilkins, 2002: 469–553.

2. Sehgal CM. Physical principles and clinical applications of Doppler echography. In: St. John Sutton MG,

Oldershaw PJ, Kotler MN, eds. *Textbook of Echocardiography and Doppler in Adults and Children*, 2nd edn. Cambridge, MA: Blackwell, 1996: 3–30.

3. American Institute of Ultrasound in Medicine Consensus Report on Potential Bioeffects of Diagnostic Ultrasound. Executive summary and associated articles. *J Ultrasound Med* 2008; **27**: 503–632.

4. Lindner JR. Microbubbles in medical imaging: current applications and future directions. *Nat Rev Drug Discov* 2004; **3**: 527–32.

5. Wood AKW, Bunte RM, Cohen JD, *et al.* The antivascular action of physiotherapy ultrasound on a murine tumor: role of a microbubble contrast agent. *Ultrasound Med Biol* 2007; **33**: 1901–10.

6. Berg WA, Blume JD, Cormack JB, Mendelson EB, Madsen EL. Lesion detection and characterization in a breast US phantom: results of the ACRIN 6666 Investigators. *Radiology* 2006; **239**: 693–702.

7. Berg WA. Rationale for a trial of screening breast ultrasound: American College of Radiology Imaging Network (ACRIN) *AJR Am J Roentgenol* 2003; **180**: 1225–8.

8. Phoon CK. Imaging tools for the developmental biologist: ultrasound biomicroscopy of mouse embryonic development. *Pediatr Res* 2006; **60**: 14–21.

9. Cohn RD, Liang HY, Shetty R, Abraham T, Wagner KR. Myostatin does not regulate cardiac hypertrophy or fibrosis. *Neuromuscul Disord* 2007; **17**: 290–6.

10. Wirtzfeld LA, Graham KC, Groom AC, *et al.* Volume measurement variability in three-dimensional high-frequency ultrasound images of murine liver metastasis. *Phys Med Biol* 2006; **56**: 2367–81.

Magnetic resonance imaging

Felix W. Wehrli

Sixty years after the first demonstration of nuclear magnetic resonance in condensed phase, and over three decades after the first cross-sectional image was published, magnetic resonance imaging (MRI) has without doubt evolved into the richest and most versatile biomedical imaging technique today. Initially a mainly anatomical and morphological imaging tool, MRI has, during the past decade, evolved into a functional and physiological imaging modality with a wide spectrum of applications covering virtually all organ systems. Today, MRI is a mainstay of diagnostic imaging, playing a critically important role for patient management and treatment response monitoring. Even though the physics of MRI is well understood, getting a grasp of the method can be challenging to the uninitiated. This brief chapter seeks to introduce the MRI novice to the fundamentals of spin excitation and detection, detection sensitivity, spatial encoding and image reconstruction, and resolution, and to provide an understanding of the basic contrast mechanisms. For an in-depth treatment of theory, physics, and engineering aspects, the reader is referred to the many excellent texts [1–3]. Applications to specific organ systems are covered in other chapters of this book.

Magnetic resonance signal

Unlike transmission techniques such as computed tomography (CT), where the attenuation of a beam of radiation is measured and an image reconstructed from multiple angular projections, the nuclear magnetic resonance (NMR) phenomenon exploits the magnetic properties of atomic nuclei, typically protons. When placed in a strong uniform magnetic field $\mathbf{B_0}$ (also referred to as the *static* or *polarizing* field), the nuclear magnetic moments μ of a sample (such as a portion of mammalian tissue containing

water) become aligned with the field so as to create a macroscopic magnetic moment, also called *magnetization*, $\mathbf{M}$. By applying a second, circularly polarized radiofrequency (RF) magnetic field, denoted $\mathbf{B_1}$, acting perpendicular to the static field, $\mathbf{M}$ is deflected into a plane transverse to the static field, precessing at a frequency $\omega_0 = \gamma B_0$, called *Larmor frequency*, and inducing a voltage in a suitably positioned receive coil (which can but need not be identical to the transmit coil that generates the $\mathbf{B_1}$ RF field). At a typical field strength of a magnetic resonance imager of 15 000 Gauss, the resonance frequency is 64 MHz.

We can describe the motion of the magnetization vector in terms of the phenomenological *Bloch equation*:

$$\frac{d\mathbf{M}}{dt} = \gamma \mathbf{M} \times \mathbf{B} - \frac{M_{xy}}{T_2} - \frac{M_z - M_0}{T_1} \qquad (7.1)$$

where γ is the *gyromagnetic ratio*, $\mathbf{B}$ the effective magnetic field, M_0 the equilibrium magnetization and T_1 and T_2 the relaxation times for the longitudinal and transverse component, respectively, of the magnetization.

Equation 7.1 forms a set of coupled differential equations, which can easily be solved for typical initial conditions by anyone familiar with just the fundamentals of vector calculus. Let us assume that the magnetization has been perturbed from equilibrium (M_0) by an RF pulse, thereby rotating it into the transverse plane, and further, that this perturbation occurred in a short time relative to the relaxation times, so that relaxation during the pulse can be neglected.

Following the rules of vector multiplication and considering further that for the static field (the only magnetic field present following brief action of the

Introduction to the Science of Medical Imaging, ed. R. Nick Bryan. Published by Cambridge University Press. © Cambridge University Press 2010.

RF field), $\mathbf{B_0} = \hat{z}H_z$, Equation 7.1 can be rewritten for the three spatial components, as:

$$\dot{M}_x = \omega_0 M_y - M_x/T_2$$
$$\dot{M}_y = -\omega_0 M_x - M_y/T_2 \qquad (7.2a–c)$$
$$\dot{M}_z = -(M_z - M_0)/T_1$$

We now see that only Equations 7.2a and 7.2b are coupled. At this stage it is useful to introduce complex notation for the transverse magnetization as $M_{xy}(t) = M_x + iM_y$. We can then express Equations 7.2a and 7.2b as follows: $\dot{M}_{xy} = M_{xy}(i\omega_0 - 1/T_2)$. By imposing the initial condition $M_{xy}(0) = M_0$, this equation is readily integrated to yield:

$$M_{xy} = M_0 e^{i\omega_0 t} e^{-t/T2} \qquad (7.3)$$

The real and imaginary components of Equation 7.3 are thus a damped cosine and sine, respectively, with frequency ω_0 and decay time constant T_2. Thus, the magnetization following an RF pulse oscillates at the

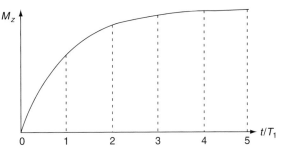

Figure 7.2. Solution to Equation 7.2c showing temporal evolution of longitudinal magnetization for initial condition $M_z(0) = 0$.

Larmor frequency and its amplitude decays exponentially with a time constant equal to the transverse relaxation time, as shown graphically in Figure 7.1. The detected signal is called *free induction decay* (FID).

Equation 7.2c, expressing the temporal evolution of the longitudinal magnetization (which cannot directly be detected), can be integrated to yield:

$$M_z(t) = M_0 + (M_z(0) - M_0)e^{-t/T1} \qquad (7.4)$$

Again assuming the same initial conditions resulting from a 90° RF pulse yielding $M_z(0) = 0$, Equation 7.4 predicts an exponential recovery of the longitudinal magnetization toward its equilibrium value with a time constant T_1, the spin-lattice or longitudinal relaxation time (Figure 7.2). We notice that the time constants for return to thermal equilibrium of the longitudinal and transverse magnetization (T_1 and T_2, respectively) are independent of one another, except that $T_1 \geq T_2$ holds. The latter is obvious, since it is clear that the magnetization cannot reach its equilibrium state as long as there is a finite transverse component. We will see later that tissue-dependent variations in the proton relaxation times are the basis of MRI contrast.

Principles of spatial encoding and reconstruction

K-space

In 1973 Lauterbur showed that the NMR method lends itself to cross-sectional imaging by spatially encoding the nuclear magnetic moments [4]. Whereas in a uniform magnetic field all nuclei resonate at the same frequency, given by the Larmor frequency, as discussed above, this is no longer the case when a small, spatially variant field (i.e., a *gradient magnetic field*) is superimposed on the

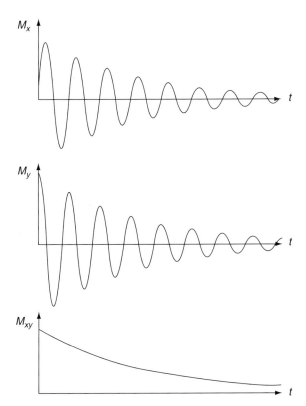

Figure 7.1. Solutions to the Bloch equations following a 90° RF pulse around the x-axis of the coordinate frame, yielding a damped sine and cosine for the imaginary and real components (M_x and M_y) and simple exponential for the magnitude of the FID (M_{xy}). The FID is damped with a time constant T_2.

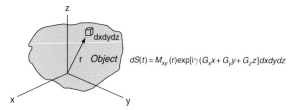

Figure 7.3. NMR signal from volume element *dxdydz* in an object of magnetization density $M_{xy}(t)$. The signal is proportional to the magnetization in the volume element *dxdydz* and a phase factor representative of the precession rate at location **r** determined by the spatial encoding gradient **G** and its duration *t*.

main field $\mathbf{B_0}$.[1] The field strength at some position **r** then becomes:

$$B(\mathbf{r}) = B_0 + \mathbf{r} \cdot \mathbf{G} \tag{7.5}$$

where **G** is the magnetic field gradient in the direction of **r**. The resonance frequency thus becomes a function of spatial location according to:

$$\omega(\mathbf{r}) = -\gamma(B_0 + \mathbf{G} \cdot \mathbf{r}) \tag{7.6}$$

Ignoring precession due to the polarizing field (first term in Equation 7.6), we see that the complex NMR signal at time *t* has a phase $\varphi = \gamma \mathbf{G} \cdot \mathbf{r}t$. Thus, we can write for the time-dependent signal d$S(t)$ in a volume element *dxdydz* (Figure 7.3):

$$dS(t) = M_{xy}(\mathbf{r}) \exp\left[i\gamma(G_x x + G_y y + G_z z)\right]dxdydz \tag{7.7}$$

However, rather than expressing the signal as a function of time, we define a variable that is conjugate to units we use for measuring object or image space. This variable is called *spatial frequency*, typically measured in reciprocal length units, e.g., cm^{-1}, versus spatial coordinates, expressed in cm:

$$\mathbf{k}(t) = \frac{\gamma}{2\pi} \int_0^t \mathbf{G}(t')dt' \tag{7.8}$$

where $\mathbf{G}(t')$ is the time-dependent spatial encoding gradient. For an object of magnetization density $M'_{xy}(\mathbf{k})$ the spatial frequency signal thus is given by:

$$M'_{xy}(\mathbf{k}) = \int_{object} M_{xy}(r)e^{-2\pi i \mathbf{k}(t)\cdot\mathbf{r}}dr \tag{7.9}$$

with integration running across the entire object. The argument of the complex exponential again is the phase of the signal, which we can now express in terms of the spatial frequency as $\varphi = 2\pi\mathbf{k} \cdot \mathbf{r}$. Pictorially, the spatial frequency may be regarded as the phase rotation per unit length of the object the magnetization experiences after being exposed to a gradient $\mathbf{G}(t')$ for some period *t*.

Notice from Equation 7.9 that $M'_{xy}(\mathbf{k})$ and $M_{xy}(\mathbf{r})$ are Fourier transform pairs and thus:

$$M_{xy}(\mathbf{r}) = \int_{k\text{-}space} M'_{xy}e^{-2\pi i \mathbf{k}(t)\cdot\mathbf{r}}d\mathbf{k} \tag{7.10}$$

Figure 7.4 shows the *k*-space signal of a point source of spin density located on the diagonal of the positive *x*- and *y*-axes of the object coordinate system after the magnetization has been subjected to encoding gradients G_x and G_y. Thus, according to Equation 7.9, the *k*-space signal is given as $dxdy \exp[2\pi i(k_x x_0 + k_y y_0)]$ and, since $x_0 = y_0$, the real component is simply proportional to $\cos[2\pi x_0(k_x + k_y)]$, i.e., a cosine wave oriented at 45°.

Data sampling and reconstruction

We have seen above that the MRI signal is sampled in the spatial frequency domain, rather than in object space. There exist a multitude of approaches for sampling the *k*-space signal, the most common involving alternate application of two or three orthogonal gradients varying in duration. This approach was originally referred to as *Fourier zeugmatography* [5]. An important modification of the latter approach consists of varying the amplitude rather than the duration of one or two of the encoding gradients (spin-warp method [6]). Here, signal detection and sampling occur in the presence of a constant gradient, G_x (also referred to as *readout gradient*), which is applied along one of the spatial encoding axes. During this period (typically lasting a few milliseconds), one line of *k*-space is sampled. Subsequent lines are obtained by applying a *phase-encoding gradient*, G_y, which is increased incrementally in each of the following RF pulse cycles. In this manner, a Cartesian grid of data is produced from which the image pixel amplitudes are obtained by discrete Fourier transform as discussed below.

The path of the spatial frequency vector during execution of the pulse sequence is determined by the time-dependent gradient wave forms. According to Equation 7.8, the location and magnitude of the

---

[1] The magnetic field gradients are with respect to the z-component of the static field, i.e., $G_x \equiv \partial B_z/\partial x$, $G_y \equiv \partial B_z/\partial y$, $G_z \equiv \partial B_z/\partial z$.

(a)

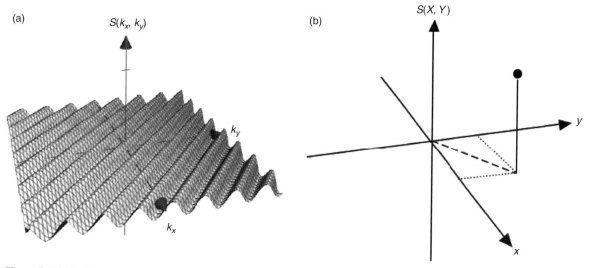

(b) $S(X, Y)$

y

x

Figure 7.4. (a) Real part of the k-space signal for a point source of spin density located at equal distance from x- and y-axes, shown in (b).

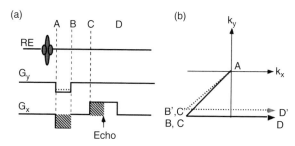

Figure 7.5. Spin-warp imaging pulse sequence (a) and k-space trajectory (b). Two pulse sequence cycles are shown. K-space coordinates k_x and k_y are determined as the (signed) area under the gradient-time curves. A-D represent distinct time points (a) and the corresponding position of the spatial frequency vector (b). The time point for which the hatched areas are equal corresponds to maximum re-phasing of the gradient echo ($k_x = 0$). Gradients G_x and G_y are called *readout* and *phase-encoding gradient*, respectively.

k-vector at some point in time are readily determined from the area under the gradient-time curve. Figure 7.5 shows a simple 2D spin-warp pulse sequence along with the trajectory of the k-vector during two successive pulse sequence cycles.

In practice, data is sampled discretely at a rate determined to satisfy the *Nyquist* criterion, which demands that at least two samples be acquired per cycle for the highest frequency present. Hence, the image is reconstructed from the k-space data with a discretized version of Equation 7.10, i.e., the integral is converted to a sum of complex exponentials in such a manner that the coefficients are measurements of the signal from $-k_{max}$ to $+k_{max}$, or $-(N/2) \cdot \Delta k_i (i = x, y, z)$ to $+(N/2) \cdot \Delta k_i$ where N is

the number of data samples (ultimately resulting in the number of pixels in the image). Noting that the highest frequency occurs at the edge of the field of view (FOV), Nyquist then demands that for the maximum number of cycles, the following relationship must be satisfied:

$$2k_{max} \cdot \text{FOV} = N \tag{7.11}$$

Since the pixel size is given as $\Delta r = FOV/N$ we can rewrite Equation 7.11 as:

$$\Delta r = \frac{1}{2k_{max}} \tag{7.12}$$

where $r = x, y, z$. This is an important relationship that conveys that the maximum spatial frequency sampled determines resolution. We can rewrite Equation 7.11 by considering that $\Delta k = 2k_{max}/N$, yielding a second important relationship:

$$\Delta k = \frac{1}{\text{FOV}} \tag{7.13}$$

Thus, the sampling interval determines the field of view.

Let us now examine the sampling process in more detail. At low values of k, the phase dispersion across the imaging object is small and thus the signal is large (recalling that the phase is given as the product of k and r). Therefore, the low-k components of the signal carry most of the image intensity and determine the gross shape of the object. However, finer spatial detail is inherent to the higher spatial frequency components. Figure 7.6 illustrates the effect

163

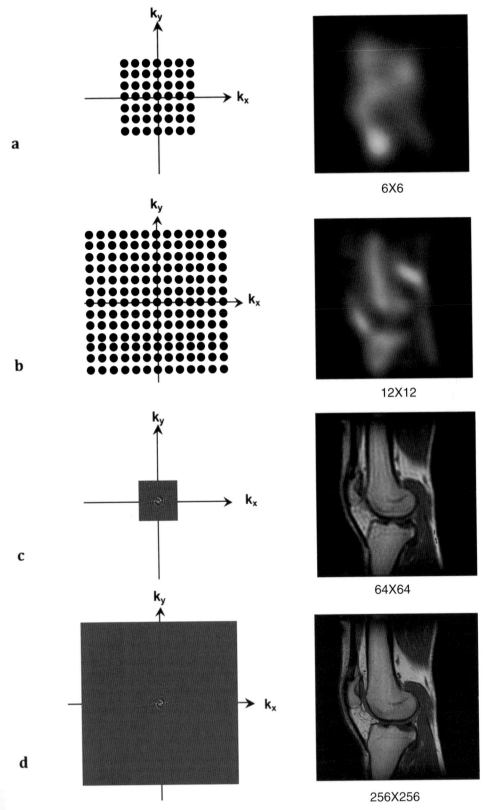

6X6

12X12

64X64

256X256

Figure 7.6. Effect of increasing *k*-space coverage for image reconstruction: (left) *k*-space, (right) image space. (a) and (b) show schematically *k*-space samples used for reconstruction, based on center 6×6 and 12×12 array; (c,d) left: actual *k*-space plots for 64×64 and 256×256 data arrays. (Images courtesy Dr. Hsiao-Wen Chung, National Taiwan University, Taiwan.)

of progressively increasing the range over which the Fourier components are summed, resulting in ever greater spatial detail in the reconstructed images.

Scan acquisition speed

Since the early 1980s, when MRI emerged as a clinical imaging modality (see [7], for example), the time needed to scan a subject has been reduced by nearly three orders of magnitude, from 10 minutes or more to less than a second for specialized applications. Shortening scan time is motivated not only by the need to contain procedure cost but also by the requirement to overcome the adverse effects of physiologic and involuntary subject motion during the examination. Clearly, once data acquisition time is lowered below the period of physiologic motion, the effect of motion unsharpness in the image data could effectively be suppressed.

Typically, the minimum time required for scanning 2D k-space in Cartesian sampling as in the previously described spin-warp imaging technique (Figure 7.5) is the product of data sampling time (time to sample one line k_x) and the number of lines sampled, N_y. However, in practice, the time between sampling successive lines is much longer, and is dictated by the spin dynamics, in particular T_1, which governs the repetition time, TR, between successive excitations. Hence, the minimum scan time for the acquisition of the data from which a 2D image can be reconstructed is $N_y \cdot TR$.

Two fundamentally different strategies have been pursued for enhancing scan acquisition rate. The first is to simply reduce the pulse repetition time, along with lowered RF pulse flip angle (the latter as a means to minimize excessive signal loss by saturation). In this manner, images can be acquired in seconds or even fractions thereof, rather than in minutes [8]. There exist multiple embodiments of this class of pulse sequences (referred to as *gradient-echo pulse sequences*) in which an echo is created by reversal of the readout gradient polarity (Figure 7.5). These pulse sequences allow for high-temporal resolution and thus have broad applications in areas where rapid physiologic motion is present, such as for imaging of the heart. There is, however, a significant trade-off in terms of signal-to-noise ratio (SNR) or resolution since the available magnetization is only a fraction of its equilibrium value (Figure 7.2). For a review of the subject, see, for example, [9,10].

An alternative class of pulse sequences seeks to acquire multiple lines in k-space from a single

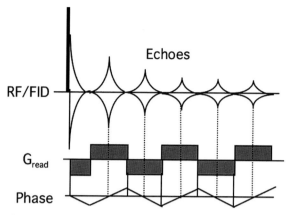

Figure 7.7. Principle of echo-planar encoding. A train of echoes is generated by periodically reversing the polarity of the readout gradient. Spin isochromats are refocused (phase $\varphi = 0$) when the condition $\int G(t)dt = 0$ is met, i.e., when positive and negative gradient areas cancel. By preceding each echo with a phase-encoding gradient (not shown in the figure), multiple lines of k-space are sampled, thereby shortening scan time in proportion to the number of echoes sampled.

excitation. A method known as *echo-planar imaging* (EPI), first conceived in 1977 [11], has in recent years become a standard technique in functional MRI of the brain and for evaluation of tissue perfusion [12] and diffusion, for example, for early detection of stroke [13], or for fiber tracking to evaluate neural pathways [14]. For in-depth coverage of EPI techniques and application, the reader is referred to the excellent text by Schmitt and co-authors [15]. In brief, the principle underlying EPI is to generate a series of echoes, rather than a single echo as in the basic spin-warp pulse sequence of Figure 7.5. This can be accomplished by alternately reversing the sign of the readout gradient. Echoes are then individually encoded with a phase-encoding gradient preceding each echo readout. Multiple lines of k-space can be acquired in this manner. Ideally, all lines needed to reconstruct an image of the desired field of view and pixel size from an echo train are generated by a single excitation (also referred to as single-shot EPI to indicate that all echoes to fill k-space were obtained from a single excitation). The latter requires that the echo train length is on the order of T_2^*, the effective transverse relaxation time, or less. The principle of generating a train of successive echoes by alternate gradient reversal is illustrated in Figure 7.7. Single-shot EPI allows for the high temporal resolution required to follow rate processes such as the study of the wash-in of a contrast agent (for example to quantify perfusion [16]). Figure 7.8 shows a series of echo-planar images to illustrate the effect of the transit

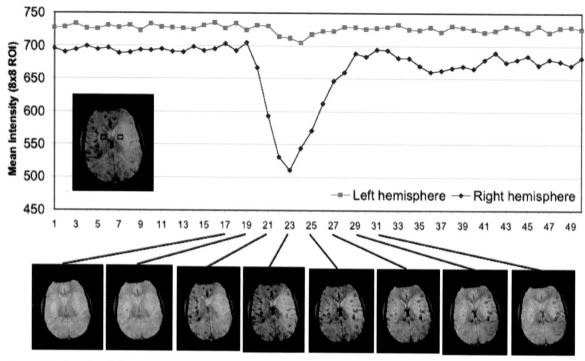

Figure 7.8. (Top) Plot of EPI signal intensity of time-series of images obtained at 1.5 second intervals from a patient with a left MCA territory infarct. (Bottom) Images representing successive time-frames 17–31 showing dip in signal intensity as the bolus traverses the brain for the right but not the left infarcted region. (Data courtesy of Dr. R. Wolf, Department of Radiology, University of Pennsylvania.)

of a bolus of Gd-DTPA causing transient signal reduction due to the agent's paramagnetism, along with a plot of signal intensity.

Signal-to-noise, contrast, and image resolution

The single most distinguishing feature of MRI (compared, for example, to x-ray-based modalities such as CT), is its extraordinarily large *innate contrast*, which, for two soft tissues, can be on the order of several hundred percent. In x-ray imaging, contrast is a consequence of differences in the attenuation coefficients for two adjacent soft-tissue structures and is on the order of a few percent at best. If it relied only on the differences in proton spin density, ρ, of various tissues, MRI contrast would be on the order of 5–20% at best, whereas in reality contrast between two regions, A and B, defined as:

$$C_{AB} = (S_A - S_B)/S_A \qquad (7.14)$$

can be several hundred percent. The reason for this discrepancy is the circumstance that the MR signal commonly is acquired under *non-equilibrium*

conditions. At the time of perturbation, the nuclear magnetic moments typically have not fully recovered from the effect of the previous pulse sequence cycle's RF pulses, nor is the signal usually detected immediately after its creation.

Typically, a spin-echo is detected as a means to alleviate spin coherence losses from static field inhomogeneity. The spin-echo signal amplitude for an RF pulse sequence $\pi/2$-τ-π-τ repeated every T_R seconds is approximately given by:

$$S(t = 2\tau) \approx \rho(1 - e^{-T_R/T_1})e^{-T_E/T_2} \qquad (7.15)$$

The above is a good approximation as long as $T_E \ll T_R$ and $T_2 \ll T_R$, in which case there is no residual transverse magnetization across successive pulse sequence cycles. In Equation 7.15 ρ is the voxel spin density and echo time $T_E = 2\tau$. Thus, the contrast between adjacent structures can be optimized by solving:

$$\partial C_{AB}(T_R, T_E)/\partial T_i = 0 \qquad (7.16)$$

for $T_i = T_R$ or T_E. In practice, however, this is not particularly useful, since the relaxation times are not known *a priori* and a multitude of tissue interfaces exist. Empirically, it is known that tissues differ in at least one of the intrinsic quantities, T_1, T_2, or ρ. It therefore suffices to acquire images in such a manner that contrast is sensitive to one particular parameter. For example a "T_2-weighted" image would be acquired with $T_E \sim T_2$ and $T_R \gg T_1$ and, similarly, a "T_1-weighted" image with $T_R < T_1$ and $T_E \ll T_2$. In a T_1-weighted image, the signal of protons with "long T_1" would be attenuated relative to that of protons with shorter T_1. A case in point is cerebrospinal fluid (CSF), which has a T_1 approximately three times longer than protons in gray or white matter, and thus appears hypointense. Similarly, in a T_2-weighted image, the signal from protons with long T_2, such as those in malignant brain tumors or ventricular

CSF, appears hyperintense relative to brain tissue, whose water protons have considerably shorter T_2. These relationships are readily apparent from Equation 7.15.

The parameters T_1, T_2, and ρ are called "intrinsic" because they are endogenous and, in general, not modifiable except when a relaxation reagent is administered. Most common among the latter are chelates of gadolinium-III that shorten T_1 of tissue water protons (see, for example, [17] and Chapter 9). Figure 7.9 shows a pair of images obtained from a patient with brain pathology, illustrating the characteristic pulse sequence parameter-dependent contrast.

T_1 relaxation times gradually increase with increasing field strength [18]. For this reason, when T_1 relaxation times are reported, the field strength must be indicated. At 1.5 tesla field strength, T_1 in soft tissues ranges from about 500 milliseconds to 1 second (Table 7.1). An exception is adipose tissue (e.g., fat in the scalp, Figure 7.10, or bone marrow and subcutaneous tissue, Figure 7.6), where the signal results from fatty-acid glyceride protons, which have much shorter T_1. Water in white matter of the corpus callosum has a shorter T_1 than water in gray matter of the brain (Figure 7.10). This difference is a consequence of the lower water content of white relative to gray matter.

Another important quantity that affects the perceived contrast is the *signal-to-noise ratio* (SNR). The smallest signal-producing element is the *voxel* (volume element), which is equal to the product of pixel area and slice thickness. Therefore, for a given hardware configuration (magnetic field strength, RF coil, and

Table 7.1. T_1 and T_2 in various mammalian tissues at 1.5 T

Tissue	T_1 (ms)	T_2 (ms)
Muscle		
skeletal	870	47
cardiac	870	57
Liver	490	43
Kidney	560	58
Spleen	780	62
Adipose	260	84
Brain		
Gray matter	920	101
White matter	790	92

T_1 was calculated using an empirical relationship for the field dependence [18]; T_2 values are from Table 12 of Reference [18].

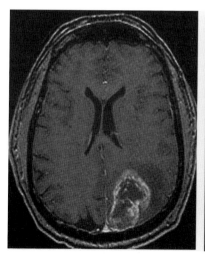 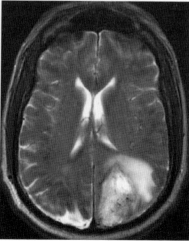

Figure 7.9. Dependence of image contrast on pulse sequence timing parameters in a patient with a high-grade glioma: (a) gadolinium contrast-enhanced T_1-weighted; (b) T_2-weighted. The tumor and surrounding edema in (a) appear hypointense except in the tumor's periphery, which exhibits high intensity caused by leakage of contrast due to blood–brain barrier disruption. In (b) both tumor and edema appear hyperintense due to prolonged T_2 relative to brain tissue. (Images courtesy of Dr. R. Wolf, Department of Radiology, University of Pennsylvania.)

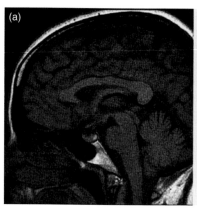
(a)

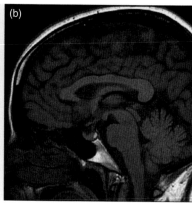
(b)

Figure 7.10. T_1-weighted sagittal images through the midline of the brain. Image (b) has twice the SNR of image (a), showing improved conspicuity of small anatomic and low-contrast detail. The two images were acquired at 1.5 T field strength using 2D imaging and identical scan parameters except for N_{av} which was 1 in (a) and 4 in (b).

receive system) the relative signal strength is proportional to voxel volume, and thus represents the numerator in the expression for SNR. The noise has a complicated dependence on various parameters, which include field strength, size and design of the radiofrequency receive coil, and the volume of tissue "seen" by the coil. We will return to this aspect below. For the time being it suffices to note that SNR can be increased by summing of the signal through repeated data collection. This is possible because of the stochastic nature of the noise, whose amplitude increases only as the square root of the number of signal samples taken, whereas the signal increases linearly. Signal averaging occurs at several levels during the k-space sampling process.

From the foregoing we obtain a simple formula for SNR per voxel of volume ΔV:

$$\begin{aligned} \mathrm{SNR} &= C \cdot \bar{\rho} \cdot \Delta V \sqrt{N_x N_y N_{av}} \\ &= C \cdot \bar{\rho} \cdot \Delta x \cdot \Delta y \cdot d_z \sqrt{N_x N_y N_{av}} \end{aligned} \quad (7.17)$$

In Equation 7.17 $\Delta x = FOV_x/N_x$, $\Delta y = FOV_y/N_y$ are the pixel dimensions given by the field of view (FOV) and the number of data samples, N_x and N_y, along x and y coordinates. The quantity d_z is the thickness of the slab selected by the slice-selective RF pulse and $\bar{\rho}$ is the spin density weighted by relaxation effects determined by relaxation times T_1 and T_2 and the pulse sequence timing parameters. Finally, N_{av} is the number of signal averages. Figure 7.10 shows two images of the human brain obtained from the same anatomic location but differing in SNR.

Lastly, the noise (essentially the standard deviation of the signal, σ_{eff}) affects the effective contrast perceived by the observer. The *contrast-to-noise ratio* (CNR) is simply the ratio of contrast divided by σ_{eff}:

$$CNR_{AB} = C_{AB}/\sigma_{\mathrm{eff}} \quad (7.18)$$

It is noted, for example, that small anatomic detail such as the stalk of the pituitary gland is better visualized in the image of Figure 7.10(b) in spite of the fact that the two images have equal contrast.

We have previously seen that resolution is determined by the area of k-space covered (Equation 7.12 and Figure 7.6). Ordinarily, the pixel size is regarded as the figure of merit for resolution. Suppose we increase the number of samples from 256 to 512, which can, for example, be achieved by doubling the frequency-encoding sampling time. In this case the k-space area is doubled, thus pixel size halved, and resolution is therefore improved by a factor of two. But now consider the situation where the pixel size is halved in image space (for example by linear interpolation). While this operation may result in a smoother image, the resolution, in terms of the observer's ability to discern small structures, is not enhanced. Similarly, if we were to double k-space without actually acquiring the high-frequency data (by zero filling those locations), we would, after Fourier reconstruction, obtain an image at half the pixel size. Even though this image would again be more pleasing to the eye, its effective resolution would not be improved. Figure 7.11 displays an axial image through the orbit, showing exquisite anatomic detail and achieved by sampling k_x- and k_y-space from -21.3 to $+21.3$ cm^{-1}.

MRI hardware

The hardware comprising an MRI system differs significantly from that of other imaging modalities such as CT or PET, discussed elsewhere in this book. A simplified functional block diagram of a typical MR imaging apparatus is given in Figure 7.12. The heart of the system is the magnet, typically a super-conducting system, to create the polarizing field. Another critical subsystem is the RF transmit/receive assembly. It consists of a transmitter and power amplifier for generating the RF voltage to be fed into the RF coil thereby creating the B_1 field for spin excitation. The resulting transverse magnetization, in turn,

induces a RF voltage in the receive coil (which may be identical by serving for both transmission and reception). The ensuing signal is then amplified in the receiver and digitized. Further unique to the MR imaging device is the gradient subsystem, which permits generation of the previously defined time-dependent gradient fields needed for spatial encoding. Both transmit/receive and gradient subsystem are under the control of a data acquisition processor, which ties in to the main computer. For more detail the reader is referred to the many excellent texts (see, for example, [1]).

Implications of magnetic field strength

We have seen previously that for a given hardware setup, the relative SNR in MRI is dictated by the scan parameters. In addition, however, the intrinsic SNR of an MRI system is significantly determined by the magnetic field strength. This recognition has substantially driven the development of MRI systems since the technology's inception. The signal strength, S, increases as the square of the resonance frequency ω (and thus field strength B_0 according to the Larmor equation). The noise, N, obeys a somewhat more complex relationship. It is determined as the square root of the total circuit resistance r that is principally made up of the receive coil and tissue resistances, r_c and r_b, which scale in proportion to ω and ω^2, respectively. Tissue resistance is caused by induced eddy currents in the electrically conductive tissues of the body. In simplified form SNR can thus be written as [19]:

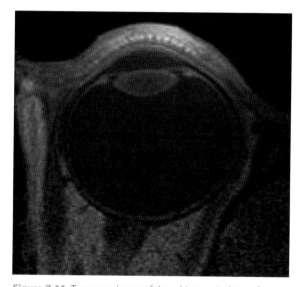

Figure 7.11. Transverse image of the orbit at a pixel size of $234 \times 234\ \mu m^2$ and a slice thickness of 3 mm. The image, obtained with a custom-built 2 cm surface coil, shows detailed architecture of the eye including anterior chamber, lens, sclera and ciliary muscle as well as the Meibomian glands in the eyelid. The image was intensity-corrected as a means to equalize overall intensity across the field of view. (Image courtesy of Dr. Samuel Patz, Brigham & Women's Hospital, Boston, MA.)

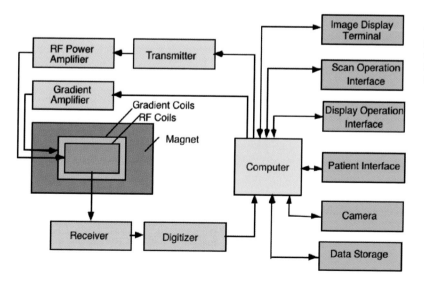

Figure 7.12. Simplified block diagram of typical MRI system. Functionally related subsystems such as transmit and receive chain, computer, and peripheral units such as patient and operator interface, are color-coded.

$$\text{SNR} = \frac{S}{N} \propto \frac{\omega^2}{\sqrt{a\omega^{1/2} + b\omega^2}} \qquad (7.19)$$

with constants a and b being a function of coil and tissue properties. In the large-sample limit and at high-magnetic field, the second noise term dominates and thus SNR scales roughly linearly with field strength (as opposed to the small-sample limit, where most of the resistance arises from the coil, in which case the first noise term dominates and SNR scales as $\omega^{7/4}$) [20].

SNR is a significant determinant of image quality (see, for example, Figure 7.10). Further, any increase in SNR can be traded for higher resolution or reduced scan time. Initially, following inception of MRI, magnet field strengths remained in the range of 0.1–0.3 T, which can be achieved with electromagnets or permanent magnets. The perfection of superconducting magnet technology (developed for laboratory NMR systems in the 1960s) subsequently drove the race toward higher magnetic field strength and, by about 1985, 1.5 T became the standard of excellence of clinical MRI.

In 1988, experimental whole-body research scanners operating at 4 T field strength emerged (see, for example, [21]). However, the high cost, uncertain clinical benefit, and technical hurdles limited diffusion of these systems to a few research centers. Toward the end of the 1990s MRI equipment manufacturers settled on the more manageable field strength of 3 T, involving integrated magnetic shielding for magnetic stray-field containment, and body-coil excitation. These systems are now in widespread use as the upper-end clinical workhorse and research platform, providing substantially improved performance in terms of SNR, and thus improved image quality [22].

In the meantime, the quest for even higher magnetic field strength continued. In 1998 Robitaille and colleagues first demonstrated the feasibility of imaging the human brain at 8 T field strength [23,24]. Another experimental head scanner operating at 7 T field strength was taken into operation shortly thereafter at the University of Minnesota [25]. The approach chosen more recently was to marry RF and gradient electronics designed for lower-field clinical systems to high-field magnets. The high cost of both equipment and installation (the latter due to the need for magnetic shielding), as well as only partially overcome technical and biological hurdles, has so far limited the spread of ultra-high-field MRI. Radiofrequency absorption, possibly causing excessive

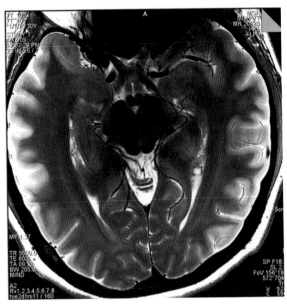

Figure 7.13. 300 MHz (7 tesla) spin-echo image of the brain in a healthy volunteer obtained at pixel size of 270 x 270 μm². (Courtesy of C. Wiggins, G. Wiggins, and L. L. Wald, Massachusetts General Hospital, Martinos Center, Boston, MA.)

tissue heating, limits the excitation schemes admissible at lower field strength. Related problems occur due to the wavelength becoming comparable to body size, thereby causing standing wave effects [22]. Nevertheless, initial results are impressive, as illustrated with the brain image in Figure 7.13.

Closing comments

Even though MRI has demonstrated its clinical utility during the past quarter of a century, the technology and its applications continue to evolve at a vigorous pace, with no end in sight. This brief introduction to the fundamentals of the methodology hopefully will create awareness and stimulate interest among physicians and biomedical scientists and prepare readers to develop a better grasp of the broader applications covered in subsequent chapters of this book. Much in this chapter has intentionally been left out or touched upon only peripherally. This includes the large array of recent developments such as the measurement and visualization of blood flow and perfusion, functional MRI of the brain, fiber tractography for the study of neuronal pathways, MR elastography for evaluation of tissue mechanical properties, and many more. Another vast field is spectroscopic imaging, making use of the chemical shift of spins, thereby allowing the study of tissue and organ metabolism. The quantum step in detection sensitivity brought about by technologies for polarizing spins several orders of magnitude above that achieved by thermal polarization is likely to revolutionize the field and lead to MR rivaling methods such as positron emission tomography.

References

1. Vlaardingerbroek MT, den Boer JA, eds. *Magnetic Resonance Imaging: Theory and Practice*. Berlin: Springer, 1996.

2. Haacke EM, Brown RW, Thompson MR, Venkatesan R. *Magnetic Resonance Imaging: Physical Principles and Sequence Design*. New York, NY: Wiley–Liss, 1999.

3. Liang ZP, Lauterbur PC. *Principles of Magnetic Resonance Imaging*. IEEE Press Series in Biomedical Engineering. New York, NY: IEEE, 2000.

4. Lauterbur PC. Image formation by induced local interactions: examples employing nuclear magnetic resonance. *Nature* 1973; **242**: 190.

5. Kumar A, Welti D, Ernst R. NMR Fourier zeugmatography. *J Magn Res* 1975; **18**: 69–83.

6. Edelstein WA, Hutchison JMS, Johnson G, Redpath T. Spin warp NMR imaging and applications to human whole-body imaging. *Phys Med Biol* 1980; **25**: 751–6.

7. Bydder GM, Steiner RE, Young IR, *et al*. Clinical NMR imaging of the brain: 140 cases. *AJR Am J Roentgenol* 1982; **139**: 215–36.

8. Haase A, Frahm J, Matthaei D, Hänicke W, Merboldt KD. FLASH Imaging: rapid NMR imaging using low flip angle pulses. *J Magn Res* 1986; **67**: 258–66.

9. Wehrli FW. *Fast-Scan Magnetic Resonance: Principles and Applications*. New York, NY: Raven, 1990.

10. Haacke EM, Tkach J. Fast MR imaging: techniques and clinical applications. *AJR Am J Roentgenol* 1990; **155**: 951–64.

11. Mansfield P. Multiplanar image formation using NMR spin echoes. *J Phys C* 1977; **10**: L55–8.

12. Detre JA, Alsop DC. Perfusion magnetic resonance imaging with continuous arterial spin labeling: methods and clinical applications in the central nervous system. *Eur J Radiol* 1999; **30**: 115–24.

13. Sorensen AG, Buonanno FS, Gonzalez RG, *et al*. Hyperacute stroke: evaluation with combined multisection diffusion-weighted and hemodynamically weighted echo-planar MR imaging. *Radiology* 1996; **199**: 391–401.

14. Conturo TE, Lori NF, Cull TS, *et al*. Tracking neuronal fiber pathways in the living human brain. *Proc Natl Acad Sci USA* 1999; **96**: 10422–7.

15. Schmitt F, Stehling MK, Turner R. *Echo-Planar Imaging: Theory, Technique and Applications*. Berlin: Springer, 1998.

16. Sorensen AG, Tievsky AL, Ostergaard L, Weisskoff RM, Rosen BR. Contrast agents in functional MR imaging. *J Magn Reson Imaging* 1997; **7**: 47–55.

17. Runge VM, Kirsch JE, Wells JW, *et al*. Magnetic resonance contrast agents in neuroimaging: new agents and applications. *Neuroimaging Clin N Am* 1994; **4**: 175–83.

18. Bottomley PA, Foster TH, Argersinger RE, Pfeifer LM. A review of normal tissue hydrogen NMR relaxation times and relaxation mechanisms from 1–100 MHz: dependence on tissue type, NMR frequency, temperature, species, excision, and age. *Med Phys* 1984; **11**: 425–48.

19. Hoult DI, Lauterbur PC. The sensitivity of the zeugmatographic experiment involving human subjects. *J Magn Reson* 1979; **34**: 425–33.

20. Edelstein WA, Glover GH, Hardy CJ, Redington RW. The intrinsic signal-to-noise ratio in NMR imaging. *Magn Reson Med* 1986; **3**: 604–18.

21. Hardy CJ, Bottomley PA, Roemer PB, Redington R. Rapid ^{31}P spectroscopy on a 4 T whole system. *Magn Reson Med* 1988; **8**: 104–9.

22. Norris DG. High field human imaging. *J Magn Reson Imaging* 2003; **18**: 519–29.

23. Robitaille PM, Abduljalil AM, Kangarlu A, *et al*. Human magnetic resonance imaging at 8 T. *NMR Biomed* 1998; **11**: 263–5.

24. Robitaille PM, Abduljalil AM, Kangarlu A. Ultra high resolution imaging of the human head at 8 tesla: 2K × 2K for Y2K. *J Comput Assist Tomogr* 2000; **24**: 2–8.

25. Yacoub E, Shmuel A, Pfeuffer J, *et al*. Imaging brain function in humans at 7 tesla. *Magn Reson Med* 2001; **45**: 588–94.

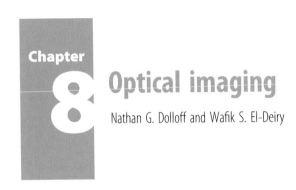

Chapter 8

Optical imaging

Nathan G. Dolloff and Wafik S. El-Deiry

Optical imaging is a ubiquitous component of biomedical research because of the applicability of fluorescent and bioluminescent proteins to a virtually infinite number of experimental assays. Green fluorescent protein (GFP), for example, can be used for tracing cell migration and protein localization, quantifying reporter gene expression and monitoring tumor growth *in vivo*, among other uses. Osamu Shimomura, Martin Chalfie, and Roger Tsien were awarded the 2008 Nobel Prize in Chemistry for their discovery and development of GFP, a contribution that has benefited all fields of biology and medicine. In the sections that follow, we discuss the natural origin and principles of bioluminescence and fluorescence, and provide examples of their application in the field of cancer research.

Bioluminescence: a historical perspective

Numerous organisms are bioluminescent or, by definition, emit light. Bioluminescent species evolved independently at least 30 times, which is evident from the lack of homology in light-producing enzymes (luciferases) and the chemical diversity of their substrates (luciferins), highlighting the evolutionary importance of this trait. The luminescence of bacteria, fungi, squid, and fish is thought to serve diverse biological functions. The firefly uses luminescent signaling to communicate with potential mates and the scale worm evades predators by producing and shedding a luminous epithelial layer that serves as a glowing decoy. The study of these intriguing behaviors has led to the identification of light-producing proteins, luciferase and GFP, which are now cornerstones of optical imaging [1].

The first natural bioluminescent system to be characterized was the jellyfish *Aequorea victoria*, which uses a two-step reaction involving the transfer of energy in the form of light from a luciferase-bound photoprotein to GFP. In its excited state, GFP emits light in the green spectrum of visible light, producing the organism's characteristic green glow. Aequorin, the photoprotein, is a stable complex of luciferase and coelenterazine, the substrate of coelenterate luciferase that exists in an inactive state in the absence of calcium. Stimuli that induce calcium release from intracellular stores, such as mechanical stretching, activate aequorin. The luciferase-driven enzymatic reaction that results is exergonic and releases energy as blue light (470 nm), which then excites the electrons of GFP, an energy-transfer acceptor, leading to the emission of green light (509 nm; Figure 8.1). The discovery of aequorin was published in 1962 [2]. The luciferase gene from the firefly *Photinus pyralis* was first cloned and ectopically expressed in bacteria in 1985, and GFP was later cloned and sequenced in 1992 [3,4]. Both proteins now serve diverse purposes in the research setting.

Bioluminescence imaging

Bioluminescence can be classified as light derived from the luciferase-driven oxidation of its substrate, luciferin. Firefly luciferase and *Renilla* luciferase from the sea pansy *Renilla reinformis* oxidize D-luciferin and coelenterazine (coelenterate luciferin), respectively (Figure 8.2). Firefly luciferase is well suited for optical imaging purposes, as D-luciferin is highly water-soluble and readily permeates cell membranes and blood barriers such as the blood–brain barrier and placenta [5]. The reaction kinetic of firefly luciferase is relatively slow and the light product is stable for approximately one hour, allowing users adequate time to acquire data. Furthermore, firefly luciferase generates light with a wavelength of approximately 560 nm,

Introduction to the Science of Medical Imaging, ed. R. Nick Bryan. Published by Cambridge University Press. © Cambridge University Press 2010.

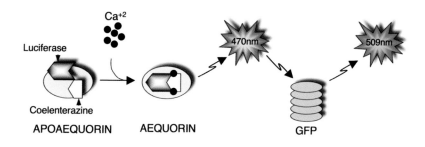

Figure 8.1. Bioluminescence in *Aequorea victoria*. The Pacific northwestern jellyfish uses a two-step reaction catalyzed by luciferase and GFP to produce green light. In the first reaction, mechanical stretching leads to the generation of calcium, which activates aequorin. The active photoprotein gives off blue light, which then excites the energy acceptor, GFP, leading to excitation and emission of green light.

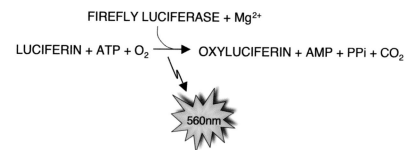

Figure 8.2. Firefly luciferase reaction. Luciferase, in the presence of magnesium, ATP, and oxygen, oxidizes its substrate D-luciferin to produce oxyluciferin, AMP, inorganic phosphate, and carbon dioxide. The reaction also generates energy in the form of light, which emits at a wavelength of ~560 nm.

making it ideal for *in vivo* applications, as higher wavelengths of light are more efficiently transmitted through tissues. Lower wavelengths of light such as the 488 nm peak emission from *Renilla* luciferase undergo considerably more absorption and scattering and therefore produce less intense and more diffuse signals. In addition, the biodistribution of coelenterazine is limited by comparison to D-luciferin. A final point is that D-luciferin firefly luciferase oxidizes D-luciferin in an ATP-dependent manner, meaning cells bearing luciferase expression must be viable in order to support the reaction and produce light. This is a critical consideration in studies that use bioluminescence imaging (BLI) to measure cell viability, such as measuring cytotoxicity or anti-tumor activity of a novel chemotherapeutic agent. By contrast, *Renilla* luciferase does not require ATP for the light-emitting reaction.

Fluorescence imaging

In contrast to luciferase, which requires a substrate to produce light, fluorescent proteins emit photons when irradiated at specific wavelengths. As an example, in the case of *Aequorea victoria*, blue light with a wavelength of 470 nm excites the electrons of GFP, propelling their rise to a higher energy level. When electrons relax and return to their ground state, photons are released. Photons emitted from GFP are of

lower energy and higher wavelength than excitation photons, a phenomenon known as the Stokes shift. Emitted light with a wavelength of ~510 nm for *A. victoria* GFP can be captured and distinguished from excitation light by using filters that permit passage of specific light wavelengths while blocking the passage of others (Figure 8.3).

The native structure of GFP was altered in many cases in order to improve its maturation and brightness at 37 °C, as well as to modify its excitation/emission spectrum [6]. This, in addition to identification of fluorescent proteins with excitation/emission spectra distinct from GFP, such as dsRed from the coral genus *Discosoma*, provides a diverse palette of fluorescent proteins from which to choose. Distinctive excitation/emission spectra allow simultaneous labeling of more than one target cell or protein. Plus, certain fluorescent molecules perform better *in vivo*, based on properties associated with their excitation/emission spectra. Of note, higher light wavelengths penetrate tissue more readily than lower wavelengths, so the incidence and emission light accompanying dsRed have superior tissue penetration compared to GFP, which undergoes significant reflection, refraction, and scattering within mammalian tissues. While the inherent fluorescent properties of dsRed are superior to GFP when considering non-invasive *in vivo* imaging, the mature dsRed protein is a tetramer that forms large and potentially toxic protein aggregates.

173

(a)

(b)

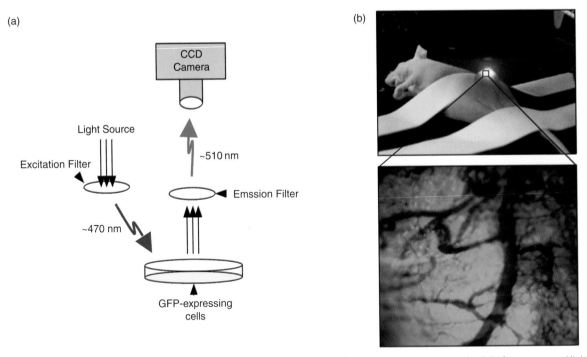

Figure 8.3. Fluorescence imaging schematic. (a) GFP, expressed by cultured cells in this example, is excited by blue light from an external light source. Green light emitted from the cells is captured and converted into a digital image by a cooled charge-coupled device (CCD) camera. A filter set is required to separate blue light from the source and green light emitted from the excitation of GFP. (b) GFP-expressing HCT116 human colon cancer xenograft tumor is imaged using a fluorescence stereomicroscope. Note the blue excitation light (top) and the lack of green fluorescence emitting from blood vessels, which derive from non-fluorescent mouse cells. Green fluorescence does not penetrate the vessels, as its photons are absorbed and scattered by tissues and proteins – hemoglobin, in particular.

Thus, multiple factors must be considered when choosing a fluorescent protein.

Optical imaging in cancer research

Optical imaging is important in many biomedical fields but has proven invaluable to the field of cancer research. It allows for non-invasive assessment of tumor growth, permitting investigation into how individual genes drive oncogenesis and accelerate tumor growth. BLI and fluorescence imaging have also facilitated measurement of tumor-supressor gene activity in real time and evaluation of how novel therapies impact tumor vasculature and apoptosis. For these reasons, the rest of this chapter will focus on applications in the field of oncology.

Monitoring tumor growth

Fluorescence and BLI provide cancer biologists the opportunity to non-invasively assess the growth of subcutaneous, orthotopic, and metastatic tumors in pre-clinical animal models. The number of photons emitted from tumors is proportional to the number of fluorescence/BLI-producing cells they contain. As detection systems are equipped with quantitative software, this offers a more reliable and objective means for measuring tumor size compared to traditional caliper measurements. As an example, BLI was used in this context to identify oncogenes that transform primary esophageal epithelial cells [7].

Studies of metastasis have perhaps benefited the most from BLI. Experimental metastatic tumors have traditionally been detected by necropsy of animals. This is a time-consuming procedure requiring surgical skill and a trained eye, and a limitation is that only the most overt tumors are easily located. Indeed, fluorescent proteins have been incorporated into this approach to assist in distinguishing tumors from mouse tissue [8–10]. However, even with the incorporation of optical reporters, the investigator must choose a region or organ to closely analyze, which introduces bias into the analysis. Using BLI, it is possible to detect as few as 100–1000 cells *in vivo* [11]. This permits the visualization of microscopic metastatic tumors in the live animal [12]. While BLI does not eliminate the need for *ex vivo* examination, it assists in identifying regions of tumor formation, which directs dissection and collection of tissue for histological processing. Another advantage associated with BLI is that growth of metastatic lesions can be observed in longitudinal studies. Otherwise, studies require multiple subjects at different time points and therefore necessitate sacrifice of large numbers of animals.

Imaging tumor vasculature

In order for tumors to grow beyond a diameter of 3 mm they must establish their own blood supply through neovascularization [13]. The dependence of tumor growth on angiogenesis has led to the development of small molecules and monoclonal antibodies aimed at interfering with angiogenesis as a strategy for slowing tumor growth in patients. The ability to image tumor vascularity non-invasively accelerates the assessment of novel anti-angiogenic drugs. This is possible in preclinical mouse models, where there is high contrast between fluorescent tumor xenografts and non-fluorescent host blood vessels. Mayes *et al.* [14] reported the use of multispectral imaging for measuring tumor vasculature in xenograft mouse models, which can be applied to testing the anti-angiogenic potential of novel cancer therapies (Figure 8.4). This approach is based on the ability of tissues – mouse blood vessels, in this case – to absorb and refract light. Light undergoes a slight spectral change when it is emitted from a fluorescent protein-expressing tumor and passes through structures that obstruct the path of photons, such as blood vessels. Multispectral imaging systems are able to measure these slight shifts in light quality, allowing measurement of relative tumor vascularity. Others have reported strategies for quantifying blood-vessel density by taking advantage of shadowing effects caused by vasculature within a fluorescent subcutaneous and metastatic tumor [15].

Hyperspectral imaging

Hyperspectral imaging, not to be confused with multispectral imaging, is a technique that has shown promise for detecting changes in vascularity. Hyperspectral imaging systems like the macroscopic Prism and Reflectance Imaging Spectroscopy System (MACRO-PARISS; LightForm Inc., Hillsborough, NJ) convert a field of view into a digitized compilation (spectral library) of spectra that span the electromagnetic spectrum from ultraviolet to infrared light. Every object or field of view is associated with its own unique spectral profile. Specimens (e.g., geological samples, tissue sections) of similar origin often have overlapping spectral characteristics, which can be used to generate a spectral signature for that class of specimen. The MACRO-PARISS was modified with a fiberoptic probe and used to develop a spectral signature specific to vascular regions of the mouse ear, which has potential in measuring vascularity/angiogenesis and could serve as a tool for measuring the efficacy of anti-angiogenic drugs (Figure 8.5, [16]). This approach was further shown to identify spectral qualities that differentiate melanoma from normal skin samples [17].

Imaging cancer stem cells

The cancer stem cell (CSC) hypothesis states that cancer arises from a small population of malignant cells that possess tumor-initiating capacity as well as self-renewal potential. This theory has been well established in hematological malignancies such as acute myeloid leukemia (AML) and has more recently gained acceptance for solid tumors [18,19]. CSCs are thought to be responsible for patient relapse, as they can evade death in the presence of anti-cancer therapy and proliferate indefinitely. Similarities exist between CSCs and normal stem cells, including the ability to efflux cellular dyes and resist cytotoxic effects of cancer therapies [20]. Additionally, CSCs express unique cell surface markers that distinguish them from non-tumor-initiating cells. Identification of CSC-specific markers allows separation of these distinct tumor-cell populations, and has facilitated the characterization of CSCs in multiple tumor types. These markers also provide the opportunity to image CSCs in real time and as part of an intact cancer-cell population rather than in isolation, which most effectively recapitulates their native environment (Figure 8.6). This ability will assist in the discovery of novel therapies that aim to eradicate CSCs as well as their non-CSC counterparts [22].

Measuring transcriptional activity

With the sequencing of the human genome and advances in DNA microarray technology, gene expression analysis is now a fundamental aspect of cancer research. Northern blotting and real-time polymerase chain reaction (RT-PCR) quantify gene transcription by

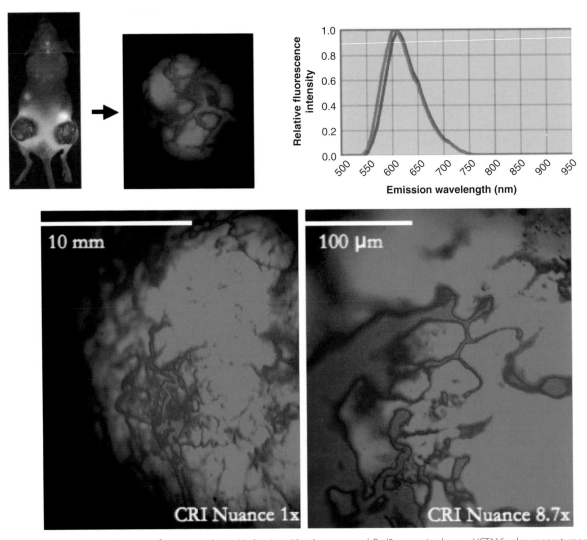

Figure 8.4. Multispectral imaging of tumor vasculature. Nude mice with subcutaneous dsRed2-expressing human HCT116 colon cancer tumors were imaged using the CRi Maestro (top left). Spectral unmixing was performed using the imaging system and related software. A 10 nm shift in emission spectra between tumor (green pseudocolor) and vasculature (red pseudocolor; top right) was detected. This technique provides a quantitative means for measuring tumor vasculature and the ability to detect microvessels (bottom) in pre-clinical cancer models. (Reproduced with permission from Mayes *et al.*, *Biotechniques* 2008; **45**: 459–60 [14].)

measuring messenger RNA levels at fixed time points. These measurements require the lysing of cells and therefore represent a static view of a gene's transcriptional activity. Optical imaging reporters circumvent this technical limitation by measuring transcriptional activity in live cells and real time. Promoter activity, representing a gene's transcriptional activity, is measured by placing the expression of an optical reporter gene under the control of that gene's promoter region. An increase in promoter activity leads to increased transcription and expression of the reporter, and thus an increase in photon generation.

Similar approaches have been applied to assess activity of transcription factors, such as the p53 tumor-suppressor gene, NF-kappa B (NFκB), hypoxia-inducible factor-1 alpha (HIF-1α), and the estrogen receptor [23–26]. Figure 8.7 illustrates a p53-inducible luciferase reporter in a high-throughput cell-based drug screen. Fluorescent proteins as gene expression reporters have the advantage of not requiring a substrate. Hence, they give a real-time report of gene transcription compared to luciferase, which is dependent on substrate biodistribution and enzyme kinetics. But again, due to its high sensitivity, in which GFP photons are absorbed or

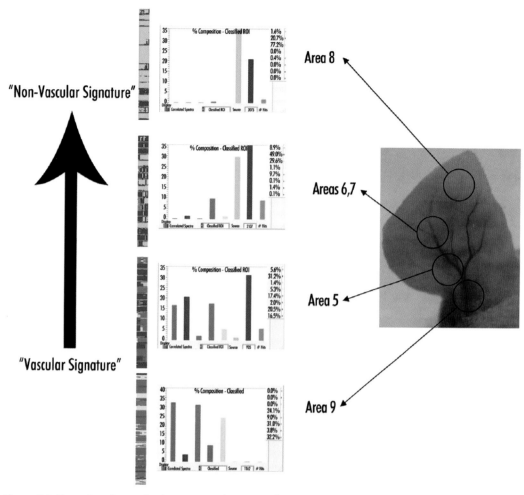

Figure 8.5. Generation of a vascular signature using hyperspectral imaging. The MACRO-PARISS hyperspectral imaging system was equipped with a fiberoptic probe that was used to analyze the spectral characteristics of vascular and avascular regions of the mouse ear. The histograms serve as examples of spectral data that are acquired using this approach and exhibit similarities that were discovered in spectra from regions of the ear with similar vascularity. (Reproduced with permission from Tumeh *et al.*, *Cancer Biology and Therapy* 2007; **6**: 447–53 [16].)

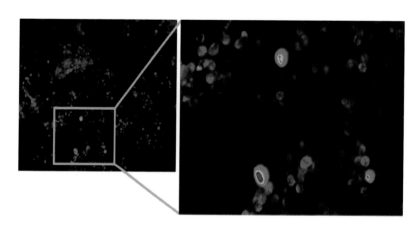

Figure 8.6. Imaging cancer stem cells (CSCs). Putative colon CSCs are imaged in live cell populations using a fluorescently conjugated antibody to CD133, a cell surface marker expressed by colon CSCs [21]. Images were captured and spectral unmixing was performed using the Nuance Multispectral Imaging System (CRi, Cambridge, MA). The green and red pseudocolors represent CD133 and Mitotracker (Molecular Probes, Eugene, OR), respectively. (Reproduced with permission from Hart and El-Deiry, *Journal of Clinical Oncology* 2008; **26**: 2901–10 [22].)

(a)

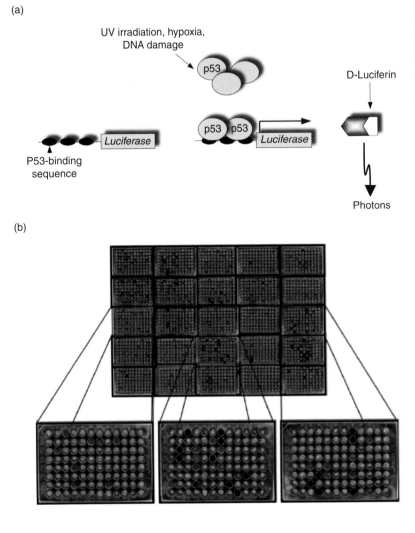

(b)

Figure 8.7. p53-induced optical reporter in drug discovery. (a) p53 transcriptional activity is induced by cellular stresses such as DNA damage, ultraviolet irradiation, and hypoxia. Stabilization and activation of p53 leads to its association with DNA binding elements within p53 target genes, leading to their subsequent transcription. p53-binding activity is measured using a luciferase reporter gene that is under the control of p53-binding domains. Thus increased p53 activity corresponds to increased expression of luciferase and generation of photons in the presence of D-luciferin. (b) The p53-responsive reporter PG13-luc was expressed in mutant p53-expressing SW480 human colon carcinoma cells and used to screen the NCI Developmental Therapeutics Program diversity set for small molecules that induce p53 transcriptional activity. Red wells indicate intense luciferase activity and therefore the highest induction of p53 transcriptional activity. (Reproduced with permission from Wang *et al.*, *Proc Natl Acad Sci USA* 2006; **103**: 11003–8 [28].)

scattered by mammalian tissues, firefly luciferase remains the better choice of reporters *in vivo*. Non-invasive visualization of gene transcription facilitates cancer research by providing insight into genetic changes that occur during cancer progression and in response to therapy. Optical imaging is also useful as a survey technique for identifying novel compounds that activate a particular transcriptional program [27]. For example, Wang *et al.* [28] identified small molecules that restore p53 transcriptional responses in p53-deficient tumor cells (Figure 8.7).

Imaging protein–protein interactions and post-translational modifications

Protein–protein interactions are critical to the activity of particular signaling networks. For example, NFκB transcriptional activity is regulated by its interaction with IκBα. Binding of NFκB subunits to IκBα results in their cytoplasmic retention and exclusion from the nucleus. Signals that activate NFκB do so by promoting proteasomal degradation of IκBα, thereby releasing the inhibition of NFκB and allowing translocation to the nucleus, where initiation of gene transcription takes place. Protein–protein interactions such as the association of NFκB and IκBα can be measured *in vivo* using reporter complementation studies, where split reporter fragments are generated with one protein of interest being ligated to the amino terminus of firefly luciferase and the other ligated to the carboxy terminus. When the proteins interact, they bring the two luciferase fragments into close proximity and reconstitute their enzymatic activity. Alternatively, interaction of two proteins of interest can be engineered to reconstitute a functional transcription factor that drives reporter expression.

(a)

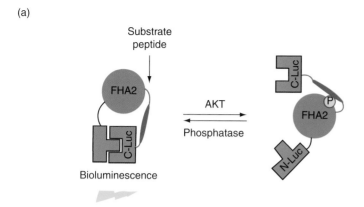

Figure 8.8. Imaging Akt kinase activity *in vivo*. (a) The schematic illustrates the split luciferase reporter system designed to detect changes in Akt activity. The "substrate peptide" is an Akt substrate consensus sequence that, in the absence of phosphorylation (lack of Akt activity), permits complementation of firefly luciferase. When the substrate linker is phosphorylated (increased Akt activity), it sterically hinders the association of the two luciferase fragments and luciferase is inactivate. (b) This Akt-responsive system was used *in vivo* to assess the efficacy and kinetic of Akt inhibitors. Note that perifosine exhibits an intense BLI signal for a prolonged period after treatment, suggesting that this compound has a longer duration of action. (Reproduced with permission from Zhang *et al.*, *Nature Medicine* 2007; **13**: 1114–19 [29].)

(b)

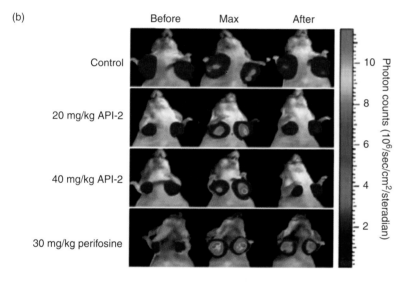

The split reporter strategy has also been employed to measure post-translational modifications, such as phosphorylation. Zhang *et al.* [29] designed an approach to measure kinase activity of the pro-survival oncogenic protein, Akt. This group constructed a complementation system where Akt phosphorylation of a peptide consensus site resulted in steric inhibition of luciferase reconstitution (Figure 8.8). Thus, in the absence of Akt kinase activity, luciferase was functional. Using this technology, they were able to image Akt activity and evaluate novel Akt inhibitors *in vivo*. Moreover, this approach was found to be useful for evaluating the pharmacokinetics of Akt inhibitors and to have utility in planning dosing schedules.

Molecular beacons

Molecular beacons are tools that can be used to image DNA or mRNA in live cells. Molecular beacons can be constructed from nucleotide sequences composed of a probe region designed to hybridize with a target mRNA or DNA sequence that is flanked on either side by two complementary nucleotide sequences. One probe-flanking region is conjugated to a quencher dye and the other to a fluorophore. In the absence of target mRNA, the beacon adopts a hairpin structure where the two flank regions hybridize, bringing the fluorophore and quencher into close proximity and quenching the fluorescent signal. When target gene expression is initiated, target mRNA is transcribed and anneals to its complementary probe sequence within the beacon. This causes unraveling of the probe and disruption of the hairpin structure. Consequently, the fluorophore is separated from the quencher, allowing light to be emitted from the fluorophore (Figure 8.9). A major limitation of this technique is its low sensitivity. As a result, efforts have been made to increase signal intensity by such

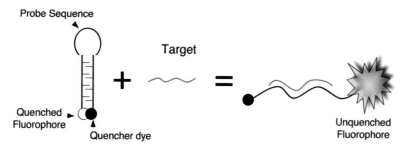

Figure 8.9. Molecular beacon structure. The probe sequence is designed to hybridize with a target mRNA sequence. In the absence of target mRNA, the beacon adopts a hairpin stem–loop structure where the quencher dye and fluorophore interact and fluorescence is quenched. Upon binding to the target, the beacon loses this hairpin conformation. The fluorophore is now removed from the quencher, and is free to emit photons.

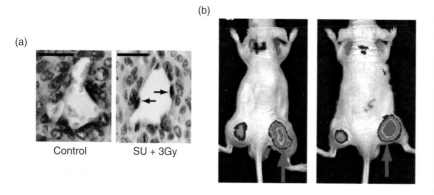

Figure 8.10. Imaging response to therapy. (a) TUNEL staining of tumor sections from control mice and mice treated with the VEGFR inhibitor SU11248 and 3 Gy radiation reveals apoptotic endothelial cells from treated tumors. (b) Phage-displayed peptides were selected for their preferential binding to irradiated tumors. These peptides were labeled with the near-infrared-emitting dye, Cy7, for *in vivo* imaging. When labeled peptides were injected into mice, they exhibited preferentially binding uptake in irradiated tumors. (Reproduced with permission from Han *et al., Nature Medicine* 2008; **14**: 343–9 [36].)

means as enzymatic amplification so that one target molecule can activate multiple beacons [30]. In addition, strategies have been introduced to accurately quantify delivered beacons and to avoid false-positive signals [31].

Imaging apoptosis

Apoptosis, or programmed cell death, is often deficient or suppressed in human cancers because of a diversity of genetic abnormalities that lead to either loss of pro-apoptotic machinery or aberrant activation of anti-apoptotic signals. Induction of cell death is the ultimate goal for all cancer therapeutics; hence the ability to image apoptosis is advantageous in the search for novel anti-cancer drugs and the evaluation of current therapies.

Apoptosis is characterized by morphological and biochemical changes. Cell-surface changes that occur during apoptosis promote recognition and clearance of dying cells by phagocytes. In the early phase of apoptosis, cells lose their membrane asymmetry and phosphatidylserine (PS) is presented on the extracellular portion of the cell membrane, whereas, under normal conditions, PS is maintained on the internal membrane face. Annexin V is a member of the annexin family of calcium-dependent phospholipid-binding proteins that specifically bind to PS and therefore specifically recognize apoptotic cells [32,33]. Conjugation of fluorescent proteins to annexin V allows the detection of apoptotic cells *in vitro*, and has also been shown *in vivo* and in *ex vivo* specimens [34,35].

There is generally high variability in response to cancer therapies. Current approaches to evaluating the effectiveness of therapy in patients may take several months, which is valuable time lost for a non-responsive patient. Imaging modalities are needed for rapid assessment of response to treatment, such that treatments can be altered if they fail to produce a favorable response. Work by Han *et al.* [36] used an *in vivo* phage selection scheme and identified peptides that preferentially bind to tumors that responded to radiation. These peptides were labeled with near-infrared light-emitting probes, thus allowing them to be traced non-invasively in mice (Figure 8.10). Strategies such as this will likely reduce the time that patients undergo ineffective treatments as well as expedite drug discovery in animal models of cancer.

Bacteriophage technology was further used to identify peptides that preferentially bind to dysplastic colonocytes compared to normal adjacent cells. Hsiung and colleagues [37] selected colon adenoma-specific phage-displayed peptides using fresh human colonoscopy biopsies. Peptides were labeled with the fluorescent dye, fluorescein, applied topically to the surface of the colon and imaged using a fibered confocal microscope that was passed through the end of a colonoscope. This study demonstrated the feasibility and potential of this approach for the early detection of colon cancer and pre-malignant lesions. It is especially noteworthy that the study was performed in human subjects. While optical imaging practices have been primarily limited to use in the laboratory, efforts similar to these are finding ways to exploit the advantages of fluorescence imaging in the clinic.

Conclusion

Optical imaging allows visualization of complex biological processes such as tumor growth, angiogenesis, gene transcription, and apoptosis. Since optical reporters are non-toxic, they are suitable for use in live cells and animals, which permits real-time investigation and longitudinal studies, thus enhancing the speed of data acquisition while driving down the cost of reagents, animals, labor, etc. Until now, optical imaging has been relegated to the pre-clinical arena due to technical limitations, such as the need to stably express reporter proteins. Nonetheless, patients have clearly benefited greatly from the translational value gained from optical imaging in pre-clinical models. Furthermore, the use of fluorescent probes and contrast dyes is currently being developed for diagnostic purposes and the evaluation of patient response to therapy.

References

1. Wilson T, Hastings JW. Bioluminescence. *Annu Rev Cell Dev Biol* 1998; **14**: 197–230.

2. Shimomura O, Johnson FH, Saiga Y. Extraction, purification and properties of aequorin, a bioluminescent protein from the luminous hydromedusan *Aequorea*. *J Cell Comp Physiol* 1962; **59**: 223–39.

3. de Wet JR, Wood KV, Helinski DR, DeLuca M. Cloning of firefly luciferase cDNA and the expression of active luciferase in *Escherichia coli*. *Proc Natl Acad Sci USA* 1985; **82**: 7870–3.

4. Prasher DC, Eckenrode VK, Ward WW, Prendergast FG, Cormier MJ. Primary structure of the *Aequorea victoria* green-fluorescent protein. *Gene* 1992; **111**: 229–33.

5. Luker GD, Luker KE. Optical imaging: current applications and future directions. *J Nucl Med* 2008; **49**: 1–4.

6. Heim R, Prasher DC, Tsien RY. Wavelength mutations and posttranslational autoxidation of green fluorescent protein. *Proc Natl Acad Sci USA* 1994; **91**: 12501–4.

7. Kim SH, Nakagawa H, Navaraj A, *et al.* Tumorigenic conversion of primary human esophageal epithelial cells using oncogene combinations in the absence of exogenous Ras. *Cancer Res* 2006; **66**: 10415–24.

8. Dolloff NG, Russell MR, Loizos N, Fatatis A. Human bone marrow activates the Akt pathway in metastatic prostate cells through transactivation of the alpha-platelet-derived growth factor receptor. *Cancer Res* 2007; **67**: 555–62.

9. Russell MR, Jamieson WL, Dolloff NG, Fatatis A. The alpha-receptor for platelet-derived growth factor as a target for antibody-mediated inhibition of skeletal metastases from prostate cancer cells. *Oncogene* 2009; **28**: 412–21.

10. Harms JF, Welch DR. MDA-MB-435 human breast carcinoma metastasis to bone. *Clin Exp Metastasis* 2003; **20**: 327–34.

11. Edinger M, Cao YA, Verneris MR, *et al.* Revealing lymphoma growth and the efficacy of immune cell therapies using in vivo bioluminescence imaging. *Blood* 2003; **101**: 640–8.

12. Jenkins DE, Hornig YS, Oei Y, Dusich J, Purchio T. Bioluminescent human breast cancer cell lines that permit rapid and sensitive in vivo detection of mammary tumors and multiple metastases in immune deficient mice. *Breast Cancer Res* 2005; **7**: R444–54.

13. Folkman J, Cole P, Zimmerman S. Tumor behavior in isolated perfused organs: in vitro growth and metastases of biopsy material in rabbit thyroid and canine intestinal segment. *Ann Surg* 1966; **164**: 491–502.

14. Mayes P, Dicker D, Liu Y, El-Deiry W. Noninvasive vascular imaging in fluorescent tumors using multispectral unmixing. *Biotechniques* 2008; **45**: 459–60.

15. Yang M, Baranov E, Li XM, *et al.* Whole-body and intravital optical imaging of angiogenesis in orthotopically implanted tumors. *Proc Natl Acad Sci USA* 2001; **98**: 2616–21.

16. Tumeh PC, Lerner JM, Dicker DT, El-Deiry WS. Differentiation of vascular and non-vascular skin spectral signatures using in vivo hyperspectral radiometric imaging. *Cancer Biol Ther* 2007; **6**: 447–53.

17. Dicker DT, Lerner J, Van Belle P, *et al.* Differentiation of normal skin and melanoma using high resolution hyperspectral imaging. *Cancer Biol Ther* 2006; **5**: 1033–8.

18. Bonnet D, Dick JE. Human acute myeloid leukemia is organized as a hierarchy that originates from a primitive hematopoietic cell. *Nat Med* 1997; **3**: 730–7.

19. Dalerba P, Cho RW, Clarke MF. Cancer stem cells: models and concepts. *Annu Rev Med* 2007; **58**: 267–84.

20. Hirschmann-Jax C, Foster AE, Wulf GG, *et al.* A distinct "side population" of cells with high drug efflux capacity in human tumor cells. *Proc Natl Acad Sci USA* 2004; **101**: 14228–33.

21. O'Brien CA, Pollett A, Gallinger S, Dick JE. A human colon cancer cell capable of initiating tumour growth in immunodeficient mice. *Nature* 2007; **445**: 106–10.

22. Hart LS, El-Deiry WS. Invincible, but not invisible: imaging approaches toward in vivo detection of cancer stem cells. *J Clin Oncol* 2008; **26**: 2901–10.

23. Carlsen H, Moskaug J, Fromm SH, Blomhoff R. In vivo imaging of NF-kappa B activity. *J Immunol* 2002; **168**: 1441–6.

24. Ciana P, Raviscioni M, Mussi P, *et al.* In vivo imaging of transcriptionally active estrogen receptors. *Nat Med* 2003; **9**: 82–6.

25. Wang W, El-Deiry WS. Bioluminescent molecular imaging of endogenous and exogenous p53-mediated transcription in vitro and in vivo using an HCT116 human colon carcinoma xenograft model. *Cancer Biol Ther* 2003; **2**: 196–202.

26. Brader P, Riedel CC, Woo Y, *et al.* Imaging of hypoxia-driven gene expression in an orthoptic liver tumor model. *Mol Cancer Ther* 2007; **6**: 2900–8.

27. El-Deiry WS, Sigman CC, Kelloff GJ. Imaging and oncologic drug development. *J Clin Oncol* 2006; **24**: 3261–73.

28. Wang W, Kim SH., El-Deiry WS. Small-molecule modulators of p53 family signaling and antitumor effects in p53-deficient human colon tumor xenografts. *Proc Natl Acad Sci USA* 2006; **103**: 11003–8.

29. Zhang L, Lee KC, Bhojani MS, *et al.* Molecular imaging of Akt kinase activity. *Nat Med* 2007; **13**: 1114–19.

30. Li JJ, Chu Y, Lee BYH, Xie XS. Enzymatic signal amplification of molecular beacons for sensitive DNA detection. *Nucleic Acids Res* 2008; **36**: e36.

31. Chen AK, Behlke MA, Tsourkas A. Avoiding false-positive signals with nuclease-vulnerable molecular beacons in single living cells. *Nucleic Acids Res* 2007; **35**: e105.

32. Thiagarajan P, Tait JF. Binding of annexin V/placental anticoagulant protein I to platelets: evidence for phosphatidylserine exposure in the procoagulant response of activated platelets. *J Biol Chem* 1990; **265**: 17420–3.

33. Koopman G, Reutelingsperger CP, Kuijten GA, *et al.* Annexin V for flow cytometric detection of phosphatidylserine expression on B cells undergoing apoptosis. *Blood* 1994; **84**: 1415–20.

34. Petrovsky A, Schellenberger E, Josephson L, Weissleder R, Bogdanov A. Near-infrared fluorescent imaging of tumor apoptosis. *Cancer Res* 2003; **63**: 1936–42.

35. Finnberg N, Kim SH, Furth EE, *et al.* Non-invasive fluorescence imaging of cell death in fresh human colon epithelia treated with 5-Fluorouracil, CPT-11 and/or TRAIL. *Cancer Biol Ther* 2005; **4**: 937–42.

36. Han Z, Fu A, Wang H, *et al.* Noninvasive assessment of cancer response to therapy. *Nat Med* 2008; **14**: 343–9.

37. Hsiung PL, Hardy J, Friedland S, *et al.* Detection of colonic dysplasia in vivo using a targeted heptapeptide and confocal microendoscopy. *Nat Med* 2008; **14**: 454–8.

Contrast agents for x-ray and MR imaging

Peter M. Joseph

Radiographic contrast

In Chapter 5, the basic physics of x-ray imaging was described. To briefly review, the x-rays are generated by the electrons in the x-ray tube striking the anode at high energy. More specifically, the energy of the electrons (in electronvolts, eV) is numerically equal to the kilovoltage applied to the anode. This creates a beam of external x-rays that has a very wide energy spectrum. The x-ray energies cover a range from (theoretically) 0 eV up to a maximum equal to the applied kilovoltage. In practice, because low-energy x-rays are much more rapidly absorbed than those with higher energies, the very lowest x-rays are absorbed in the glass envelope of the x-ray tube. More to the point, x-ray tubes are always operated with an additional metallic layer covering the opening port. This is called the "filter" and is intended further to raise the minimum x-ray energy. Because lower-energy x-rays are also absorbed by the human body more readily than those of higher energy, the absorption of the low-energy rays will contribute ionization dose to the patient's tissues without significantly contributing to image contrast, which is undesirable. Thus the radiologist can vary the so-called "effective energy" of the beam, usually by adjusting the applied kV, or occasionally by adding more metal as filter. The exact technique used depends on various factors, including the thickness of the body part being imaged and the nature of the pathology expected.

The most important concept in x-ray imaging is the *linear attenuation coefficient* (μ), as shown in Figure 9.1. The μ, whose units are inverse centimeters, represents numerically the fraction of x-rays that will be "attenuated" on passing through one centimeter of tissue. Diagnostic imaging works because various healthy and pathological tissues cause differing amounts of attenuation and therefore contrasting degrees of brightness or darkness on the image. Figure 9.2 illustrates this contrast effect graphically, comparing tissue with $\mu = 0.2\,\text{cm}^{-1}$ to tissue with $\mu = 0.4\,\text{cm}^{-1}$.

An extremely important factor that influences the attenuation coefficient is the average atomic number (not necessarily atomic weight) of the elements comprising the tissue. Higher atomic number means more rapid absorption for a given density. For example, bone is always more attenuating than soft tissue because of its high calcium and phosphorus content. Indeed, radiologists often can diagnose a disease that has abnormal calcification by observing the contrast of the calcium as seen on the radiograph. One well-known example is in diagnosis of breast cancer based on the observation of abnormal calcifications in the breast.

X-ray contrast agents

However, there arise many situations in which there are insufficient differences between tissue attenuation coefficients to permit tissue discrimination. In that case, an artificial substance whose atomic number is much larger than that of tissue and whose presence (or absence) can easily be judged from the radiograph can be introduced. There are two substances that are widely used as x-ray contrast agents: barium and iodine. The atomic number of barium is 56 and that of iodine is 53, which are far greater than that of any substance normally found in the body.

Barium, in the form of an insoluble salt, such as barium sulfate, is commonly used to examine the digestive system (both upper and lower). For many years large quantities of the contrast agent were used to make the intestines essentially opaque to x-rays. However, in recent years a new version called *double-contrast barium enema* was developed in which lesser

Introduction to the Science of Medical Imaging, ed. R. Nick Bryan. Published by Cambridge University Press. © Cambridge University Press 2010.

Attenuation of photons

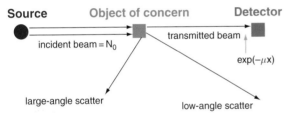

Figure 9.1. X-ray photons are attenuated (reduced in number) on passing through any type of material, including human tissue. The two major mechanisms are *photoelectric absorption* (PEA) and *scatter*. In the PEA process the photon is totally absorbed by a single atom, and so will cast a shadow on the image receptor. PEA is the dominant process that contributes to visualization of anatomic details. Scatter means that the x-ray photons change their direction. Some of the scattered photons will land on the image receptor in a place unrelated to the position of the original beam. Such photons will reduce image contrast and produce an inferior image quality.

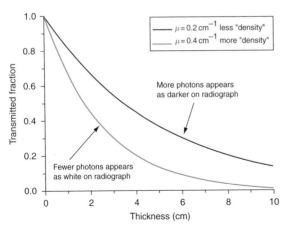

Figure 9.2. Radiographic "density" is due to differing attenuation coefficients in different tissues. Tissues that absorb more heavily, such as bone or contrast agent, have increased linear attenuation coefficient. This figure shows the effect for two different kinds of tissue, one with $\mu = 0.2\,cm^{-1}$ (less dense) and the other with $\mu = 0.4\,cm^{-1}$ (more dense). Radiographic density is dependent on the mass density (grams/cm^3) but is also dependent on atomic number. Radiographic contrast agents, such as I or Ba, are chosen because their higher atomic numbers produce increased PEA.

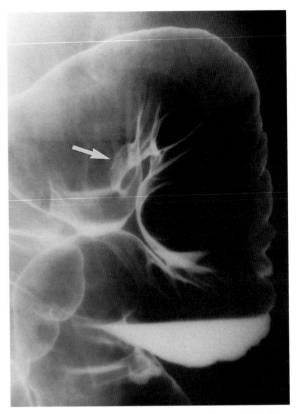

Figure 9.3. Upright right posterior oblique double-contrast barium enema spot image. The barium is seen as a horizontal surface due to gravity. A subtle plaque-like lesion (arrow) is seen in the splenic flexure. (Reproduced with permission from Levine *et al.*, *Radiology* 2000; **216**: 11–18 [1].)

amounts of barium were used together with air. That is, the air itself was considered a "negative" contrast agent. The barium tends to stick to the intestinal surface, making the surface visible. Figure 9.3 shows a typical double-contrast barium enema image using the negative contrast of air and the positive contrast of barium to outline the mucosa of the colon [1].

Intravenous iodine is usually used in soluble form to study blood vessels, tissue perfusion, or renal excretion. Figure 9.4 demonstrates a radiopaque stone in one kidney on a radiograph of the abdomen after contrast has been injected. After intravenous injection of an iodinated contrast agent, accumulation of iodine in the collecting systems of both kidneys can be easily seen. The iodine accumulation is dependent on perfusion and excretory function of the kidney, and shows the morphology of the renal pelvis and ureter.

While the use of iodinated contrast agents in radiology has become essential, their use does not come without risk. One never can inject pure iodine; it must be complexed to some organic molecule to avoid serious toxicity. However, the use of such iodinated complexes can occasionally lead to serious, even fatal, anaphylactic shock in individuals who are allergic to the substance. More common than anaphylaxis, but less life-threatening, are rapid alterations in blood chemistry and physiology, especially with agents of high osmolality. Since the late 1980s a new class of non-ionic agents has been developed that have low physics of x-ray attenuation. However, rather than single (or few) projections of the patient's anatomy, the machine measures a large number (many hundreds) of view projections. The machine physically rotates in a plane transverse to the patient's body to measure many such views. *Measured* means that more than pure geometry is involved. The machine measures that numerical factor by which each individual beam in each view is attenuated; that is, it measures (essentially) the average value of attenuation coefficient along each path. The numerical projection (*P*) values are processed by the computer to obtain an axial image of a narrow slice through the patient's body. A CT image is literally an image composed (numerically) of the attenuation values at each point in the transverse slice. In clinical CT images, the attenuation values are integers, called *Hounsfield units* (HU). Many contiguous slices are generally obtained, resulting in a 3D volume of images.

Because CT is basically another form of x-ray imaging, all contrast agents that can be used for projection radiography can be and are used for various CT examinations. Because CT is far more sensitive to subtle changes in attenuation coefficient, it is especially good at detecting abnormal contrast-agent concentrations. For example, CT of the brain using iodine contrast agent very clearly demonstrates many tumors, due to the fact that the neovascularity of tumors allows more contrast agent to extravasate into the extravascular space. This technique is especially useful in the brain because of the so-called blood–brain barrier (BBB). The BBB relates to cerebral blood vessels whose endothelial cells are tightly adhered, preventing the iodinated contrast agent from passing into brain tissue. Figure 9.6 shows an example of a contrast-enhancing brain tumor that lacks a normal BBB [3].

MRI contrast agents

Chapter 7 has described the basic physics of MRI, which is imaging using the phenomenon of nuclear magnetic resonance (NMR). To briefly review, NMR is based on the fact that certain atomic nuclei, especially hydrogen, possess a small but permanent magnetic moment. That is, each proton in water acts as a tiny permanent magnet. When placed in a fixed external magnetic field, $\mathbf{B_0}$, the protons can acquire a certain energy level due to the interaction of the magnetic moment and the external field. When the patient's body is first placed into the magnet, the protons in the body quickly achieve their lowest possible energy

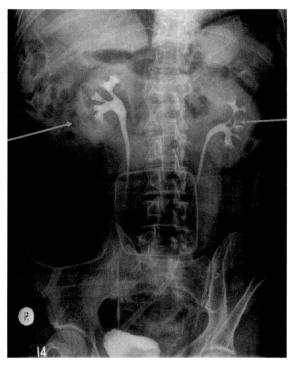

Figure 9.4. AP abdominal film shows urinary system, including kidneys, ureters, and bladder, because of IV iodine contrast agent. The right kidney is normal and shows the renal parenchyma (arrow) and the collecting system. The left has a stone in a renal calyx (arrow) so that the collecting system is not as well enhanced as it should be.

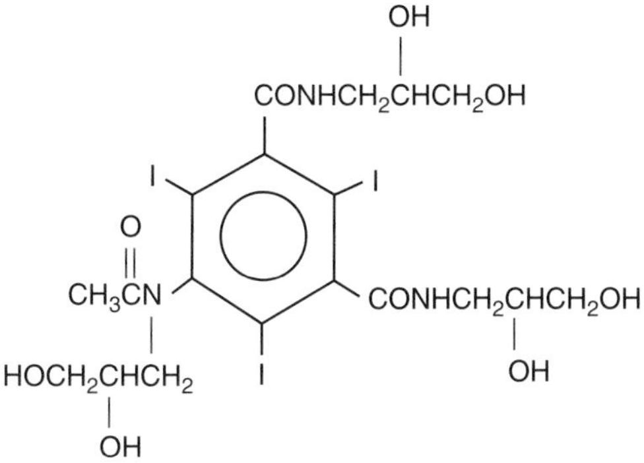

Figure 9.5. Chemical structure of iohexol, one commonly used iodinated non-ionic x-ray contrast agent. This molecule is non-ionic and does not dissociate in water, which lessens its toxic effects. In healthy tissues it is mostly intravascular and is excreted by the kidneys.

osmolality and are considered safer than the older ionic agents, and these are now in general use. One common example is iohexol (Figure 9.5). For a review see Costa [2].

The physics of computed tomography scanning has been presented in Chapter 5. To briefly review, CT is basically a more sophisticated use of the basic

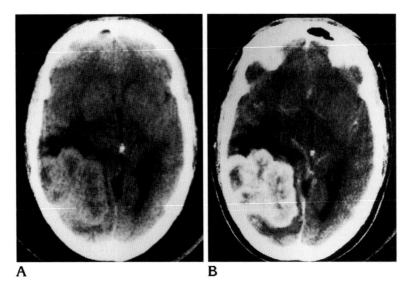

A   **B**

Figure 9.6. Pair of images of a malignant brain tumor with and without iodine contrast. The tumor enhances far more than normal brain tissue due to breakdown of the blood–brain barrier in the tumor. (Reproduced with permission from Chiechi et al., *AJNR Am J Neuroradiol* 1996; **17**: 1365–71 [3].)

state, a state that is stable and can emit no electromagnetic energy. However, when in the scanner the patient's body is surrounded by a specially tuned coil of wire (called the RF coil) that can be energized by a radiofrequency (RF) current carefully adjusted to the natural resonance frequency of the protons. This has two immediate effects: (1) the protons can absorb energy from the RF field being irradiated, and (2) they can immediately re-radiate electromagnetic energy at the same frequency. MRI works by employing a complex series of RF and magnetic pulses, designed to induce and detect radiant energy from the irradiated protons. Obviously, the strength of the signal from any given voxel will, at the least, be dependent on the concentration of protons in that voxel; this is called the *proton density* effect. However, the clinical value of MRI depends not only on the strength of signals received, but on how quickly they return to the base energy level. There are two such time constants, called T_1 and T_2, that can be influenced by pathological changes in tissues. MRI is also capable of more sophisticated types of signal analysis, such as the rate of diffusion of water and the flow of blood. However, in this chapter we shall mainly be concerned with contrast agents that alter the T_1 or T_2 (or both) of tissues to enhance the ability to differentiate tissues and diagnose clinical conditions. The main distinction between T_1 and T_2 imaging involves the concept of *echo time*. *Echo* refers to any process where, at some time interval after excitation in which the NMR signal has appeared to disappear (due to dephasing), the

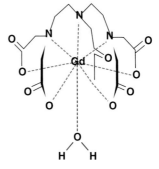

Figure 9.7. Chemical structure of Gd-DTPA, one commonly used T_1 contrast agent for MRI. The chemical binding of the Gd ion to the chelate DTPA is very strong so that the body never sees free GD, which is very toxic. That is, the chelation makes the Gd non-toxic.

signal is made to regenerate by the application of some suitable (usually RF) pulse. The time interval between the initial excitation and the appearance of the echo is called "echo time," abbreviated T_E. Typical values of T_E can range from submilliseconds to hundreds of milliseconds. The basic principle is that the longer the T_E the more dependent the signal strength is on T_2, rather than on T_1.

We shall discuss two very different types of MRI contrast agents. One is a chelated form of gadolinium called Gd-DTPA (Figure 9.7). Gadolinium itself is highly toxic. However the chelation in Gd-DTPA is very strong and so the body never sees free gadolinium. Gd-DTPA is considerably safer than iodinated x-ray contrast agents. The second MRI contrast agent consists of small particles of iron oxide.

Gadolinium

Gadolinium in the ionic state Gd^{3+} has an unusually strong magnetic moment. This magnetism is due to the structure of the electrons in the atomic orbits, and is not due to any magnetism in the nucleus, which is much weaker and essentially irrelevant. Gadolinium belongs to a class of substances called *paramagnetic*, which means that the atom is not naturally magnetized but becomes magnetized when placed in an external magnetic field (such as the B_0 of the MRI magnet). In that case, each gadolinium atom becomes a magnet several thousand times stronger than that of a proton. This means that each gadolinium atom creates a magnetic field around itself that can and does "perturb" the magnetic state of nearby protons. This perturbing effect is illustrated in Figure 9.8. Note how the magnetic field created by the gadolinium passes through the proton and so changes its magnetic energy. The effect of this tumbling magnetic field is to *accelerate* the *transition* of the proton to its ground (unexcited) energy level. That is, it works to shorten both T_1 and T_2 of the protons. Figure 9.8 should not be interpreted to mean that a single gadolinium ion can, by itself, return the proton to its ground state. To the contrary, the reduction of T_1 and T_2 takes place over milliseconds, during which the proton will feel the effects of literally thousands of similar Gd ions.

The effect of Gd on the T_1 and T_2 time constants can be written in a simple equation involving a so-called *relaxivity* constant. More precisely, we can very simply relate the change in the *inverse* of T_1 or T_2, known as the *relaxation rates* R_1 and R_2, as follows:

$$R_1(\text{Gd}) = 1/T_1(\text{Gd}) = 1/T_1(0) + r_1 * [\text{Gd}] \quad (9.1)$$

$$R_2(\text{Gd}) = 1/T_2(\text{Gd}) = 1/T_2(0) + r_2 * [\text{Gd}] \quad (9.2)$$

where $T_1(0)$ is the T_1 time constant with no gadolinium, and $T_1(\text{Gd})$ is the (shorter) T_1 constant when gadolinium is present, and [Gd] is the concentration of gadolinium in a given tissue. This simple equation is really quite plausible; the greater the tissue concentration of gadolinium the greater is the shortening of T_1 and T_2. In this equation r_1 and r_2 are constants that do not depend on the concentration of gadolinium, but do depend on the details of the interaction between the chelated gadolinium and the surrounding water molecules. That is, there are various choices of chelate other than DTPA, and different chelates will have (slightly) different values of r_1 and r_2.

In terms of physics, the values of r_1 and r_2 for Gd-DTPA are very similar (r_2 is slightly larger). However, in clinical practice Gd-DTPA is used under conditions in which the effect is mainly to shorten T_1 with little effect on T_2. This is due to the fact that most solid tissues have T_2 values that are much shorter than the T_1 values; typical values might be $T_1 = 800$ ms and $T_2 = 80$ ms. Because the $T_2(0)$ is so small, its inverse as it appears in Equation 9.2 is much larger, so the additive effect of $r_2 * [\text{Gd}]$ on

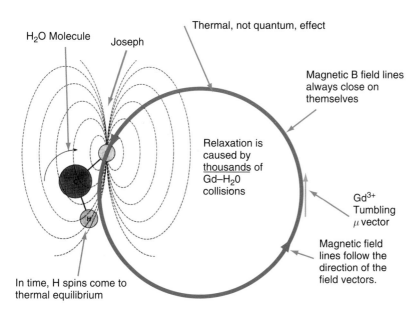

H₂O Molecule

Joseph

Thermal, not quantum, effect

Magnetic B field lines always close on themselves

Relaxation is caused by thousands of Gd–H₂0 collisions

Gd^{3+} Tumbling μ vector

Magnetic field lines follow the direction of the field vectors.

In time, H spins come to thermal equilibrium

Figure 9.8. Cartoon of the interaction between the gadolinium ion and a water molecule. The magnetic field from the Gd ion penetrates through the water molecule and alters the internal energy of the protons. Over the course of thousands of such collisions of the water molecules with different gadolinium ions, the protons in the water molecule relax back to their equilibrium state.

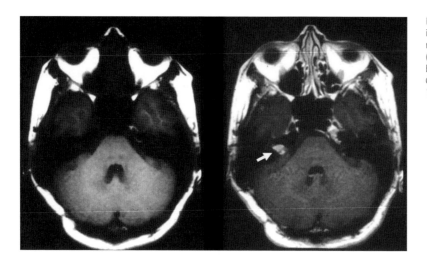

Figure 9.9. Pre- and post-Gd contrast injection T_1 MRI of enhancing acoustic neuroma with tumor enhancement (arrow) due to abnormal blood–brain barrier. (Reproduced with permission from Chiechi et al., AJNR Am J Neuroradiol 1996; **17**: 1365–71 [3].)

R_2 is relatively small. This means that Gd is normally used with a T_1-weighted pulse sequence that emphasizes changes in T_1 and de-emphasizes changes in T_2. Only in exceptional cases with extremely large concentrations of Gd will T_2 be materially shortened.

Gd-DTPA can be used clinically in almost exactly the same ways that iodinated contrast agents are used in x-ray imaging. Once the contrast agent is injected intravenously, its physiologic distribution is almost identical to that seen with x-ray contrast agents. The main difference between the use of contrast agents in MRI versus x-ray is that, at least for projection radiography, the exposure times are very short, typically only a few milliseconds. However, some MRI pulse sequences are much longer, perhaps hundreds of milliseconds, so that the radiologist has to give careful thought to the time-dependent dynamics of the contrast agent. Figure 9.9 shows a brain tumor imaged with and without Gd, based on the same physiology as the x-ray image in Figure 9.6.

However, the physics of MRI is far more complex and subtle than that of x-ray imaging, and by clever manipulation of the pulse sequence one can either suppress or enhance various kinds of tissue contrast. One common application of Gd-DTPA is called *MR angiography* (MRA). In this case one first *suppresses the signal* from stationary tissue by using a very short T_R, where T_R is the time interval between repetitions of the RF pulses. Reducing the value of T_R will always reduce the strength of the signal, since we are then giving the irradiated tissue less time to recover. The degree of recovery is obviously related to the T_1 of the tissue in question. However, when the organ is perfused with Gd-DTPA of sufficiently high

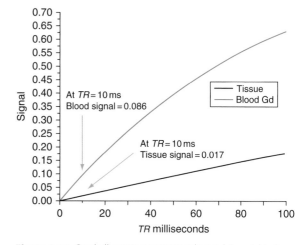

Figure 9.10. Graph illustrating contrast-enhanced T_1-weighted MRA that combines very short TR with high concentration of Gd contrast agent injected as a bolus. This combination of pulse sequence and Gd suppresses signal from poorly perfused tissues while enhancing the signal in blood vessels.

concentration, the T_1 of the perfused tissue is shortened by an amount that depends on the degree of Gd perfusion. Hence, the signals are enhanced to the extent that they are perfused. The physics of this process is illustrated in the graph in Figure 9.10. Here one sees the strength of the MRI signal as it depends on the value chosen for T_R. For the tissue both with and without Gd the signal strength is reduced as T_R is shortened. However, by utilizing a short T_R of only 10 ms, the presence of the Gd greatly increases the signal strength over that seen without the Gd. Figure 9.11 illustrates the imaging of abdominal arteries with an IV infusion of Gd-DTPA [4]. Figure 9.12 compares the results of an invasive

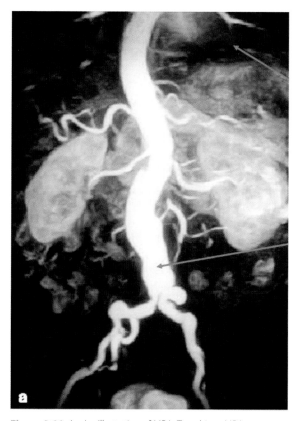

Figure 9.11. *In vivo* illustration of MRA. To achieve MRA we must both suppress signal from tissues with poor perfusion (upper arrow) and enhance signal of blood vessels containing a high concentration of Gd (lower arrow). The physiology is identical to that for iodinated x-ray contrast agents. (Reproduced with permission from Vosshenrich and Fischer, *Eur Radiol* 2002; **12**: 218–30 [4].)

procedure (intra-arterial contrast injection, x-ray digital subtraction angiogram; DSA) with the non-invasive (intravenous) MRA procedure [5].

While Gd-DTPA generally has fewer major and minor side effects, it, like any drug, can adversely affect the patient. Acute allergic and physiologic reactions are rare, but recently a chronic and potentially severe reaction called nephrogenic systemic sclerosis has been related to the intravenous administration of Gd chelates in patients with chronic renal failure [6]. The use of Gd compounds is now contraindicated in these patients.

Iron oxide

The second kind of MR contrast agent that we will discuss involves small, solid, iron oxide particles. These can shorten both T_1 and T_2 but, unlike Gd-DTPA, the effect on T_2 is usually stronger than on T_1. To discuss this we need to review the concept of spin dephasing in MRI.

As stated in Chapter 7, the NMR signal is generated by inducing a rotation of the magnetization vector for a voxel; the vector is spinning at the Larmor (resonant) frequency. The key concept is that magnetization is a vector quantity having two components that are rotating in the *x,y* (transverse) plane. The physics of this process is greatly simplified if we view the vector in the so-called *rotating frame of reference* (RFR). If we chose the RFR frequency to be the Larmor frequency, then (ideally) the magnetization vector will appear stationary in the RFR. This assumes, of course, that we <u>exactly</u> match the frequency of the RFR to the Larmor frequency. In practice,

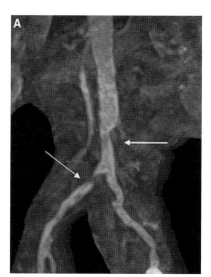
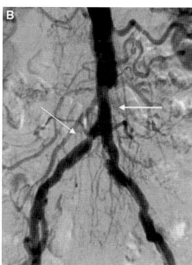

Figure 9.12. Both (a) maximum-intensity projection of gadopentetate dimeglumine-enhanced MRA and (b) x-ray DSA in left anterior oblique projections reveal a stenosis > 50% in the infrarenal abdominal aorta (bold arrow) and an occlusion of the left internal iliac (arrow). (Reproduced with permission from Schaefer *et al., Cardiovasc Interventional Radiol* 2007; **30**: 376–82 [5].)

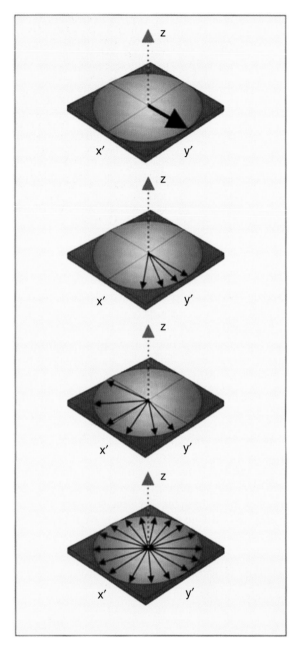

Figure 9.13. T_2 decay is due to gradual *dephasing* of the *x,y* components of the magnetization vector as viewed in the rotating frame of reference. The dephasing is induced by slight differences in Larmor frequency for protons in different parts of the voxel of tissue. Rinck, *Magnetic Resonance in Medicine*, Blackwell.

itself. The implication of this inhomogeneity is that, within any given voxel, some protons are above the Larmor frequency and some are below. This implies that some protons are spinning clockwise in the RFR and some are spinning counterclockwise. The angle that the spins make with the *x*-axis in the RFR is called the *phase angle*. This means that even if all spins are initially excited to the same phase angle, the spins will gradually accumulate different phase angles due to local magnetic-field inhomogeneities. This process, called *dephasing* is illustrated in Figure 9.13. The signal strength is determined by the net magnetization in the voxel, so that particles pointing in opposite directions tend to cancel one another out. That is, dephasing will always lead to a reduction in MR signal strength.

Iron oxide, in the form of magnetite (Fe_3O_4), is classified as *superparamagnetic*. That is, the material shares the paramagnetism of Gd ions, but is many orders of magnitude stronger. This concept is illustrated in Figure 9.14 [7]. This effect is due to the unique structure of magnetite in the solid state. Iron ions dissolved in water (such as iron in hemoglobin), while paramagnetic, do not have the same strength as superparamagnetic magnetite.

The main effect of using solid iron oxide particles for contrast is to accelerate the dephasing effect in a way dependent on the concentration of the particles in any given voxel. That is, it will have the effect of shortening T_2, so that in a T_2-weighted image the signal will appear darker in tissues with higher concentrations of iron oxide particles. For such purposes particle size plays a crucial role. To emphasize T_2, rather than T_1, the particles must not be too small. Typical particle sizes are on the order of one micron, no smaller than 0.3 microns. If the particle size is much smaller, say less than 0.1 micron, then the T_2 effect is diminished and the T_1 effect is augmented. The physics of this changeover is due to the frequency of tumbling of the particles in the aqueous milieu. The T_1 relaxation becomes prominent when the tumbling frequency is comparable to the Larmor frequency; i.e., it is possible for the particles to transfer energy to the protons and so decrease T_1. The T_2 effect does not require such a frequency match, and in fact the magnetite can dephase the spins even when tumbling at much lower frequencies. The frequency of tumbling is inversely related to particle size; i.e., the larger particles have more mass and tend to move more slowly than the smaller particles. Hence large particle size gives greater T_2 and less T_1 effect than is seen with smaller-size

such an exact match is impossible, mainly because there are natural inhomogeneities in the magnetic field within any realistic voxel. These inhomogeneities are partly due to imperfections in the main $\mathbf{B_0}$ field, and are partly induced by magnetization of the tissue

(a)

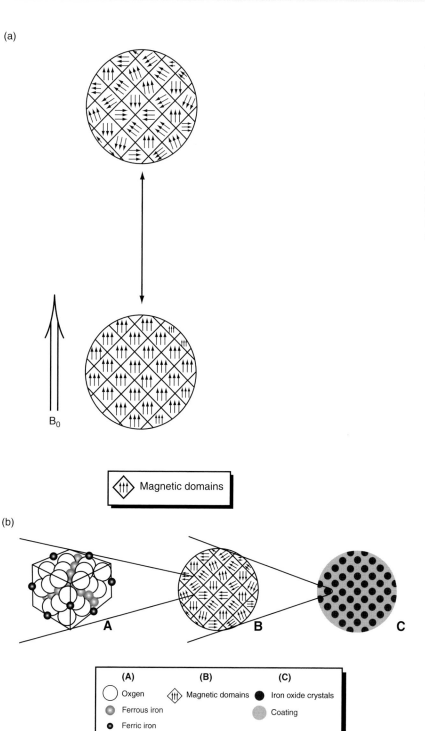

B_0

◇↿↿↿ Magnetic domains

(b)

A B C

(A)	(B)	(C)
◯ Oxgen	◇↿↿↿ Magnetic domains	⬤ Iron oxide crystals
◉ Ferrous iron		◉ Coating
⬤ Ferric iron		

Figure 9.14. Ferromagnetic material, such as magnetite, is composed of many microscopic "domains" (a). Within each domain all of the molecules are magnetically aligned, although those in various domains have a random orientation in the absence of an external magnetic field. An external magnetic field, **B_0**, will cause all of the domains to lie parallel to the field direction, thus producing a very strong magnetization which will, in turn, create a new magnetic field outside of the particles (b). The new field will induce dephasing in nearby tissues, thus shortening T_2. (Adapted with permission from Wang *et al.*, *Eur Radiol* 2001; **11**: 2319–31 [7].)

particles. There has evolved a variety of magnetite particles that are commercially available. The most important parameter is the size of the particle. The largest size have a diameter of 0.3 microns or larger, and are usually given orally; they are commonly abbreviated as SPIO (superparamagnetic iron oxide). The liver will rapidly absorb those particles, so they can be used for liver imaging. The next size range is abbreviated SSPIO, with diameters in the range 60–150 nanometers (nm). The smallest size are called ultra-small (USPIO), with particle diameters about 20–40 nm.

The major effect of particle size is to alter the ratio of r_2/r_1, which is always greater than 1. The largest size have the most effect on T_2 with minimal effect on T_1, e.g., a r_2/r_1 ratio of about 7. Such particles are used only with a T_2-weighted image technique (such as fast spin echo) so the effect of the contrast agent is to reduce signal strength. The ultra-small particles have r_2/r_1 ratio of about 2, and these are usually used with a T_1-weighted MR pulse sequence. For example, by choosing both T_R and T_E to be as small as possible (typically a few milliseconds) one emphasizes the T_1 effect and de-emphasizes the T_2 effect. Increased signal strength will be seen in tissues that accumulate more iron oxide particles.

The larger-size particles are absorbed by macrophages or other cells in the reticuloendothelial system. If given orally, these particles are commonly absorbed in the liver, assuming that the liver is functioning normally. However, if there is a tumor in the liver that cannot absorb the magnetite, it will appear bright on a T_2-weighted image, relative to the surrounding normal liver cells. This effect is illustrated in Figure 9.15 [8].

However, for some purposes rapid absorption of the particles by the liver is a disadvantage. Absorption by the liver can be partially inhibited by (1) using much smaller particles, ~ 0.1 micron, and (2) applying a biochemical coating, such as dextran. Such a particle has been described by Weissleder *et al.*, and has a half-life in blood of 81 minutes, much longer than the six minutes found with previous particles [9]. The particles can be injected intravenously, since they will pass through capillaries, and can enter the lymphatics, where they can be absorbed by normal lymph nodes. An example of this technique, using T_2-weighted imaging, for the detection of metastatic disease from prostate cancer is shown in Figure 9.16 [10].

Another particle formulation called ferumoxytol is a USPIO that has a blood lifetime of several days, allowing the patient to be scanned several times over the course of several days without re-injection. Figure 9.17 shows images of the uptake of the particles in a case of glioblastoma multiforme [11]. Due to its long half-life and slow tumor accumulation, the USPIO agent demonstrates a larger portion of the tumor than does the Gd contrast agent.

Perhaps the most exciting development in the use of SPIO particles is the possibility of attaching them to monoclonal antibodies (mAb) so that highly selective biological targeting is possible. Figure 9.18 shows an example of attaching a SPIO particle to a monoclonal antibody directed at the HER-2 receptor on the surface of a cell [12]. HER (human endothelium receptor) is involved with cell proliferation and is often overexpressed on the membranes of cancerous cells. Another possible target is the transferrin

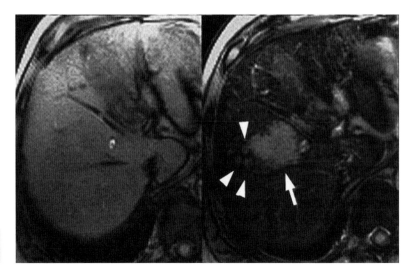

Figure 9.15. Clinical example of the use of magnetite particles to diagnose hepatocellular carcinoma. The left image shows the liver image without the contrast agent; there is little indication of a tumor. The right image with magnetite shows that most of the healthy liver has lost signal due to absorbing the particles (normal hepatic function). However, the tumor cells cannot absorb the particles so the tumor appears brighter on the T_2-weighted image (arrow and arrowheads). (Reproduced with permission from Tanimoto and Kuribayashi, *Eur J Radiol* 2006; **58**: 200–16 [8].)

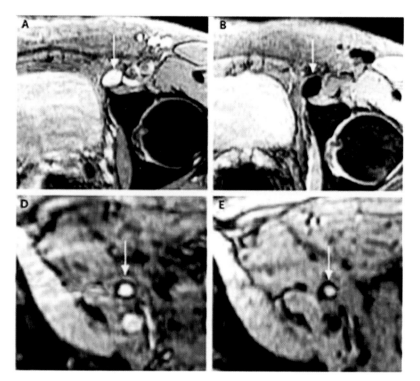

Figure 9.16. One kind of magnetite particle is coated with materials that inhibit rapid absorption by the liver, but is picked up by the reticuloendothelial cells in lymph nodes. This can be used to diagnose lymphatic spread of cancer cells. The upper left image shows a normal node with no magnetite; it is bright in the T_2-weighted image. The upper right image shows that the normal mode turns dark due to the (normal) absorption of the particles. The two lower images show a node partially filled with cancer cells. The diagnosis is based on the fact that the node retains a central bright core, indicating that the cells there are not normal and cannot absorb the particles. (Reproduced with permission from Harisinghani *et al.*, *N Eng J Med* 2003; **348**: 2491–9 [10].)

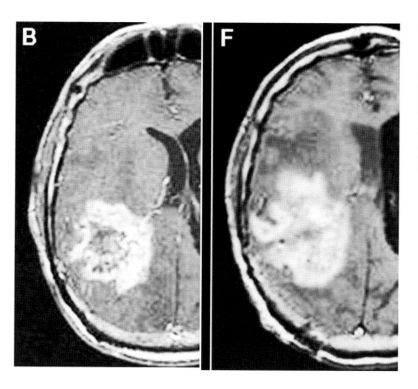

Figure 9.17. Clinical example of using ultra-small magnetic particles with very long vascular lifetime for T_1-weighted image of brain tumor. Left figure (B) shows enhancement of the tumor using Gd, as discussed previously. Right image (F) was done 4–6 hours after injection of ultra-small magnetic particles. Note that the particle contrast agent shows larger tumor volume than that seen with the gadolinium. (Reproduced with permission from Neuwelt *et al.*, *Neurosurgery* 2007; **60**: 601–11 [11].)

receptor, which also regulates cell division and is often overexpressed in cancer cells. This is true for a wide variety of human cancer cells including leukemia, colorectal cancer, breast adenocarcinoma, mesothelioma, and liver carcinoma [13]. One investigator injected nude mice with two different cell lines of 9L gliosarcoma, differing in the level of transferrin expressed [14]. As shown in Figure 9.19, the SPIO-antibody technique dramatically decreased T_2 signal within the antigen-bearing portion of the tumor. Furthermore, the two strains of gliosarcoma were distinguishable by quantitative analysis of the amount of T_2 reduction. As of 2009 these monoclonal antibody techniques were still in the embryonic stage. Hopefully they will evolve into useful clinical diagnostic tools.

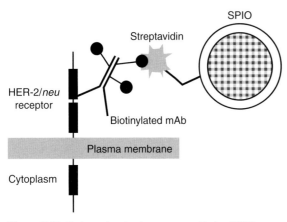

Figure 9.18. Cartoon showing how one can attach a SPIO to an antibody that attaches to the HER-2 receptor, commonly found on the surface of cancerous cells. This results in highly specific targeting of pathological tissue. (Reproduced with permission from Raman *et al., NMR Biomed* 2007; **20**: 186–99 [12].)

References

1. Levine MS, Rubesin SE, Laufer I, Herlinger H. Diagnosis of colorectal neoplasms at double-contrast barium enema examination. *Radiology* 2000; **216**: 11–18.

2. Costa N. Understanding contrast media. *J Infus Nurs* 2004; **27**: 302–12.

3. Chiechi MV, Smirniotopoulos JG, Mena H. Intracranial hemangiopericytomas: MR and CT features. *AJNR Am J Neuroradiol* 1996; **17**: 1365–71.

4. Vosshenrich R, Fischer U. Contrast-enhanced MR angiography of abdominal vessels: is there still a role for angiography? *Eur Radiol* 2002; **12**: 218–30.

5. Schaefer PJ, Schaefer FKW, Mueller-Huelsbeck S, *et al.* Value of single-dose contrast-enhanced magnetic resonance angiography versus intraarterial digital subtraction angiography in therapy indications in abdominal and iliac arteries. *Cardiovasc Intervent Radiol* 2005; **30**: 376–82.

6. Thomsen HS. Nephrongenic systemic fibrosis: a serious late adverse effect of gadodiamide. *Eur Radiol* 2006; **16**: 2619–21.

7. Wang YX, Hussain SM, Krestin GP. Superparamagnetic iron oxide contrast agents: physicochemical characteristics and applications in MR imaging. *Eur Radiol* 2001; **11**: 2319–31.

8. Tanimoto A, Kuribayashi S. Application of superparamagnetic iron oxide to imaging of hepatocellular carcinoma. *Eur J Radiol* 2006; **58**: 200–16.

9. Weissleder R, Elizondo G, Wittenberg J, *et al.* Ultrasmall superparamagnetic iron oxide: characterization of a new class of contrast agents for MR imaging. *Radiology* 1990; **175**: 489–93.

10. Harisinghani MG, Barentsz J, Hahn PF, *et al.* Noninvasive detection of clinically occult lymph-node metastases in prostate cancer. *N Engl J Med* 2003; **348**: 2491–9.

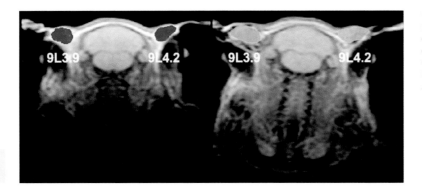

Figure 9.19. SPIO attached to monoclonal antibodies to two slightly different strains of glioblastoma with differing expressions of HER-2 receptors. (Reproduced with permission from Hogemann-Savellano *et al., Neoplasia* 2003; **5**: 495–506 [14].)

11. Neuwelt EA, Varallyay CG, Manninger S, *et al.* The potential of ferumoxytol nanoparticle magnetic resonance imaging, perfusion, and angiography in central nervous system malignancy: a pilot study. *Neurosurgery* 2007; **60**: 601–11.

12. Raman V, Pathak AP, Glunde K, Artemov D, Bhujwalla ZM. Magnetic resonance imaging and spectroscopy of transgenic models of cancer. *NMR Biomed* 2007; **20**: 186–99.

13. Daniels TR, Delgado T, Helguera G, Penichet ML. The transferrin receptor part II: targeted delivery of therapeutic agents into cancer cells. *Clin Immunol* 2006; **121**: 159–76.

14. Hogemann-Savellano D, Bos E, Blondet C, *et al.* The transferrin receptor: a potential molecular imaging marker for human cancer. *Neoplasia* 2003; **5**: 495–506.

Nuclear molecular labeling

Datta Ponde and Chaitanya Divgi

The tracer principle, articulated by the Hungarian chemist Georg de Hevesy (1885–1966) while in Rutherford's Manchester laboratory, remains the cornerstone of molecular imaging. de Hevesy discovered that a suitably marked small ("trace") quantity of a compound could be used to observe the behavior of the compound in the living system. In other words, a small amount of glucose labeled with radioactive carbon can be administered to study the behavior of glucose in the body; a small amount of hyperpolarized carbon-labeled pyruvate can be administered to study pyruvate metabolism. An important feature of the principle is that the amount of tracer should be small enough not to perturb the milieu. For these insights, de Hevesy was awarded the 1943 Nobel Prize in Chemistry. In this chapter, we will focus on radioactive tracers used for evaluating biochemical processes *in vivo*.

Molecular labeling fundamentals

Attachment of radioactive isotopes to compounds of interest has increasing applications in nuclear medicine and modern drug discovery. There are several challenges one faces in the attachment of isotopes to molecules, including the intended final diagnostic/ therapeutic application of the molecule.

Radiopharmaceuticals are radioactive compounds used for the diagnosis and treatment of many diseases, and utilized most often at very low molar concentrations that do not have pharmacologic effects on the body. *Radioligand* generally refers to any radiopharmaceutical that binds to a receptor on or in a cell. We will use the terms *radiotracer* and *radioligand* interchangeably to refer to radiopharmaceuticals without pharmacologic effects and used non-therapeutically. Radioligands used therapeutically may have pharmacologic effects, and

in those cases the term radiotracer is no longer appropriate.

Diagnostic imaging agents are designed to localize in specific organs or tissue types. An ideal imaging agent should rapidly and avidly localize in the organ/ tissue of interest, should remain there for the duration of study, and be quickly excreted from the remainder of the body. In designing a radiotracer for imaging purposes, various factors such as selection of isotope, type of decay of isotope, position of labeling within the molecule (dependent on its metabolic behavior), size and charge of labeling molecule, specific activity, stability, and solubility need to be considered. In addition, the final radiopharmaceutical should be produced in a reasonable amount of time (shorter for shorter-lived radioisotopes) and with favorable radiochemical yield (amount of radiotracer produced as a fraction of the overall tracer used for radioconjugation) sufficient for human nuclear medicine studies.

The half-life of an isotope plays a very important role in determining the type of study for which it may be used. Every radionuclide has a unique physical half-life ($t_{1/2}$), defined as the time to reduce its initial radioactivity or disintegration rate by half. The half-life is a function of the decay constant λ of a radionuclide, and is related by

$$\lambda = 0.693/t_{1/2} \qquad (10.1)$$

The biologic half-life of the compound being studied is also important, and is defined by the period to reduce its concentration in the body by half. From an imaging standpoint, the effective half-life is critical. The optimum effective half-life should be about 1–1.5 times the study period. Effective half-life may be calculated as follows:

Introduction to the Science of Medical Imaging, ed. R. Nick Bryan. Published by Cambridge University Press. © Cambridge University Press 2010.

$$[t_{1/2}]1/\text{Effective } t_{1/2} = \left[1/\text{Biologic } t_{1/2} \right.$$
$$\left. +1/\text{Physical } t_{1/2}\right] \quad (10.2)$$

There are various mechanisms by which radio-tracers can localize in the organ/tissue of interest; the most common is by binding to membrane surface receptors. After transport (active or passive) across the cell membrane, there may be a metabolic trapping of radiotracer by enzyme activity, by binding to either DNA or RNA, or proteins with consequent accumulation of radioactivity in the target area. Since these are critical considerations in designing novel radiopharmaceuticals, care should be taken to ensure radio-conjugate stability in the presence of enzyme activity and protein degradation, to name two important issues.

Specific activity (amount of radioactivity per unit mass of a pharmaceutical), also plays a very important role, especially when the target is a receptor, but even more so when the pharmaceutical has a potential pharmacologic effect. The specific activity should be as high as possible to avoid pharmacologic effects and to ensure maximal binding of the radioligand to the receptor.

An important point to be considered in designing a radiopharmaceutical is its water or organic solubility. This is usually designated by a partition coefficient. In general, the higher the partition coefficient, the more soluble the agent is in organic solvents. Lipophilicity is particularly important for radiopharmaceuticals intended to cross cell membranes and barriers like the blood–brain barrier (BBB). Another important factor for consideration is affinity for target. In general, agents with high affinity (i.e., low dissociation coefficients, or K_D) are preferred since targeting can be achieved at lower, sub pharmacologic mass amounts. There is debate about the role of affinity for macromolecular targeting, with some groups believing that low-affinity macromolecules are preferable since the low affinity permits penetration into tissue.

Positron emission tomography (PET) and single photon emission computed tomography (SPECT) radiotracers are distinguished mainly by the type of radioisotope incorporated in the tracer. SPECT studies use radiopharmaceuticals labeled with a single photon emitter, a radioisotope that emits gamma rays during radioactive decay. Some commonly used single photon emitters are technetium-99 m (^{99m}Tc), thallium-201 (^{201}Tl), iodine-123 (^{123}I), indium-111 (^{111}In), and gallium-67 (^{67}Ga). Many of these nuclides also have

Table 10.1. Physical properties of commonly used SPECT isotopes

Nuclide	Half-life	Decay mode	Photons (MeV)
^{67}Ga	3.26 days	Electron capture	0.093, 0.185, 0.300
^{99m}Tc	6 h	Isomeric transition	0.140
^{111}In	2.8 days	Electron capture	0.171, 0.245
^{113m}In	1.66 h	Isomeric transition	0.392
^{123}I	13.2 h	Electron capture	0.159

positron isotopes (e.g., ^{94m}Tc, ^{124}I, ^{110m}In, ^{68}Ga). Positron emitters, as the term implies, emit positrons during radioactive decay. The positrons, being antimatter, annihilate with an electron and this annihilation results in the discharge of two photons of identical energy in opposite directions.

SPECT agents

General principles of SPECT agents

SPECT isotopes are produced in a cyclotron or a reactor. Isotopes produced in a reactor are generally either products of the fission reaction or are produced by neutron bombardment of a stable isotope. Purification of the desired radioisotope can be costly and difficult, limiting specific activity. In a cyclotron, various charged particles such as protons, deuterons, alpha particles, and helium particles are accelerated in a circular path and then irradiated on a target of stable elements to produce radioisotopes. For cyclotron-produced isotopes, the isotope produced depends on the irradiating particle, its energy, and the target nuclei. The nuclides produced by charged-particle nuclear reactions are not isotopes of the target nuclide. Consequently, chemical separation of product and target nuclides is possible and a high-specific-activity product can be achieved. The most common SPECT isotopes made in cyclotrons are ^{67}Ga, ^{123}I, and ^{111}In (Table 10.1).

Technetium-99m (^{99m}Tc)

Technetium-99m is the most widely used radioisotope in nuclear medicine. The technetium isotope ^{99m}Tc is unusual in that it has a half-life for gamma emission of 6.03 hours. This is extremely long for an electromagnetic decay – more typical is 10^{-16} seconds. With such a long half-life for the excited state leading to this decay, this state is called a *metastable state*, and hence the designation 99m. ^{99m}Tc is easily available, since it can be produced daily by elution from a generator. In addition to the advantage of its short half-life, its low-energy (140 KeV) gamma emission is not accompanied by beta emission, decreasing radiation burden and consequently permitting administration of greater amounts of radioactivity.

^{99m}Tc is produced in radionuclide generators (from molybdenum-99, obtained from a nuclear reactor). These generators are constructed on the principles of the decay–growth relationship between a long-lived parent radionuclide and its short-lived daughter radionuclide. It is very important that the chemical property of the daughter nuclide be distinctly different from that of the parent nuclide, so that the former can be readily separated. The useful life of a generator depends on the parent half-life. A generator provides a supply of short-lived daughter radionuclides as needed until the parent activity is depleted. These radionuclide generators are easily transportable, and serve as sources of short-lived radionuclides in institutions far from the site of any cyclotron. The most commonly generator-produced SPECT isotopes are ^{99m}Tc and ^{113}In.

Technetium-99m is produced by bombarding molybdenum ^{98}Mo with neutrons. The resultant ^{99}Mo decays with a half-life of 66 hours to the metastable state of ^{99m}Tc. This process permits the production of ^{99m}Tc for medical purposes. Since ^{99}Mo is a fission product of ^{235}U fission, it can be separated from the other fission products and used to generate ^{99m}Tc. For medical purposes, the ^{99m}Tc is used in the form of pertechnetate, TcO_4^-.

Since its beginnings in 1958, technetium-99m, a radioactive isotope of the man-made element technetium, has become the most widely used radioisotope for diagnosing diseased organs. Technetium-99m is the favored choice of the medical profession because the type of radiation it emits allows the practitioner to image internal body organs without causing radiation damage. Its half-life of six hours is long enough for a medical examination and short enough to allow a patient to leave the hospital soon afterwards. For instance, technetium-99m is used in 20 million diagnostic nuclear medical procedures per year, half of which are bone scans while the other half are roughly divided between kidney, heart, and lung scans. Approximately 85% of diagnostic imaging procedures in nuclear medicine use this isotope.

Figure 10.1 depicts various chelating agents used for attaching technetium to agents. The resulting radiolabeled compounds are used for imaging a variety of tissue structures, providing information on a variety of pathophysiologic processes, notably hydroxyapatite turnover in bone (used to detect a variety of bone and joint diseases), bilirubin metabolism in the liver (to evaluate gallbladder function), and mitochondrial function in the myocyte (for assessment of coronary artery disease).

Bone imaging remains the most common non-cardiac nuclear imaging study. Figure 10.2 is an example of a patient imaged with ^{99m}Tc-MDP. The phosphonate is incorporated in hydroxyapatite, and areas of increased turnover (darker areas), in this case the surrounding metastatic deposits, are clearly visualized.

Figure 10.3 illustrates other technetium-labeled radiopharmaceuticals currently in use in the clinic. ^{99m}Tc-MAG3 is used routinely for assessment of renal function, particularly in renal transplants [1]. $^{99;m}$Tc-methoxyisobutylisonitrile, also known as sestamibi, is used primarily for detection of myocardial perfusion abnormalities, particularly for detection of myocardial ischemia and infarcts [2]. ^{99m}Tc-sestamibi is also used in the evaluation of breast nodules [3].

Indium-111 and other radiometals

Some molecules do not lend themselves to attachment of ^{99m}Tc. In such cases, radioactive metals may be an attractive option. Moreover, many radioactive metals have attractive imaging characteristics, including suitable physical decay and an abundance of photons. The most widely used radioactive metal is indium-111 (^{111}In). Indium-111 is an electron capture nuclide, i.e., it does not emit a beta particle but instead captures one of the orbital electrons (usually the K electron) in the indium atom. Following the capture of this electron, the resulting cadmium nucleus is left in an excited state and gives off this excess energy by emitting gamma-ray photons.

^{111}In-oxine-labeled leukocytes remain the gold standard for intra-abdominal infection detection [4]. Both platelets and leukocytes can be labeled with ^{111}In-oxine [5]. The primary use of ^{111}In-leukocytes is in the detection of inflammatory diseases and other infections. The In-labeled platelets are used for detecting deep-vein thrombi. ^{111}In-DTPA is most commonly used in cisternography [6, 7].

Indium-111, by virtue of its approximately three-day half-life, particularly lends itself to the study of

Diethylene triamine pentaacetic acid (DTPA)

Pyrophosphoric acid

Tc-labeling core

Methylene diphosphonic acid (MDP)

Figure 10.1. ^{99m}Tc chelating agents.

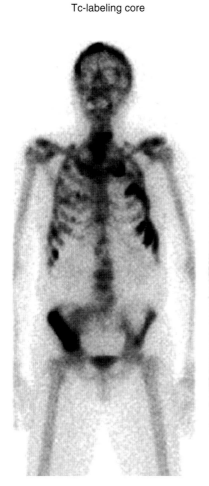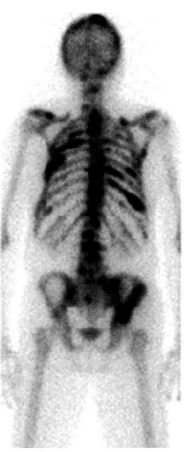

Figure 10.2. ^{99m}Tc-MDP bone scan of skeletal metastasis.

macromolecules that have a long residence time in the body, e.g., antibodies. Figure 10.4 shows an example of a SPECT scan obtained three days after injection of an indium-111 labeled antibody. Targeting of the (radio-active) antibody (arrow, top panel) to disease in the bone (depicted on CT, middle panel, arrow) in this patient with small-cell lung cancer is evident (the bottom image is the SPECT/CT fusion); examination of serial images permits estimates of clearance and uptake characteristics of this macromolecule.

Gallium is another metal that has radioactive iso-topes suitable for imaging. The earliest isotope of gallium to be used was gallium-67 (^{67}Ga). Like other metals, gallium has a high affinity for transferrin, and gallium citrate was found to be useful in evaluating lymphoma as well as identifying sites of infection.

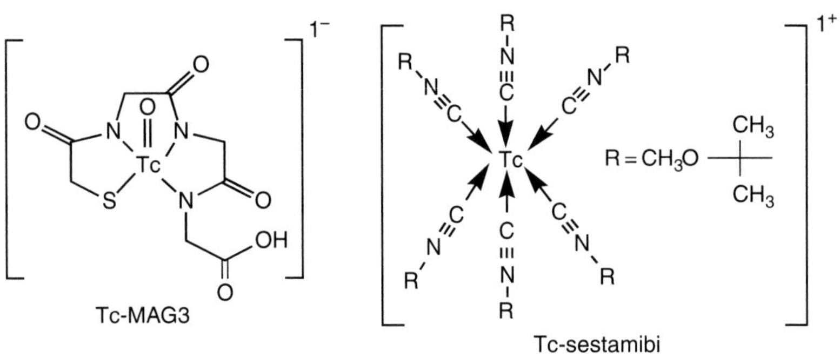

Tc-MAG3

Tc-sestamibi

$R = CH_3O$

Figure 10.3. ^{99m}Tc-labeled radiopharmaceuticals currently in use.

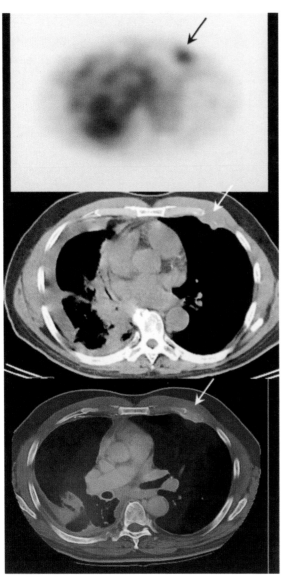

Figure 10.4. ^{111}In-radiolabeled antibody scan of bone metastasis from lung cancer. See text for details.

While its use in lymphoma staging and evaluation has been supplanted by FDG-PET (see below), it remains the gold standard for the imaging of *Pneumocystis carinii* pneumonia (PCP) infection. Figure 10.5 is an example of an image of the head and chest of a patient with PCP. Diffuse uptake of radioactivity in the lungs – characteristic of PCP – is clearly appreciated in the images obtained two days after intravenous injection of gallium-67 citrate.

Two isotopes of gallium, ^{67}Ga and ^{68}Ga, are commonly used. SPECT isotope ^{67}Ga is cyclotron-produced, while PET isotope ^{68}Ga is generator-produced (from a germanium-68 generator).

The chemistry of gallium and indium is similar. Chelating agents commonly used to stabilize indium and gallium at a higher pH *in vitro* include citrate, oxine, DTPA, and EDTA. The Ga^{3+} and In^{3+} undergo ligand exchange from weaker complexes to transferrin in plasma. The chemistry of Ga^{3+} cation is similar to that of indium, and it can form stable complexes with small organic molecules or macromolecules. It is established that macrocyclic chelator, 1,4,7,10-tetraazacyclododecanetetraacetic acid (DOTA), either free or coupled to macromolecules, forms very stable complexes with ^{68}Ga.

Iodine

Radioiodine's importance in nuclear medicine stems from its diverse chemistry and the availability of several isotopes with different physical properties. While iodine-125 is widely used for pre-clinical studies, its relatively weak photon emission precludes its widespread use in the clinic. Iodine-123 is used widely for the evaluation of thyroid disorders. When given orally, iodide accumulates in the thyroid (where it is conjugated to tyrosine to eventually form a thyroid hormone). Iodine-131 has been used as the iodide clinically for several decades, in the detection and therapy of thyroid disorders. Iodine-131, conjugated to a variety of proteins and peptides, is used extensively for imaging biodistribution as well as for therapy.

Sodium iodide ^{123}I is an odorless compound, freely soluble in water. ^{123}I is produced in an accelerator by bombardment of enriched xenon-124 with protons [^{124}Xe (p,2n) ^{123}Cs → ^{123}Xe → ^{123}I]. ^{123}I is well suited for imaging because its gamma energy (159 KeV) is abundant and efficiently detected by sodium iodide crystals. Figure 10.6 is an example of iodine-123 images in a patient with thyroid cancer. The thyroid gland in this patient was surgically removed. An iodine-123 image after surgery revealed small amounts of thyroid tissue in the neck and there was excellent targeting of therapy with ^{131}I, as depicted in an image taken a week after therapy. Note that at this time all radioiodine from normal tissues has cleared, and thus there is no visualization of any other tissue.

Iodination of a molecule is governed primarily by the oxidation state of iodine. In the oxidized form, iodine binds strongly to numerous molecules. Commonly available iodine can be oxidized to I$^+$ by various oxidizing agents. In protein iodination, the phenolic ring of tyrosine is the primary site of iodination. Most of protein iodination occurs between pH 7 and 9.

Iodinated compounds can be prepared by several methods, including isotope exchange, nucleophilic substitution, electrophilic substitution, addition to double bonds, iododemetalation, and conjugation labeling with prosthetic groups. While direct iodination methods are commonly used, there has been increasing development of conjugation labeling, which also increases the stability of a tracer *in vivo*.

Figure 10.7 shows commonly used iodinated radiopharmaceuticals in the clinic. ^{123}I 2-([2-([di-methyl-amino]methyl)phenyl]thio)-5-[^{123}I] iodophenyl-amine (ADAM) is a serotonin transporter radioligand used for neuropsychiatric studies. The primary use of

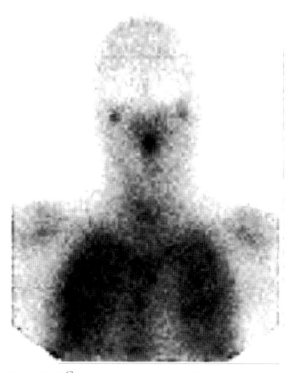

Figure 10.5. ^{67}Ga-citrate scan of pulmonary *Pneumocystis carinii* infection.

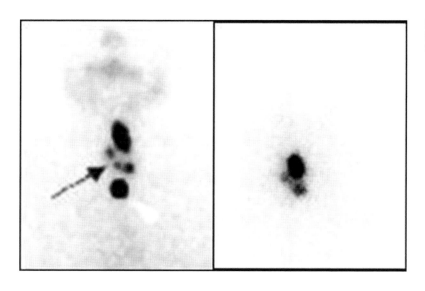

Figure 10.6. ^{123}I diagnostic scan of thyroid cancer (arrow, left) and ^{131}I post-therapeutic scan one week later (right).

Table 10.2. Physical properties of commonly used PET isotopes

Radionuclide	Half-life	Decay modes (%)	Max. β^+ energy (MeV)	Production method
^{11}C	20.4 min	β^+(100)	0.96	^{14}N(p,α)^{11}C
^{13}N	9.96 min	β^+(100)	1.19	^{16}O(p,α)^{13}N
^{15}O	2.03 min	β^+(100)	1.73	^{14}N(d,n)^{15}O
^{18}F	109.8 min	β^+(97) EC (3)	0.635	^{18}O(p,n)^{18}F
^{124}I	4.2 days	β^+(25) EC (75)	2.13	^{124}Te(p,n)^{124}I
^{64}Cu	12.7 h	β^+(19) EC (41)	0.656	^{64}Ni(p,n)^{64}Cu

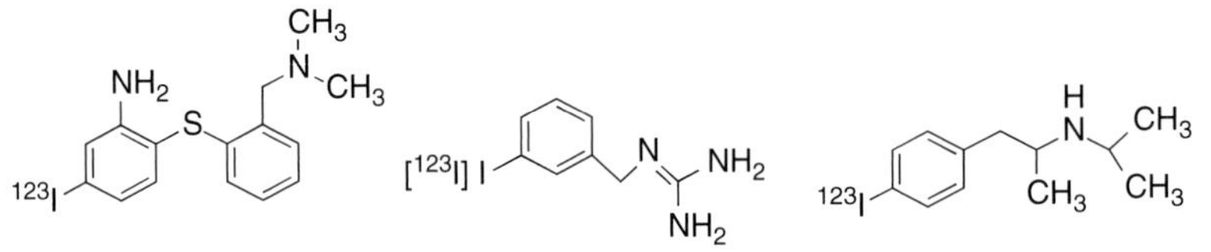

[^{123}I] ADAM

[^{123}I] MIBG

[^{123}I] IMP

Figure 10.7. Common clinical iodinated radiopharmaceuticals.

radioiodinated MIBG is in the detection of pheochromocytoma [8]. ^{123}I-MIBG has also been used in the diagnosis of neuroblastoma followed by treatment with its ^{131}I analog [9]. ^{123}I-d,l-N-Isopropyl-p-iodoamphetamine hydrochloride (IMP) is useful in the evaluation of stroke and similar neurological deficits in the brain [10].

PET agents

General principles of PET agents

PET is a quantitative, non-invasive tool for measuring metabolic and transport processes in the body. The basis of the technique is that a chemical compound of interest is radiolabeled with a short-lived positron-emitting isotope such as ^{11}C or ^{18}F. The compound is then injected into the patient and the distribution of the isotope can be followed as a function of time by detection of the coincident gamma rays emitted when the positron combines with an electron and is annihilated. Some commonly used positron emitters are ^{11}C, ^{13}N, ^{15}O, and ^{18}F (Table 10.2). These are atoms that are found in most biologic agents, thus enabling imaging of *in vivo* distribution. Positron-emitting nuclides lie on the proton-rich side of the line of beta stability and are usually produced by accelerators that bombard targets with charged particles, rather than by using nuclear reactors as a source of neutrons to irradiate targets. A few isotopes used for imaging are also produced by generator-based systems (e.g., rubidium-82, gallium-68).

Fluorine-18 (^{18}F)

Fluorine-18 is the archetypal PET nuclide, much as ^{99m}Tc is for SPECT. The 110-minute half-life of ^{18}F is very convenient for radiopharmaceutical synthesis and for imaging. The half-life further enables centralized production of radiotracers, minimizing the need for in-house cyclotron production. ^{18}F-Fluorodeoxyglucose (FDG) is the most widely used PET tracer and, in the United States, most FDG used clinically is provided by commercial manufacturers. The radionuclide can be produced in two chemical forms, high-specific-activity ^{18}F-fluoride ion and moderate-specific-activity gaseous ^{18}F-fluorine ([^{18}F] F$_2$).

From a purely physical perspective, ^{18}F has the most favorable nuclear properties for imaging with PET. The half-life (110 minutes), high percentage of β^+ emission (97%), and relatively low positron energy (0.635 MeV) make this the ideal PET isotope for high-resolution images. Other favorable features of ^{18}F are that the fluorine atom is small, that it can accept a hydrogen bond, and that the carbon–fluorine bond is very strong.

The chemistry of fluorine-18, however, presents several difficulties. First of all, replacement labeling of molecules that contain fluorine in their structure is uncommon. More common is substitution for another atom by fluorine-18, and this may result in a change of biologic behavior of the molecule. The best-known example of atomic substitution is FDG, which enters the cell in a manner analogous to glucose but does not proceed further down the glycolytic pathway after phosphorylation. Fluorodeoxyglucose-6-phosphate thus

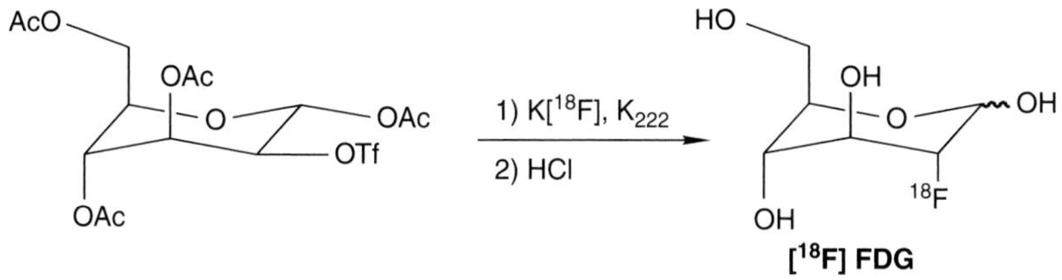

Figure 10.8. An example of nucleophilic conjugation, FDG is the most commonly used PET imaging agent, and has gained increasing acceptance as a cancer detection tool.

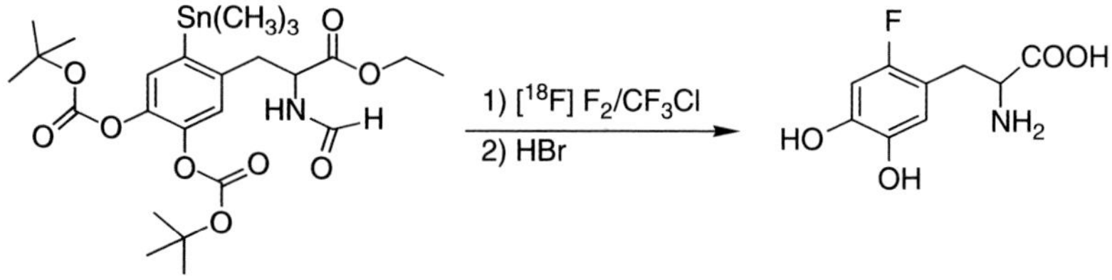

[18F] FDG

Figure 10.9. An example of electrophilic substitution, ^{18}F-DOPA is used for evaluation of Parkinson's disease.

accumulates in the cell, the extent of accumulation being proportional to glycolysis. Thus, fluorine-labeled compounds should not be expected to behave analogously to their parent molecules, and careful biodistribution studies are necessary for such tracers.

Fluorine-18 is produced in two chemical forms with very different behavior. The fluoride for nucleophilic conjugations such as FDG synthesis is obtained via ^{18}O (p,n)^{18}F (Figure 10.8). The target consists of enriched oxygen-18 water (isotopic abundance 0.1%), and the reaction produces large amounts of high-specific-activity ^{18}F. The nuclear reaction ^{20}Ne (d, α) ^{18}F provides fluorine [^{18}F]F$_2$, an extremely reactive electrophilic form obtained with the addition of fluorine-19 carrier in the target (which decreases the specific activity). Such synthesis, as for ^{18}F-DOPA, requires the production of F$_2$ gas, which, in turn, requires deuterons, available only in specialized cyclotrons (Figure 10.9). Specific activity of such compounds is also much lower than that of tracers produced with nucleophilic methods. Other compounds of potential interest as PET imaging agents include thymidine (to measure proliferation) [11], fluoro hydroxyl butyl guanine (for imaging gene expression) [12], fluoro estradiol [13], and testosterone (to measure hormone receptors) [14]. FDG is by far the most common clinical PET radionuclide in use and is used extensively for the evaluation of cancer, many types of which are characterized by high glucose metabolic rates (Figure 10.10).

Carbon-11 (^{11}C)

Carbon-11 has a 20-minute half-life. Labeling of molecules by ^{11}C does not change molecular behavior, thus allowing the drug to be studied in its natural state. The target product for ^{11}C is ^{11}C-CO$_2$, which can either be used directly as a labeling reagent or incorporated in a large number of synthetic precursors such as methyl iodide, methyl triflate, hydrogen cyanide, nitromethane, carbon monoxide, methyl cuprates, and methyl lithium. ^{11}C-methyl iodide is especially valuable because of the large number of molecules that can be labeled by methylation. Figure 10.11 shows representative examples of electrophilic and nucleophilic labeling. The formation of ^{11}C-choline is a typical electrophilic reaction. In nucleophilic reactions, ^{11}C-HCN is generated as a nucleophile for C-C bond formation. Most ^{11}C amino acids are synthesized in this manner. Given its short half-life, radiosynthesis using ^{11}C needs to be rapid, since the specific activity (radioactivity per unit mass) of the final radiopharmaceutical decreases with time. Among other compounds that have been labeled with ^{11}C and studied clinically has been thymidine, a nucleoside analog. Thymidine incorporation is widely considered to be a marker of cell proliferation (Figure 10.12).

Specific activity plays an extremely critical role in radiotracers of agents that have pharmacologic action. A good example is ^{11}C-carfentanil (Figure 10.13). ^{11}C-Carfentanil is routinely used in human studies of opioid dependence, and for investigation of pain [15]. A decrease in specific activity can result in either inadequate radioactivity for satisfactory imaging or administration of mass amounts that cause symptoms of opioid toxicity.

Nitrogen-13 (^{13}N)

The proton irradiation of ^{16}O-water results in formation of ^{13}N in a variety of chemical forms. The desired form, ^{13}N-ammonia, represents only a fraction of the total ^{13}N radioactivity that is produced. ^{13}N-ammonia is formed when ^{13}N atoms abstract hydrogen from water. However, radiolytic oxidation also occurs during cyclotron irradiation of water, and ^{13}N-ammonia is

converted to a large extent to anions such as 13-nitrate or nitrite (up to 85% of total ^{13}N radioactivity [16]. By replacing naturally occurring amines with ^{13}N, researchers have studied their distribution and function, with special emphasis on synthesis of radiolabeled amino acids, and then determined their protein synthesis rate in tumors. Clinically, ^{13}N-ammonia PET is used in the evaluation of myocardial and other tissue perfusion; its very short half-life precludes its use other than in centers with in-house cyclotrons.

Oxygen-15 (^{15}O)

Because of the short half-life of ^{15}O, PET radiopharmaceuticals that are labeled with this nuclide are produced online. Although ^{15}O-oxygen can be used as a PET radiopharmaceutical for measuring tissue oxygen consumption, it is more commonly used to synthesize ^{15}O-water for blood flow imaging (by irradiation of hydrogen and oxygen) or ^{15}O-carbon monoxide for oxygen metabolism. Oxides of nitrogen can also be produced by irradiating mixtures of nitrogen and oxygen.

Iodine-124

Iodine-124 is an isotope of iodine that has suitable characteristics for PET imaging. Its four-day half-life in particular makes it suitable for use as an imaging agent conjugated with macromolecules, in particular antibodies. Figure 10.14 is an example of tumor targeting of ^{124}I-labeled antibody in a patient with a clear-cell kidney cancer.

Radiometals

As outlined above, radiometal-conjugated tracers are frequently used to image biologic processes. The most commonly used metal isotopes for PET imaging are ^{62}Cu, ^{64}Cu, ^{68}Ga, and ^{82}Rb. Except for ^{64}Cu, all of these isotopes are generator-produced and offer the possibility of providing positron emitters for PET scanning

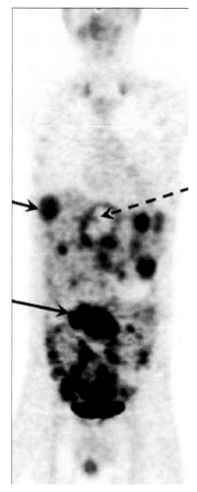

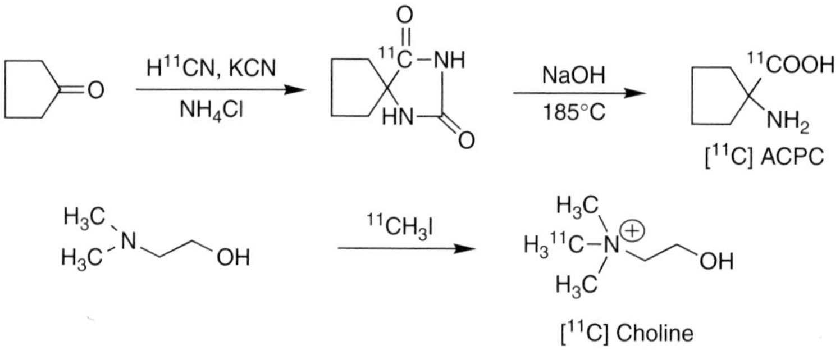

Figure 10.10. Coronal FDG-PET image of a patient with a gastrointestinal stromal tumor. Note the accumulation of FDG in disease in the liver and bowel (arrows). Note also that there is no accumulation of radioactivity in the necrotic central portion of the tumor (broken arrow).

Figure 10.11. ^{11}C nucleophilic labeling of the amino acid, aminocyclopentane-carboxylic acid (ACPC) (top), and electrophilic labeling of choline (bottom). Both compounds are used for imaging tumor metabolism.

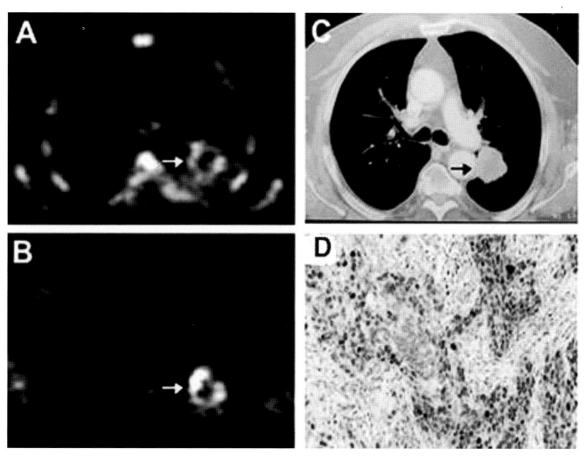

Figure 10.12. (a) Transaxial PET image through a lung tumor demonstrating increased uptake of C-11 thymidine (arrow). Corresponding CT slide (b); and FDG PET (c). (d) Ki-67 immunohistochemistry of the tumor demonstrstes tumor cell proliferation. (Images kindly provided by Anthony Shields, MD, PhD, Karmanos Cancer Institute, Detroit, MI.).

Figure 10.13. ^{11}C-Carfentanil.

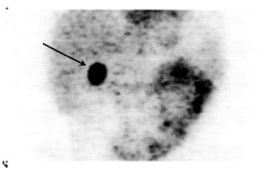

Figure 10.14. ^{124}I-labeled antibody PET scan of kidney cancer (arrow).

in the absence of a cyclotron. A generator containing ^{68}Ge (half-life 287 days) is used for production of the positron emitter ^{68}Ga (half-life 68 minutes), which is formed following electron-capture decay of the parent nuclide, is readily available on demand, and decays by 89% through positron emission, resulting in images with high resolution and potentially accurate quantification.

^{64}Cu has a half-life of 12.701 ± 0.002 hours and decays 17.86 (± 0.14)% by positron emission, 39.0 (± 0.3)% by beta decay, 43.075 (± 0.500)% by electron capture, and 0.475 (± 0.010)% by gamma radiation/ internal conversion. Copper (II) forms mononuclear complexes that are paramagnetic and prefers ligands of

205

sulfur and nitrogen. Using a biomedical cyclotron the $^{64}Ni(p,n)^{64}Cu$ nuclear reaction can produce large quantities of the nuclide with high specific activity. The shorter half-lives and higher positron decay fractions of ^{60}Cu and ^{62}Cu make them suitable for characterizing the faster kinetics of smaller tracer molecules such as copper-diacetyl-bis(N^4-methylthiosemicarbazone) (Cu-ATSM), which is preferentially taken up by hypoxic cells, and copper-pyruvaldehyde-bis(N^4-methylthiosemicarbazone) (Cu-PTSM), a perfusion radiotracer [17]. The longer half-lives of ^{61}Cu and ^{64}Cu are better suited to studying the slower kinetics of labeled peptides, antibodies, and cells.

Strontium (^{82}Sr, half-life 25 days) decays to rubidium (^{82}Rb). Rubidium-82 decays by positron emission and associated gamma emission with a physical half-life of 75 seconds. Rubidium-82 chloride is a myocardial perfusion agent that is useful in the evaluation of blood flow and is used increasingly in the evaluation of myocardial blood flow in patients with coronary artery disease.

Summary

The exponential growth of positron emission tomography has led to an expanding interest and growth in the application of radiotracers in the study of biologic processes *in vivo*. Single-photon-emitting radioligands are also increasingly being used, and their use will continue to grow with the further development of hybrid SPECT/CT devices. Radioligand development is hampered by the constraints on the production of isotopes in cyclotrons, necessitating highly precise controlled physical reactions. Radiochemistry development, while significant, is also constrained by the need to conjugate and purify as well as carry out quality control of the radioligand in a short time period, as determined by the half-life of the radionuclide. Despite these limitations, the growth and development of radioligands has been impressive, leading to an explosion in the non-invasive study of biologic processes *in vivo* using radiopharmaceuticals.

References

1. Kobayashi Y, Usui Y, Shima M. Evaluation of renal function after laparoscopic partial nephrectomy with renal scintigraphy using 99 m-technetium-mercaptoacetyltriglycine. *Int J Urol* 2006; **13**: 1371–4.

2. Tangari A, Fernandes GS, Cattani CAM, *et al.* 99mTc-Sestamibi dipyridamole myocardial perfusion single-photon emission tomography and coronary computed tomography angiography scanning in detection of allograft coronary artery disease after heart transplantation. *Circulation* 2008; **118**: E318–19.

3. Rajkovaca Z, Vuleta G, Matavulj A, Kovacevic P, Ponorac N. 99 m Tc-sestamibi scintimammography in detection of recurrent breast cancer. *Bosn J Basic Med Sci* 2007; **7**: 256–60.

4. Carter NJ, Eustance CN, Barrington SF, O'Doherty MJ, Coakley AJ. Imaging of abdominal infection using 99 mTc stannous fluoride colloid labelled leukocytes. *Nucl Med Commun* 2002; **23**: 153–60.

5. Thakur ML, Riba AL, Gottschalk A, et al. Canine and rabbit platelets labeled with In-111 oxine. *J Nucl Med* 1980; **21**: 597–8.

6. Brusa A, Claudiani F, Meneghini S, Mombelloni P, Piccardo A. Progressive supranuclear palsy and In111 DTPA cisternography. *J Neurol Neurosurg Psychiatry* 1984; **47**: 1238–40.

7. Bai J, Yokoyama K, Kinuya S, *et al.* Radionuclide cisternography in intracranial hypotension syndrome. *Ann Nucl Med* 2002; **16**: 75–8.

8. Havekes B, Lai EW, Corssmit EP, *et al.* Detection and treatment of pheochromocytomas and paragangliomas: current standing of MIBG scintigraphy and future role of PET imaging Q *J Nucl Med Mol Imaging* 2008; **52**: 419–29.

9. DuBois SG, Matthay KK. Radiolabeled metaiodobenzylguanidine for the treatment of neuroblastoma. *Nucl Med Biol* 2008; **35**: S35–48.

10. Ohkuma H, Tanaka M, Kondoh I, Suzuki S. Role of ^{123}I-IMP SPET in the early diagnosis of borderline chronic hydrocephalus after aneurysmal subarachnoid haemorrhage. *Eur J Nucl Med* 2000; **27**: 559–65.

11. Oyama N, Ponde DE, Dence CS, *et al.* Monitoring of therapy in androgen-dependent prostate tumor model by measuring tumor proliferation. *J Nucl Med* 2004; **45**: 519–25.

12. Ponde DE, Dence CS, Schuster DP, Welch MJ. Rapid and reproducible radiosynthesis of [F-18] FHBG. *Nucl Med Biol* 2004; **31**: 133–8.

13. Linden HM, Stekhova SA, Link JM, *et al.* Quantitative fluoroestradiol positron emission tomography imaging predicts response to endocrine treatment in breast cancer. *J Clin Oncol* 2006; **24**: 2793–9.

14. Zanzonico PB, Finn R, Pentlow KS, *et al.* PET-based radiation dosimetry in man of 18F-fluorodihydrotestosterone, a new radiotracer for imaging prostate cancer. *J Nucl Med* 2004; **45**: 1966–71.

15. Jewett DM, Kilbourn MR. In vivo evaluation of new carfentanil based radioligands for the mu opiate receptor *Nucl Med Biol* 2004; **31**: 321–5.

16. Parks NJ, Krohn KA. The synthesis of ^{13}N labeled ammonia, dinitrogen, nitrite and nitrate using a single cyclotron target system. *Int J Appl Radicat Isot* 1978; **29**: 754–6.

17. Padhani A. PET imaging of tumour hypoxia. *Cancer Imaging* 2006; **6**: S117–21.

Image analysis
Human observers

Harold L. Kundel

Image quality

Image quality has a commonsense meaning that most people understand but it is difficult to find agreement about a precise technical definition. Most people rate image sharpness as the most desirable features of a high-quality image, but in medical imaging there is a general consensus that the final arbiter of image quality is diagnostic performance. A high-quality image is one that enables accurate diagnosis by an intelligent observer. There is also general agreement that it is important to be able to evaluate imaging systems objectively in order to set performance standards, optimize system parameters for maximum effectiveness, and determine which of two or more competing systems is best. The concept of task-dependent image quality is very important. The task provides a common ground for the comparison of imaging systems. For example, the performance of two systems that produce images with very different physical properties, such as magnetic resonance imaging and computed tomography, can be compared as long as the diagnostic task is the same.

The two components of an imaging system

It is convenient to think of imaging systems as having two major components: the first converts a radiant signal received from the patient under study into a detected image, and the second consists of image processing devices that convert the detected image into a displayed image with an appearance that is matched to the intelligent decision maker, which for the most part is a human observer. Image quality evaluation starts with measurements of the fidelity of transferring information from the patient to the detected image. Image fidelity depends upon the reproduction of

contrast and detail and the interference of noise. These fundamental system properties are commonly measured as the large-scale transfer characteristic, the spatial resolution properties, and the noise properties [1]. The properties are typically expressed as a signal-to-noise ratio (SNR). Once the physical parameters are determined, the task-dependent performance of the system is evaluated by using observers.

The fundamental properties of contrast and resolution can also be measured using psychophysical techniques, but such measurements, although easily performed, are difficult to use quantitatively because of human bias and variability in reporting the results.

Physical measurement of image quality

The large-scale system transfer characteristic

The large-scale system transfer characteristic determines how the intrinsic contrast in the radiant signal obtained from the object is rendered in the output image. Contrast can be measured in different ways, and when discussing contrast the definition should be made clear. In imaging physics, contrast (C) is usually defined as the difference in the intensity of two regions (I_1 and I_2) divided by the average intensity:

$$C = \frac{I_2 - I_1}{(I_2 + I_1)/2} \qquad (11.1)$$

An example of a large area transfer characteristic is shown in Figure 11.1. In x-ray imaging, the input, shown as the x-coordinate, is the log of the image receptor exposure and the output, shown as the y-coordinate, is the log of the light intensity of the image, which in x-ray film is density. The input–output contrast shown in

---

Introduction to the Science of Medical Imaging, ed. R. Nick Bryan. Published by Cambridge University Press. © Cambridge University Press 2010.

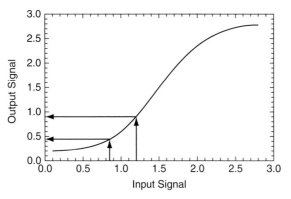

Figure 11.1. An input–output transfer characteristic curve.

Figure 11.1 is not constant because the curve is not linear. At the place shown by the arrows, the contrast is 0.4 for the input (Equation 11.2) and 0.68 for the output (Equation 11.3), indicating a lower image contrast for the contrast in the incoming radiant signal:

$$C_{input} = \frac{1.2 - 0.8}{(1.2 + 0.8)/2} = \frac{0.4}{1.0} = 0.4 \quad (11.2)$$

$$C_{output} = \frac{0.9 - 0.45}{(0.9 + 0.45)/2} = \frac{0.45}{0.675} = 0.68 \quad (11.3)$$

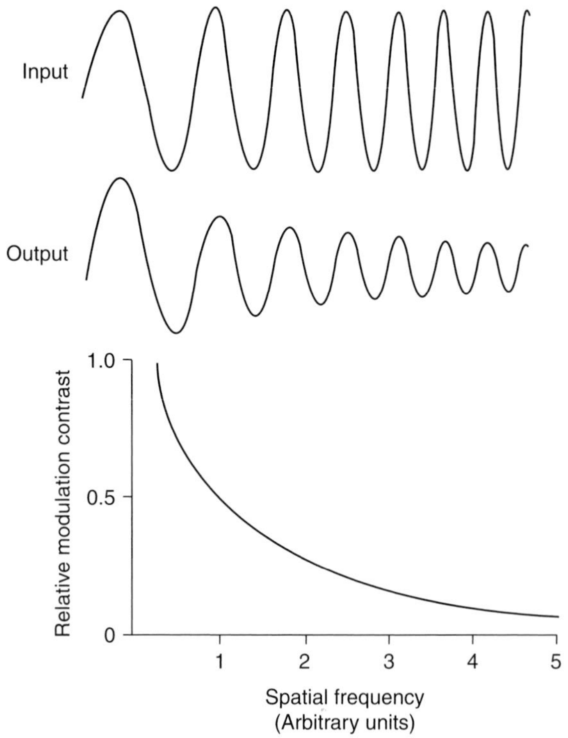

Figure 11.2. Illustration of the modulation transfer function. Input: a sine wave input signal of increasing frequency. Output: the sine wave modulated by passing through the imaging system. Graph: a plot of the modulation of contrast as a function of increasing frequency.

Spatial resolution properties

In medical imaging, spatial resolution is the ability to separate two high-contrast lines. This is expressed as the number of line pairs per millimeter that can be imaged. A line pair consists of a black line and a white space and constitutes one cycle. Thus, spatial resolution is expressed as a frequency with units of cycles per mm. In most imaging systems, the contrast of the signal decreases as the frequency increases. The dependence of the relative contrast or modulation of the signal is expressed as the modulation transfer function (MTF). An example of an input signal consisting of a sine wave of decreasing frequency with the same amplitude at all frequencies and a theoretical output with the amplitude decreasing as the frequency increases is shown in Figure 11.2. The MTF that results from plotting relative amplitude against frequency is shown at the bottom of the figure.

Calculating the MTF of real imaging systems is complicated but easily done in a well-equipped laboratory.

Noise properties

Noise is the random variation in the intensity of the signal from place to place. It is introduced at each stage of the imaging system and is generally cumulative. Noise interferes with both the contrast and the resolution of an imaging system. Imaging noise has a frequency distribution, large-scale perturbations that are low-frequency noise, and fine-grain variations that are high frequency. The noise is usually described as a frequency spectrum called the noise power spectrum (NPS). The presence of noise at one small location in an image (like a pixel in a digital image) may influence the noise in adjacent locations. This effect, known as correlation, must also be considered when noise is measured.

Signal-to-noise ratio (SNR)

When using the basic physical properties to characterize an imaging system, the signal has to be described using the same units as the MTF and the NPS. This means that a relatively simple signal has to be chosen. Nodular masses are very popular because they are easily modeled mathematically and are important clinically as manifestations of cancer. The signal properties and the system properties can be expressed as an SNR, which is shown in narrative style in Equation 11.4, where S is the signal properties expressed in terms of spatial frequency, G is the slope of the large-scale transfer characteristic, MTF is the modulation transfer function, and NPS is the noise power spectrum:

$$SNR^2 = \int \frac{S^2 \, G^2 \, MTF^2}{NPS} \qquad (11.4)$$

This SNR is useful because it can be used to compare different imaging modalities and it is compatible with the SNR derived from measures of the performance of observers detecting the signal in real images [2].

Subjective measures of image quality

Expert opinion

The simplest way to compare image quality is to ask an expert to decide which of two or more images is better. Having experts rank-order images may be a useful simple method for evaluating image quality [3]. However, experts disagree. In fact, when decisions become more difficult because images are similar or ambiguous, they disagree a lot. A consensus panel of experts can produce more reliable results, but the method of arriving at a consensus can drastically change the outcome.

Measures based on visibility

Spatial resolution can be expressed as the number of line pairs per mm visible in a test pattern such as the one shown in Figure 11.3. This value can be deceptive

because, as the bars get closer together, the displayed contrast decreases as illustrated in Figure 11.2.

G. C. E. Burger, a pioneer imaging physicist, tried to overcome this problem by making a test phantom that produced a pattern consisting of disks of decreasing diameter and decreasing contrast, as shown in Figure 11.4(a). An imaging system that added noise would produce a display that looked like Figure 11.4 (b). The noise interferes with the visibility of the disks. Rose [4], who proposed a psychophysical equation that would relate contrast, detail, and noise, used images like those in Figure 11.4(b), and the phantom has been called the Rose phantom or, to give proper credit, the Rose–Burger phantom.

A contrast–detail diagram shown in Figure 11.5 is constructed by asking an observer to indicate the contrast at which a disk of each size is "just visible."

Task-dependent system performance

Imaging tasks

Medical images have many uses, including screening for new disease, following the progress of a known

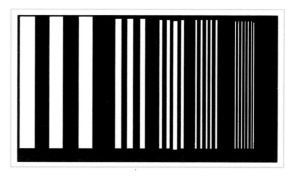

Figure 11.3. An example of a bar pattern used for estimating the threshold spatial resolution of an imaging system. Notice the decrease in contrast as the bars get closer together.

(a)

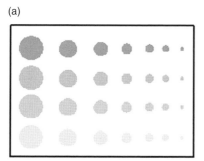

(b)

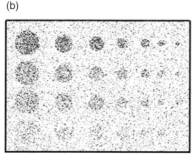

Figure 11.4. The output display of a Rose–Burger phantom. (a) The disks decrease in size and contrast against a basically noise-free background. (b) The same disks with Gaussian noise added to the disks and the background.

disease, and treatment planning. In the context of assessing image quality on the basis of performance, tasks can be divided into estimation and discrimination. Estimation tasks consist of determining the value of some image property such as size, shape, or intensity. Discrimination is the ability to tell two stimuli apart, and this is the task that is specifically addressed by signal detection theory. A list of discrimination tasks is shown in Table 11.1.

Measurement of discrimination

The signal detection theory model

Signal detection theory had its origins in psychology and engineering in the 1950s as an outgrowth of statistical decision theory. It was introduced into diagnostic medicine in the 1960s [5], and only recently has it made its way into the mainstream of biostatistics [6]. The theory is based on a binormal statistical model [7], and is fundamentally a method for quantifying an observer's ability to identify an object with known properties (the signal) that is embedded in a randomly

varying background (the noise). The methodology includes experimental procedures and data analysis, and produces indices of diagnostic performance that separate decision factors from sensory factors.

In its simplest form, the decision maker is presented with a stimulus and must determine if it is noise only or signal plus noise. The decision maker is usually a human, but the theory applies equally to computer decision algorithms. In terms of medical imaging, there is a known disease that is embedded in an anatomical surround; when presented with an image, the decision maker must decide if it contains the disease or is disease-free. This is known as a yes–no decision. Alternatively, the observer is shown two images side-by-side, one with noise only and the other with the signal plus noise and is asked to pick the one with the signal. This is known as a two-alternative forced choice (2AFC) situation. Both methods are used to obtain data that can be analyzed using the signal detection model [7]. The yes–no methodology is used most often in studies of imaging technology and is not restricted to reporting an image as positive or negative but more commonly uses either a continuous or a rating scale. The yes–no situation results in four possible decision outcomes, as shown in Table 11.2.

The fraction of cases in each of the four outcome categories is determined by dividing each outcome by the number of disease or disease-free images, as shown in Table 11.3. For example:

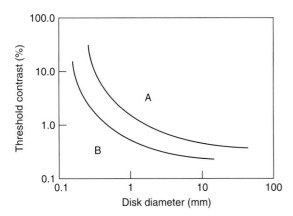

Figure 11.5. Contrast–detail diagram. The graph shows the results obtained from an observer viewing a phantom that produces an image similar to the one shown in Figure 11.4. System B has a contrast–detail performance that is superior to system A.

Table 11.1. Typical discrimination tasks

Task	Description
Detection	Determine if a known stimulus is present
Recognition	Select a particular stimulus among multiple candidates
Identification	Assign a name to a stimulus
Classification	Sort the stimuli into classes
Location	Determine the physical location of a stimulus

Table 11.2. The four elementary decision outcomes

		Response		
		Disease	**Disease-free**	**Number of images**
True state of the image	**Disease**	True positive (TP)	False negative (FN)	Disease images
	Disease-free	False positive (FP)	True negative (TN)	Disease-free images

Table 11.3. The four elementary decision outcomes given the true state of disease

		Response		
		Disease	Disease-free	Total
True state of the image	**Disease**	True positive fraction (TPF)	False negative fraction (FNF)	1.0
	Disease-free	False positive fraction (FPF)	True negative fraction (TNF)	1.0

Table 11.4. Variations in terminology used in decision-making articles

Decision Theory	**Engineering**	**Biostatistics**
True positive fraction	Hit	Sensitivity
True negative fraction	Correct rejection	Specificity
False positive fraction	False alarm	1−Specificity
False negative fraction	Miss	none

Table 11.5. The performance of observers given the task of detecting pneumoconiosis on a set of 200 screening radiographs arranged in order of increasing true positive percentage

	Observer						
	E	C	A	F	G	D	B
True positive percent	57	81	83	85	90	93	94
False positive percent	2	9	9	3	13	18	14

$$\text{True positive fraction (TPF)}$$
$$= \frac{\text{True positive responses (TP)}}{\text{Number of disease images}} \qquad (11.5)$$

A note about terminology

There is a great deal of sometimes confusing terminology in the field of decision making. Statistical decision theory was developed by psychologists studying acoustics and visual perception and by engineers developing radar receivers. Medical decisions were also described independently by biostatisticians. The terminology used, sometimes interchangeably, by the different disciplines is shown in Table 11.4.

The receiver operating characteristic (ROC) curve

The receiver operating characteristic (ROC) curve is a plot of the true positive fraction (TPF) against the false

positive fraction (FPF). It is so central to the analysis of signal detection that the methodology for analyzing decision outcome data is commonly called ROC analysis.

The data in Table 11.5 are taken from a report of a group of seven observers interpreting a series of 200 test films for pneumoconiosis.

Figure 11.6 is a plot of the TPF against the FPF showing the seven data points fitted with a smooth curve. The points are the decision cutoff points between normal and abnormal and are sometimes called "operating points." The curve was not drawn arbitrarily but was fitted to the data points by a computer program using a technique called maximum likelihood estimation. The program computes the parameters necessary for plotting the curve as well as some summary parameters including the area under the curve, which is referred to as AUC or Az (pronounced A sub z by aficionados). The area under the curve or Az for the data in Table 11.5 is 0.95 with a standard error of 0.013 and 95% confidence levels of 0.92 to 0.98.

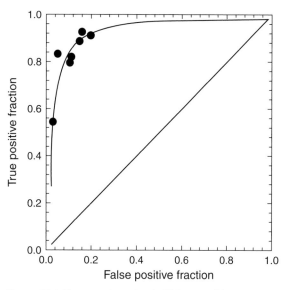

Figure 11.6. The operating points in ROC space of the seven observers whose data are given in Table 11.5, and the ROC curve that best fits the points.

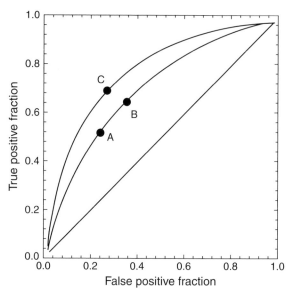

Figure 11.7. Illustration of detectability and bias on ROC curves. Two ROC curves and the operating points of three observers are shown. Observers A and B have the same detectability (AUC = 0.7) but are biased toward positive decisions. Observer A uses decision criteria more stringently than observer B. Observer C has superior detectability (AUC = 0.8) and the same bias as observer B but uses decision criteria more leniently than observer A.

The conclusion that can be drawn from the ROC analysis is that the ability of the observers to discriminate between normal and pneumoconiosis on a chest radiograph is roughly equivalent but that they apply decision criteria very differently. Observer E, with an FPF of 0.02 and a TPF of 0.57, applies criteria very stringently, while observer B, with an FPF of 0.14 and a TPF of 0.94, is more lenient. Observer F, with an FPF of 0.03 and a TPF of 0.85, is an exception who may be operating on a different ROC curve and actually performing better than the rest. The principle is shown in Figure 11.7. A change in performance from point A to point B represents equal detectability but a shift to the application of less stringent decision criteria. A change in performance from point B to point C is an improvement in detectability without a change in the application of decision criteria, while a change from point A to point C represents a change in both. The advantage of the ROC analysis over an analysis of TPF and FPF or of sensitivity and specificity separately is that a single parameter can be used as a summary of performance.

ROC methodology

Most observer performance studies using ROC analysis can be classified as either laboratory tests or field tests. Laboratory tests are most common, and many of them take the form of system stress tests, where a

particular abnormality is chosen to stress some imaging-system property. For example, lung nodules or breast masses have been used to stress contrast discrimination, and the fine linear features of interstitial fibrosis or breast microcalcifications have been used to stress spatial resolution. Field trials usually involve specific diseases, and may be used to compare different imaging modalities. Both types of study require that the diseased images be proven by a method independent of the imaging system being studied. This is clearly more difficult in field tests than in laboratory tests. Once the study objective has been defined, a test set of proven images must be assembled and viewed by a group of trained observers. The observer interprets the case and indicates the diagnosis, either using a rating scale such as definitely abnormal, probably abnormal, possibly abnormal, probably normal, definitely normal, or alternatively using a sliding scale from 1 to 100. The data are then analyzed using one of the available computer programs. The most powerful program is called multi-reader multi-case (MRMC) and uses both the maximum likelihood method to develop ROC curves and an analysis of variance (ANOVA) to compute the final statistics [8].

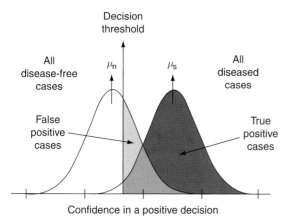

Decision threshold

All disease-free cases

μ_n μ_s

All diseased cases

False positive cases

True positive cases

Confidence in a positive decision

Figure 11.8. The signal detection model. The distribution of diseased and disease-free cases is shown as the decision confidence is varied. The area under the curves to the right of the decision threshold is the TPF and FPF. A plot of the TPF and FPF pairs that result as the decision threshold sweeps along the *x*-axis is a ROC curve. Two normal distributions of equal variance are shown here but are not required.

ROC analysis is limited by the need to have independent proof of the diagnosis, which is often difficult and forces investigators to use expert panels that may not be entirely reliable. It can also deal with just one lesion per image and does not take location accuracy into consideration. Current research is addressing these issues.

The ideal observer

Performing observer studies is expensive and difficult. A mathematical model that predicts performance would be extremely useful for evaluating new equipment, image processing, or methods of computer-aided diagnosis. Although the goal of predicting performance has not as yet been achieved, considerable progress has been made [9]. Signal detection theory is based on a model in which two overlapping normal distributions represent the distribution of noise (disease-free cases) and signal (disease cases) over the confidence in a positive decision (Figure 11.8).

In simple imaging situations where the signal and background noise are known exactly, the properties of the distributions can be calculated. One property in particular, an index of detectability called d' (*d*-prime), has the form of a signal-to-noise ratio:

$$d' = \frac{\mu_s - \mu_n}{\sigma} \tag{11.6}$$

where μ_s is the signal mean, μ_n is the noise mean, and σ is the standard deviation. An ideal observer has full

knowledge of the distributions and uses a decision strategy that maximizes the true positives and minimizes the false positives. An index of detectability for a human observer can be calculated from the output of the ROC analysis. Comparison of the human observer with an ideal observer is an indication of the efficiency of human decision making, and can also show how much room there is for improvement. The index of detectability for the ideal observer and for the human observer can also be compared with the SNR. A fully satisfactory method for the objective assessment of medical imaging performance using human or machine observers has not been developed but there is active research in the field and the modeling approach appears to be the most promising [10].

References

1. Cunningham I. Applied linear systems theory. In: Beutel J, Kundel HL, Van Metter RL, eds. *Handbook of Medical Imaging*. Vol. 1. Bellingham, WA: SPIE Press, 2000: 79–159.

2. Wagner RF, Brown DG. Unified SNR analysis of medical imaging systems. *Phys Med Biol* 1985; **30**: 489–518.

3. Rockette HE, Li W, Brown ML, Britton CA, Towers JT, Gur D. Statistical test to assess rank-order imaging studies. *Acad Radiol* 2001; **8**: 24–30.

4. Rose A, ed. *Vision: Human and Electronic*. New York, NY: Plenum Press, 1973.

5. Lusted LB. Signal detectability and medical decision making. *Science* 1971; **171**: 1217–19.

6. Zhou XH, Obuchowski NA, McClish DK. *Statistical Methods in Diagnostic Medicine*. New York, NY: Wiley, 2002.

7. Macmillan NA, Creelman CD. *Detection Theory: a User's Guide*, 2nd edn. Mahwah, NJ: Lawrence Erlbaum, 2005.

8. Dorfman DD, Berbaum KS, Metz CE. Receiver operating characteristic analysis: generalization to the population of readers and patients with the jackknife method. *Invest Radiol* 1992; **27**: 723–31.

9. Burgess A. Image quality, the ideal observer, and human performance of radiologic detection tasks. *Acad Radiol* 1995; **2**: 522–6.

10. Eckstein MP, Abbey CK, Bochud FO. A practical guide to model observers for visual detection in synthetic and natural noisy images. In: Beutel J, Kundel HL, Van Metter RL, eds. *Handbook of Medical Imaging*. Vol 1. Bellingham, WA: SPIE Press, 2000: 593–628.

Digital image processing: an overview

Jayarama K. Udupa

Characteristics of digital image data

Images produced by most of the current biomedical imaging systems, right from the signal capture and transduction level, are digital in nature. The main purpose of processing such images is to produce qualitative and quantitative information about an object/object system under study by using a digital computer, given multiple, multimodality biomedical images pertaining to the object system under study. As described in other chapters, currently many imaging modalities are available that capture morphological (anatomical), physiological, and molecular information about the object system being studied. The types of objects studied may include rigid (e.g., bones), deformable (e.g., soft-tissue structures), static (e.g., skull), dynamic (e.g., lungs, heart, joints), and conceptual (e.g., activity regions in PET and functional MRI, isodose surfaces in radiation therapy) objects.

Currently, two- and three-dimensional (2D and 3D) images are ubiquitous in biomedicine, e.g., a digital or digitized radiograph (2D), and a volume of tomographic slices of a static object (3D). Four-dimensional (4D) images are also becoming available which may be thought of as comprising sequences of 3D images representing a dynamic object system, e.g., a sequence of 3D CT images of the thorax representing a sufficient number of time points of the cardiac cycle. In most applications, the *object system* of study consists of several static objects. For example, an MRI 3D study of a patient's head may focus on three 3D objects: white matter, gray matter, and cerebrospinal fluid (CSF).

An n-dimensional image will be represented by a pair $I = (C, f)$. In this notation, C is an n-dimensional rectangular array of image elements called the *domain* of I, which constitutes a digitization of the region of the body that is imaged, while f, called the *intensity function* of I, is a mapping that assigns to each element of C an intensity value from a set of numbers, $L = [L_1, L_2]$. The image elements are called *pixels* when $n = 2$ and voxels when $n > 2$. For any voxel $c \in C, f(c)$ represents an estimate of an aggregate value of a specific imaged property of the tissue that is within the region represented by voxel c.

In the above description, the image elements have a single (scalar) value, and hence the image is scalar. When multiple property values are estimated at each element, the intensity function becomes vector-valued and I becomes a vectorial image. For example, in MRI, if T_1-, T_2-, and proton-density-weighted intensity values can be estimated at each voxel for a body region, then we obtain a three-element vectorial image of the body region. Similarly in dual-source CT, I becomes a two-element vectorial image.

Image processing algorithms have to contend with various artifacts appearing in the image arising from imperfections of the imaging device. These may manifest themselves in such a manner as to influence image intensities in a *local* or *global* manner. Some of the common local artifacts are random noise, such as thermal noise in MRI, speckle in ultrasound, scatter in CT, and partial volume effects caused by voxels containing multiple tissues – especially when they are in the boundaries of objects. The common global artifacts are beam hardening streak artifacts in CT, background image non-uniformities arising from magnetic field inhomogeneities in MRI, and varying intensity of gray scales observed in MRI even under the same imaging protocol.

For a given subject under consideration, a variety of images may be acquired for the same body region. In addition to the various artifacts, the resolution of the different images may vary, their intensities may have different meanings, and their voxels may not constitute the same anatomic location. The challenge and goal of image processing are to overcome these

Introduction to the Science of Medical Imaging, ed. R. Nick Bryan. Published by Cambridge University Press. © Cambridge University Press 2010.

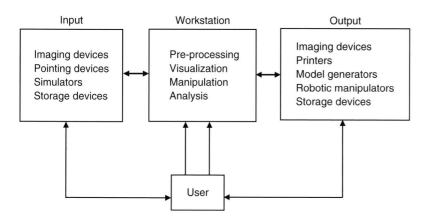

Input | Workstation | Output

Imaging devices
Pointing devices
Simulators
Storage devices

Pre-processing
Visualization
Manipulation
Analysis

Imaging devices
Printers
Model generators
Robotic manipulators
Storage devices

User

Figure 12.1. A schematic representation of CAVA (computer-aided visualization and analysis) systems.

hurdles and to derive qualitative (visualizable) and quantitative (measurable) information that can effectively help in studying the disease condition of the imaged body region of a particular subject.

Classification of image operations

Operations on images may be broadly classified into four groups: pre-processing, visualization, manipulation, and analysis. The *pre-processing* operations either enhance object information captured in a given image or explicitly define boundaries of objects in the image in the form of geometric models. Common pre-processing operations include interpolation, filtering, registration, and segmentation. The *visualization* operations are for viewing and comprehending the object system. The operations include various forms of 2D, 3D, and 4D displays such as slice display, surface rendering, volume rendering, maximum intensity projection, and animated displays to show the dynamic nature of the object system. The *manipulation* operations aim at altering the object models and carrying out virtual surgery and interventions. The goal of *analysis* operations is to derive quantitative information about the objects for depicting their morphology, architecture, physiology, and function. These four groups of operations are highly interdependent. For example, some form of visualization is essential to facilitate the other three groups of operations. Similarly, object definition through an appropriate set of pre-processing operations is vital to the effective 3D visualization, manipulation, and analysis of the objects. The four groups of operations will be collectively referred to as CAVA (computer-aided visualization and analysis) operations throughout this chapter.

The monoscopic or stereoscopic video display monitor of a computer workstation is presently the most commonly used viewing medium to facilitate CAVA operations. However, other media, such as holography and head-mounted displays, are also available. Unlike the 2D computer monitor, holography offers a 3D medium for viewing. The head-mounted displays are basically two miniature monitors presented in front of the two eyes through a helmet-like device that is worn over the head. This offers the sensation of being free from our natural surrounding and immersed in an artificial environment. The computer monitor, however, is by far the most commonly used viewing medium, mainly because of its superior flexibility, speed of interaction, and resolution over other media.

A generic representation of CAVA systems is shown in Figure 12.1. A workstation with appropriate software implementing CAVA operations forms the core of the system. Depending on application, a wide variety of input/output devices are utilized. Considering the core of the system (independent of input/output), the following categorization of CAVA systems can be made: (1) display consoles/workstations provided by imaging device (scanner) vendors; (2) image processing/visualization workstations supplied by other independent vendors; (3) CAVA software provided by software vendors; (4) open-source and controlled open-source software freely available via the Internet. In the rest of this chapter, the commonly used CAVA operations under pre-processing and visualization are described in detail, while those under manipulation and analysis are briefly summarized.

Pre-processing

Given an image $I = (C, f)$ or, a pair of images $I_1 = (C_1, f_1)$ and $I_2 = (C_2, f_2)$, these operations output either a new image $I_o = (C_o, f_o)$ that facilitates creating a computer object model or, more directly, a computer object model S. The commonly used operations are *interpolation*, *filtering*, *registration*, and *segmentation*.

Interpolation

This operation converts a given image $I = (C, f)$ to another image $I_o = (C_o, f_o)$ such that C and C_o cover roughly the same body region and f_o constitutes an "interpolant" of f. Its purpose is to change the level of discretization (sampling) of the input image. Interpolation becomes necessary in the following situations: (1) to change the non-isotropic discretization of the input image to an isotropic or to a desired level of discretization; (2) to represent longitudinal image acquisitions of a patient in a registered common image coordinate system; (3) to represent multimodality images in a registered common image coordinate system; (4) in reslicing the given image. Two classes of methods are available: *image-based* and *object-based*.

Image-based

The intensity of a voxel v in image I_o is determined based on the intensity of voxels in the neighborhood of v in image I. Methods differ in how the neighborhoods are determined and in the form of the functions of the neighboring intensities used to estimate the intensity of v [1]. The simplest situation in 3D interpolation is to estimate new slices between slices of image I keeping the pixel size of image I_o the same as that of I. This leads to a 1D interpolation problem: to estimate the image intensity of any voxel v in image I_o from the intensities of voxels in image I on the two sides of v in the z direction (the direction orthogonal to the slices). In nearest-neighbor interpolation, v is assigned the value of the voxel that is closest to v in image I. In linear interpolation, two voxels v_1 and v_2 on the previous and next adjoining slices, with the same x,y coordinates as that of v, are considered. The value of v is determined based on the assumption that f changes linearly from $f(v_1)$ to $f(v_2)$. In higher-order (such as cubic) interpolations, more neighboring voxels on the two sides of v are considered. When the size of v in I_o is different in all its dimensions from that of voxels in I, the situation becomes more general than that described above. Now, intensities are assumed to vary linearly or as a higher-order polynomial in each of the three directions in I. These operations can be generalized to 4D images as well as to vectorial images.

Object-based

Object information derived from images is used in guiding the interpolation process. In one extreme [2], I is first converted to a "binary" image by a segmentation operation (described later). The idea is that the 1-valued voxels represent the object of interest and the 0-valued voxels denote the rest of the image domain. The "shape" of the region represented by the 1-valued voxels (the object) is then utilized to create an output binary image I_o with similar shape via interpolation. This is done by first converting the binary image back into a gray-valued image by assigning to every voxel in this image a value that represents the shortest distance of the voxel to the boundary between 0- and 1-valued voxels. The 0-voxels are assigned a negative distance value and the 1-voxels are assigned a positive distance. This image is then interpolated using an image-based technique and subsequently converted back to a (interpolated) binary image I_o by setting a threshold at 0. At the other extreme, the shape of the intensity profile of I is itself considered as an "object" to guide interpolation so that this shape is retained as best as possible in I_o [3]. To interpolate a 2D image by this method, for example, it is converted into a 3D surface of intensity profile wherein the height of the surface represents pixel intensities. This (binary) object is then interpolated using the object-based method just described. Several methods in between these extremes exist [4]. The object-based methods have been shown to produce more accurate results than the commonly used image-based methods.

Figure 12.2 shows an example of binary object-based (shape-based) interpolation of a child's skull at "coarse" and "fine" levels of discretization derived from CT data. The original 3D image was first thresholded to create a binary image. This binary image was then interpolated at coarse (Figure 12.2a) and fine (Figure 12.2b) levels and then surface-rendered. A major challenge in interpolation is to identify specific object information and to incorporate the information into the interpolation process to improve its accuracy.

Filtering

This operation converts a given image $I = (C, f)$ to another image $I_o = (C_o, f_o)$ such that $C_o = C$ and f_o represents a filtered version of f. Its purpose is to enhance wanted (object) information and to suppress unwanted (noise/artifact/background/other object) information in the output image. Two classes of filtering

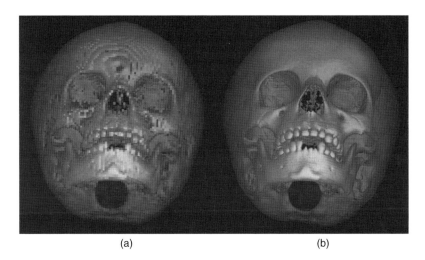

Figure 12.2. Shape-based interpolation. A CT image of a child's skull was thresholded to create a binary image first. (a) This image was then interpolated via the shape-based method at a coarse resolution and was surface-rendered. (b) The binary image was interpolated (shape-based) at a fine resolution and then surface-rendered.

(a)　　　　　　　　　　　　(b)

operations are available: (1) *suppressing*, in which unwanted information is suppressed, hopefully without affecting wanted information, and (2) *enhancing*, in which wanted information is enhanced, hopefully without affecting unwanted information.

The most commonly used suppressing filter is a smoothing operation mainly used for suppressing noise. Here, a voxel v in I_o is assigned an intensity $f_o(v)$ which is a weighted average of the intensities of voxels in the neighborhood of v in I [1]. Methods differ as to how the neighborhoods are determined and how the weights are assigned. One commonly used method is median filtering. In this method, $f_o(v)$ is simply the middle value (median) of the intensities of the voxels in the neighborhood of v in I when they are arranged in an ascending order. In another method [5], a process of diffusion and flow is considered to govern the nature and extent of smoothing. The idea here is that in regions of low rate of change of intensity, voxel intensities diffuse and flow into neighboring regions. This process is prevented, or reduced considerably, by voxels at which the rate of change of intensity is high. The parameter of the conductance function controls the extent of diffusion that takes place. The method is quite effective in overcoming noise and yet sensitive enough not to suppress subtle details and blur edges.

The most commonly used enhancing filter is an edge enhancer [6]. Here, $f_o(v)$ is the rate of change of $f(v)$ or the magnitude of the gradient $\nabla f(v)$ of $f(v)$. Since $f(v)$ is not known in analytic form, various digital approximations of the gradient operator are used to estimate the magnitude of $\nabla f(v)$. The gradient has a magnitude (the rate of change) and a direction in which this change is maximum. For filtering, the direction is usually ignored, although it is used in operations relating to creating three-dimensional renditions depicting surfaces and tissue interfaces portrayed in I. Methods differ in how the digital approximation is arrived at, which is extensively studied in computer vision [6].

Filtering methods have also been developed for reducing the influence of other artifacts referred to earlier, such as intensity non-uniformities, gray-scale non-standardness, streak artifacts, and partial volume effects. These corrective operations may be grouped under either suppressive or enhancive filters.

Figure 12.3 shows an example of a smoothing filter, an edge-enhancing filter, and a non-uniformity correction filter applied to an axial slice of an MR image of a human head, and a sagittal abdominal MRI slice. Most existing suppressing filters often suppress object information, and enhancing filters enhance unwanted information. To minimize these effects, explicit incorporation of object knowledge into these operations becomes necessary, and still remains a challenge.

Registration

This operation takes as input two images I_1 and I_2 or two objects S_1 and S_2 and outputs a transformation T which, when applied to the second image or second object, matches it as best as possible to the first. Its purpose is to combine image/object information from multiple images/modalities/protocols, to determine change, growth, motion, and displacements of objects, and to aid in object identification.

217

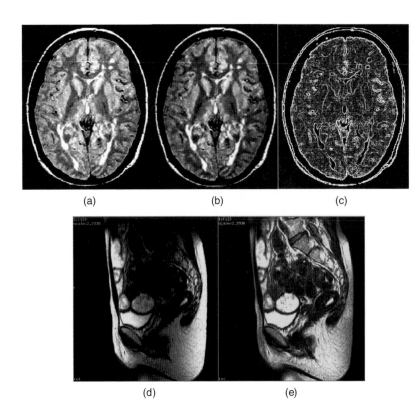

Figure 12.3. Illustration of suppressing and enhancing filtering operations. (a) A proton-density-weighted MRI slice of a human head. (b) The slice in (a) after applying a smoothing diffusion filter [5]; note that noise is suppressed in regions of uniform intensity but edges are not blurred. (c) The slice in (a) after applying an edge-enhancing filter; note that regions of uniform intensity are not enhanced since the gradient in these regions is small. However, the boundaries are enhanced. (d) An abdominal MRI slice with non-uniformity of severe intensity. (e) The image in (d) after filtering to correct for these non-uniformities.

The dimensionality of I_1 and I_2 may not be the same. For example, 2D to 3D matching problems arise in several situations, such as matching a 2D radiographic projection image to a 3D tomographic image. The transformation T may be rigid, described by translations and rotations only. Or it may be affine, involving additional scaling and shear in each of the dimensions. It may also be more complex, involving elastic deformations described by a deformation field which indicates how each voxel of I_2 should move to match with a voxel in I_1. Often T may be an admixture of these different forms of transformations, such as in the situation involving the movement of bones (rigid), connective tissues such as ligaments and tendons (perhaps affine), and soft tissues and fluids (elastic). For a more detailed discussion of registration methods, see Chapter 13.

Segmentation

Given an image I, this operation outputs a set of geometric objects $S_1, \ldots, S_n$ which constitute computer models of object information captured in I. Segmentation consists of two related tasks: *recognition* and *delineation*.

Recognition is the process of determining roughly the whereabouts of the objects in the image. This does not involve the precise specification of the region occupied by the object or of its boundary location. It is a high-level act of indicating, for example, in an MR image of a human brain, "this is the white-matter object, this is the gray-matter object, this is the CSF object, etc." Human-assisted recognition can be accomplished, for example, by using the mouse cursor to point at object regions or to specify seed points, seed curves, or seed surfaces.

Delineation involves determining the object's precise spatial extent and composition, including gradation in the image. If bone is the object system of interest in an image of the knee, for example, then delineation consists of defining the spatial extent of the femur, tibia, fibula, and patella *separately*, and for each voxel in each object specifying an objectness value. Once the objects are defined separately, they can be individually or compositely visualized, manipulated, and analyzed.

Object knowledge usually facilitates its recognition and delineation. Ironically, this implies that segmentation is required for effective object segmentation. As we have observed, segmentation is needed for carrying out most of the pre-processing operations in an optimum fashion since object information, if made available, can enhance those operations. Segmentation is an essential operation for most visualization, manipulation, and analysis tasks also. It is, therefore, the most crucial among all CAVA imaging operations and also the most challenging.

Knowledgeable humans usually outperform computer algorithms in the high-level task of recognition. However, carefully designed computer algorithms outperform humans in precise, accurate, and efficient delineation. Clearly, human delineation that can account for graded object composition (which comes from natural-object material heterogeneity, noise, and various artifacts such as partial volume effects) is impossible. Most of the challenges in completely automating segmentation may be attributed to the shortcomings in computerized recognition techniques, and to the lack of delineation techniques that can incorporate recognition techniques that work synergistically with delineation strategies.

Approaches to recognition

Two classes of methods are available for recognition: automatic and manual.

Automatic (knowledge- and model-based) – Artificial intelligence methods are used to represent knowledge about objects and their relationships [7]. Preliminary delineation is usually needed by these methods to extract object components and to form and test hypotheses related to whole objects. A carefully created "atlas" consisting of a complete description of the geometry and relationship of objects is often used [8]. Some delineation of object components in the given scene is necessary for these methods. This information is used for determining the mapping needed to transform voxels or other geometric elements from the scene space to the atlas. The information is also used in the opposite direction, to deform the atlas so that it matches the delineated object components in the scene. Alternatively, statistical shape models have also been used to facilitate recognition [9].

Human-assisted – Often a simple human assistance is a sufficient recognition aid in solving the recognition problem. This assistance may be in the form of specification of several "seed" voxels inside the 3D region occupied by the object or on its boundary; or indication of a box (or other simple geometric shapes as seed objects) that just encloses the object and that can be quickly specified; or a click of a mouse button to accept a real object (say a lesion) or to reject a false object.

Approaches to delineation

A variety of methods are available for delineation, a number of which have been studied for nearly five decades [10]. Often, delineation is itself considered to be the total segmentation problem and, as such, its solutions are considered to be equivalent to solutions to the entire segmentation problem. It is, however, helpful to distinguish between recognition and delineation for understanding and hopefully solving the difficulties encountered in segmentation. Approaches to delineation can be broadly classified as boundary-based, region-based, and hybrid. *Boundary-based* methods output an object description in the form of a boundary surface that separates the object from the background. The boundary description may be as a hard set of primitives – points, polygons, surface patches, voxels, etc. – or as a fuzzy set of primitives such that each primitive has a grade of "boundariness" associated with it. *Region-based* methods produce an object description in the form of the region occupied by the object. The description may be simply as a (hard) set of voxels, in which case each voxel in the set is considered to contain 100% object material, or as a fuzzy set, in which case membership in each voxel may be any number between 0% and 100%. Prior information about object classes is more easily captured via boundaries than in region description. *Hybrid methods* attempt to combine information about boundaries and regions in seeking a solution to the delineation problem. If we combine the approaches for recognition and delineation, there are 12 possible classes of approaches to segmentation from automatic, hard, boundary-based methods to human-assisted, hybrid, fuzzy strategies. We will now examine some of these strategies briefly.

Hard, boundary-based, automatic methods – The most common technique in this class is *thresholding* and *isosurfacing* [11,12]. A threshold scene intensity is specified, and the surface that separates voxels whose intensity is above the threshold from those whose intensity is below the threshold is computed. Methods differ in how the surface is represented and computed, and in whether or not connectedness of the surface is taken into account. The surface may be represented in terms of voxels, voxel faces, points, triangles, and other surface elements.

219

Fuzzy, boundary-based, automatic methods – Concepts related to fuzzy boundaries, such as connectedness, closure, and orientedness, which are well established for hard boundaries, are difficult and not yet developed. However, computational methods that identify only those voxels of the scene that are in the vicinity of the object boundary and that assign to them a grade of boundariness have been developed [13]. These use image intensity and/or intensity gradient to determine boundary gradation.

Hard, boundary-based, human-assisted methods – The degree of human assistance in these methods ranges from fully manual boundary tracing (manual recognition and delineation) to specifying just a point inside the object or on its boundary (i.e., manual recognition and automatic delineation) [14]. There are many user-assisted methods that fall in between the extremes indicated above and that require different degrees of human assistance for each scene to be segmented [15–17]. In view of the inadequacy of the minimally user-assisted methods referred to above, much effort has been focused on doing recognition more-or-less manually and delineation more-or-less automatically. These methods go under various names: active contours or snakes [15], active surfaces [16], and live-wire/live-lane [17].

In *active contour/surface* methods, an initial boundary is specified, for instance by indicating a rectangle or a rectangular box close to the boundary of interest. The boundary is considered to have certain stiffness properties. Additionally, the given image is considered to exert forces on the boundary dependent on intensity gradients. Within this static mechanical system, the initial boundary deforms and eventually arrives at a shape for which the combined potential energy is the minimum. Unfortunately, the steady-state shape is usually impossible to compute. Further, whatever shape is accepted as an alternative may not match with the desired boundary. In this case, further correction of the boundary may be needed. In *live-wire/live-lane* methods, every pixel edge is considered to represent two oriented and directed edges whose orientation is opposite to each other. The "inside" of the boundary is considered to be to the left of the directed edge, and its "outside" to the right. A cost is assigned to every directed edge based on several factors, such as intensity to the left (inside) and to the right (outside), and intensity gradient and its direction at the edge. The user initially selects a point (pixel vertex) v_o on the boundary of interest. The computer now shows a "live-wire"

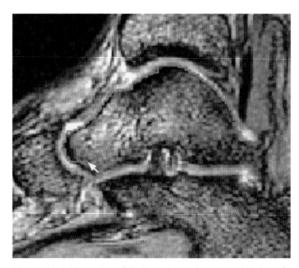

Figure 12.4. Illustration of the live-wire method on an MR slice of a foot. The boundary of interest is the cortical boundary of the talus bone. The contour shown represents one live-wire segment from the first point on the far right to the second point on the far left (arrow).

segment from v_o to the current mouse cursor position v, which is an oriented path (a connected sequence of directed pixel edges) whose total edge cost is the smallest of all paths from v_o to v. As the user changes v through mouse movement, the optimal path is computed and displayed in real time. In particular, if v is on or close to the boundary, the live wire snaps onto the boundary (Figure 12.4). v is now deposited and becomes the new starting point, and the process continues. Typically 2–5 points are sufficient to segment a boundary. This method and its derivatives are shown to be 2–3 times faster and more repeatable than manual tracing. Note that, in this method, recognition is manual but delineation is automatic.

Active shape/appearance model-based methods [9] have gained popularity recently. They differ from active contour methods in an essential way in that statistical information about the boundary geography and shape, their variation, the intensity pattern in the vicinity of the boundary, and its variation are all captured in the model to assist in segmentation. A statistical model is built first from a set of training images by identifying the same homologous set of landmark points on the boundaries and by creating a mean boundary shape from the landmarks, and also by quantifying the variation of the training boundaries around this mean shape. Subsequently, to segment a given image, the model is utilized to search for a location where the model would best fit the image

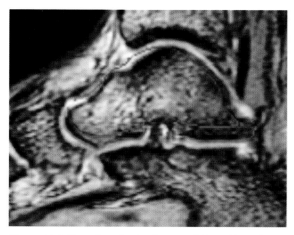

Figure 12.5. Illustration of active shape model-based boundary segmentation of the MR slice of Figure 12.4. The two contours shown represent the initial model contour (red) and the final delineated boundary (green).

evidence for a similarly shaped boundary, and then the mean boundary is deformed locally by moving its landmarks so that the deformed mean boundary matches the local boundary intensity pattern as best as possible. This local adjustment is done in such a way that the deformed mean boundary still falls within the boundary variation observed in the training images and captured in the model. Figure 12.5 illustrates segmentation of the talus in the MR image of Figure 12.4 by using the active shape method.

Hard, region-based, automatic methods – The most common among these methods is *thresholding*. A voxel is considered to belong to the object region if its intensity is at or above a lower threshold and at or below an upper threshold. If the object is the brightest in the scene (e.g., bone in CT images), then only the lower threshold needs to be specified. Another commonly used method is *clustering*. Suppose we determine multiple values associated with every voxel, say the T_2 and proton density (PD) values through MR imaging of the head of a patient, thereby creating a vectorial image. Consider a 2D histogram (often called a scatter plot) of these values – a plot of the number of voxels in the given 3D image for each possible (T_2, PD) value pair. Figure 12.6a shows a pair of T_2, PD slices and Figure 12.6b shows such a histogram. The 2D space of all possible (T_2, PD) value pairs is usually referred to as a *feature space*. The idea in clustering is that feature values corresponding to the objects of interest cluster together in the 2D histogram (feature space). To segment an object, therefore, we need to just

identify and delineate this cluster. In other words, the problem of segmenting the image is converted into the problem of segmenting the 2D image representing the 2D histogram. For the cluster indicated in Figure 12.6b, the object segmented is shown in Figure 12.6c. In addition to the (T_2, PD) values at every voxel, we may also use computed features such as the rate of change of T_2 and of PD values at every voxel or texture measures. In this case, our feature space would be four-dimensional. There is a well-developed body of techniques in the area of pattern recognition for automatically identifying clusters [18], and these have been extensively applied to medical images.

One of the popular cluster identification methods is the *k*-nearest neighbor (*k*NN) technique [18]. Suppose our problem is segmenting the white-matter (WM) region in a 3D MR image of a patient's head, wherein we have imaged for each voxel the T_2 and the PD value. The first step in this method is to identify two sets – X_{WM} and X_{NWM} – of points in the 2D feature space, corresponding to WM and non-WM regions. These will be used as the basis for determining whether or not a voxel in the given image to be segmented belongs to WM. These sets are determined through a "training" set of images. Suppose we previously segmented manually one or more images. Each voxel in the WM and non-WM regions in each image contributes a point to the respective set X_{WM} or X_{NWM}. The next step is to select a value for k, say $k = 7$; k is a parameter in the method and remains fixed. For each voxel v in the given image to be segmented, its location P in the feature space is determined. Then seven points that are "closest" to P from the sets X_{WM} and X_{NWM} are determined. If a majority of these (> 4) are from X_{WM}, then v is considered to be in WM; otherwise v does not belong to WM. Note that thresholding is essentially clustering in a 1D feature space. All clustering methods have parameters whose values need to be somehow determined. If these are fixed in an application, the effectiveness of the method in routine processing cannot be guaranteed, and usually some user assistance becomes necessary eventually for each study.

Fuzzy, region-based, automatic methods – The simplest among these methods is *fuzzy thresholding* [19], which is a generalization of the thresholding idea. It requires the specification of four intensity thresholds, $t_1 \leq t_2 \leq t_3 \leq t_4$, for indicating a trapezoidal function. If the intensity of a voxel v is less than t_1 or greater than t_4, objectness of voxel v is 0. Its objectness

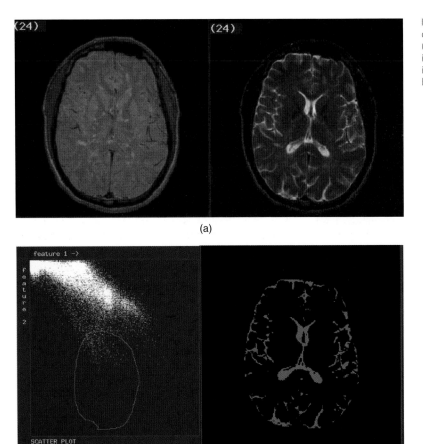

(a)

(b)   **(c)**

Figure 12.6. (a) A T_2 and a PD slice of an MR image of a patient's head. (b) The scatter plot of the slices shown in (a) together with a cluster outline indicated for CSF. (c) The segmented binary slice showing CSF.

is 1 (100%) if its intensity lies between t_2 and t_3. For other intensity values, objectness takes on in-between values. Other functional forms such as a Gaussian have also been used.

Many of the clustering methods can be generalized to output fuzzy object information. For example, in the kNN method described previously, if m out of k points closest to P are from X_{WM}, then the objectness (white-matterness) of v may be set to m/k. The above fuzzy generalization of thresholding is a form of fuzzy clustering. One approach to more generalized fuzzy clustering is the *fuzzy c-means* method [18]. Roughly, the idea is as follows. Suppose that there are two types of tissues to be segmented, say WM and GM, in a 3D MR image, and let the feature space be 2D (T_2 and PD values). Actually, we need to consider three classes: WM, GM, and everything else. In the 2D scatter plot of the given image, therefore, our task is to define three clusters, corresponding to these three classes. The set X of points to which the given image maps in the feature space can be partitioned into three clusters in a large

(although finite) number of ways. The idea in the *hard c-means* method is to choose that particular cluster arrangement for which the sum (over all clusters) of squared distances between points in each cluster and the cluster center is the smallest. In the *fuzzy c-means* method, additionally, each point in X is allowed to have an objectness value that lies between 0 and 1. Now the number of cluster arrangements is infinite. The distance in the criterion to be minimized is modified by the objectness value. Algorithms have been described for both methods to find clusters that approximately minimize the criterion described above.

Hard, region-based, human-assisted methods – The simplest among these techniques is *manual painting* of regions using a mouse-driven paintbrush [20]. This is the region dual of manual boundary tracing. In contrast to this completely manual recognition and delineation scheme, there are methods in which recognition is manual but delineation is automatic. *Region growing* is a popular method in this group. At the start, the user specifies a "seed" voxel within the object region, say by using a mouse pointer on a slice display. A set of criteria for inclusion of a voxel in the object is also specified. For example, (1) the image intensity of the voxel should be within an interval t_1 to t_2; (2) the mean intensity of voxels included in the growing region at any time during the growing process should be within an interval t_3 to t_4; (3) the intensity variance of voxels included in the growing region at any time during the growing process should be within an interval t_5 to t_6. Starting with the seed voxel, its 3D neighbors are examined for inclusion. Those that are included are marked so that they will not be reconsidered for inclusion later. The neighbors of the voxels selected for inclusion are then examined, and so on. The process continues until no more voxels can be selected for inclusion. If we use only criterion (1), and if t_1 and t_2 are fixed during the growing process, then this method outputs essentially a connected component of voxels satisfying a hard threshold interval. Note that, for any combination of criteria (1) to (3), or if t_1 to t_6 are not fixed, it is not possible to guarantee that the set of voxels (object) $O(v_1)$ obtained with a seed voxel v_1 is the same as object $O(v_2)$, where $v_2 \neq v_1$ is a voxel in $O(v_1)$. This lack of theoretical robustness is a problem with many region-based methods.

Fuzzy, region-based, human-assisted methods – An example in this group is the *fuzzy connectedness* technique. In this method, recognition is manual and involves pointing at an object in a slice display. Delineation is automatic and takes into account both the characteristics of intensity gradation and how these gradations hang together in an object. It has been effectively applied in several large applications [21]. In this method, every pair (v_1, v_2) of nearby voxels in an image is assigned a *fuzzy affinity* relationship which indicates how v_1 and v_2 hang together locally in the same object. The strength of this relationship (varying between 0 and 1) is a function of how close v_1 and v_2 are spatially, how similar their intensity values are, and how close these intensities are to an intensity expected for the object. Affinity expresses the degree to which voxels "hang together" locally. The real "hanging-togetherness" of voxels in a global sense is captured through a fuzzy relationship called *fuzzy connectedness*. To any pair of voxels (v_1, v_2) in the image that may not be nearby, a strength of connectedness is assigned as follows. There are numerous possible paths between v_1 and v_2. A path from v_1 to v_2 is a sequence of voxels starting from v_1 and ending on v_2, the successive voxels being nearby. The "strength" of

a path is simply the smallest of the affinities associated with pairs of successive voxels along the path. The strength of connectedness between v_1 and v_2 is simply the largest of the strengths associated with all possible paths between v_1 and v_2. A *fuzzy object* is a pool of voxels held together with a membership (between 0 and 1) assigned to each voxel that represents its "objectness." The pool is such that the strength of connectedness between any two voxels in the pool is greater than a threshold value, and the strength between any two voxels, one in the pool and the other not in the pool, is less than the threshold value. A wide variety of application-specific knowledge of image characteristics can be incorporated into the affinity relation. Figure 12.7 shows an example of fuzzy-connected segmentation (in 3D) of a contrast-enhanced MRA dataset and a rendition of the 3D fuzzy-connected vessel tree with the arteries and veins separated.

Hybrid strategies – These methods (e.g., [22]) try to synergistically combine the strengths of boundary-based and region-based methods, with the hope of overcoming the individual weaknesses of each by the strengths of the other. The current trend seems to be toward combining model-based (such as active shape) methods with region-based methods.

The challenges in the variety of approaches and methods of delineation are to: (1) develop general segmentation methods that can be easily and quickly adapted to a given application; (2) keep the human assistance required on a per-image basis to a minimum; (3) develop fuzzy and statistical methods that can realistically handle uncertainties in data and prior knowledge about object families; (4) assess the efficacy of segmentation methods.

Visualization

Given an image I or a set of objects $S_1, ..., S_n$, these operations create renditions which are 2D images depicting the object information captured in I or in $S_1, ..., S_n$. Their purpose is to facilitate the visual perception of object information portrayed in the given image or objects. Two classes of approaches are available: *image-based* and *object-based*.

Image-based methods

In this approach, renditions are created directly from the given image I. Two further subclasses may be identified: *slice mode* and *volume mode*.

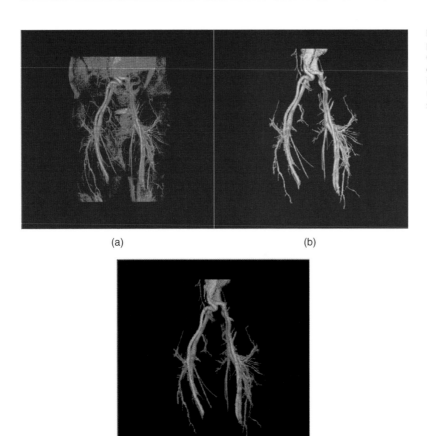

(a) (b)

(c)

Figure 12.7. (a) A maximum-intensity projection 3D rendition of an MRA image. (b) A volume rendition of the 3D fuzzy-connected vessels detected from the image rendered in (a). (c) A volume rendition of the arteries and veins separated via fuzzy connectedness.

Slice mode

Methods differ based on *what* is considered to constitute a "slice" and *how* this information is displayed. *What*: natural slices (axial, coronal, sagittal), oblique/curved slices; these various forms of "slices" are computed from *I* via interpolation. *How*: montage, roam through/fly through, gray-scale/pseudo-color display; the computed "slices" are then displayed in one of these forms.

As an example of the slice mode of display, Figure 12.8 shows a pseudo-color display of the "same" MR slice of a multiple sclerosis patient's brain obtained at two different longitudinal time instances (and subsequently registered). The two slices corresponding to the two time instances are assigned red and green hues. Where the slices match perfectly or where there has been no change (in, say, the lesions), the display shows yellow because of the combination of red and green. At other places, either red or green is observed.

Volume mode

In this mode, *what* is displayed and *how* it is done are as follows. *What*: surfaces, interfaces, intensity distributions. *How*: maximum intensity projection (MIP), surface rendering, volume rendering. Surfaces and interfaces are not explicitly computed from *I* as an intermediate object, but are displayed directly from *I* on the fly.

In any of these methods, a technique of *projection* is needed to go from the higher-dimensional scene to the 2D screen of the monitor. Two approaches are pursued: *ray casting*, which consists of tracing a line perpendicular to the viewing plane from every pixel in the viewing plane into the image domain, and *voxel projection*, which consists of directly projecting voxels encountered along the projection line from the image onto the viewing plane. Either of these projection methods may be used in the rendering methods described below. Voxel projection is generally considerably faster than ray casting.

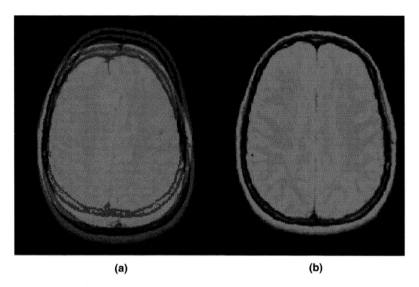

(a)   (b)

Figure 12.8. (a) Illustration of pseudo-color display. Approximately the same MR slice of a patient's head taken at two different times, one displayed in green and the other in red. Where there is a match, the display appears yellow. Green and red indicate mismatch. (b) The same slice displayed after registration. Now green and red indicate either a registration error or change in an object such as a lesion between the two time instances.

Maximum intensity projection (MIP) – In these methods [23], the intensity assigned to a pixel in the rendition is simply the maximum of the scene intensity encountered along the projection line. Figure 12.7 shows its application to MRA. This is the simplest 3D rendering technique. It is most effective when the objects of interest are the brightest in the image, they have simple 3D morphology, and they have minimal gradation of intensity values. Contrast-enhanced CT angiography and MRA are ideal applications for this method. By appropriately mapping the image intensity onto a new gray scale, so that the intensities in the object of interest appear with the highest intensity in the new scale, irrespective of whether they are intermediate or low value in the given image, the MIP idea can be generalized to render objects of any intensity. The main advantage of MIP is that it requires no segmentation. However, the ideal conditions mentioned earlier frequently go unfulfilled due to the presence of other bright objects such as clutter from surface coils in MR angiography, bone in CT angiography, or other obscuring vessels that may not be of interest. Consequently, some segmentation eventually becomes necessary.

Image-based surface rendering – In these methods [24], object surfaces are portrayed in the rendition directly from the given image. A threshold interval must be specified to indicate the object of interest in the given image. Clearly, the speed of rendering is of utmost importance here since the idea is that object renditions are created interactively directly from the image as the threshold is changed. Instead of thresholding, any automatic, hard boundary- or

region-based segmentation method can be used. However, in this case, the parameters of the method will have to be specified interactively, and segmentation and rendition should be at sufficient speed for this mode of visualization to be useful. Although at present rendering based on thresholding can be accomplished in about 0.01–0.1 seconds on a 2 GHz Pentium PC using appropriate algorithms in software [20], more sophisticated segmentation methods (such as kNN) may not offer interactive speed.

The actual rendering itself consists of the following three basic steps: *projection, hidden-part removal,* and *shading*. These are needed to impart a sense of three-dimensionality to the rendered image that is created. Additional cues for three-dimensionality may be provided by techniques such as stereoscopic display, motion parallax by rotation of the objects, shadowing, and texture mapping. If ray casting is the method of projection chosen, then *hidden-part removal* is done by stopping at the first voxel encountered along each ray that satisfies the threshold criterion. The value (shading) assigned to the pixel (in the viewing plane) corresponding to the ray is determined as described below. If voxel projection is used, hidden parts can be removed by projecting voxels from the furthest to the closest (with respect to the viewing plane) and always overwriting the shading value, which can be achieved in a number of computationally efficient ways.

The *shading* value assigned to a pixel p in the viewing plane is dependent on the voxel v that is eventually projected onto p. The faithfulness with which this value reflects the shape of the surface around v depends to a large extent on the surface normal vector estimated at v.

225

Two classes of methods are available for this purpose: *object-based* and *image-based*. In object-based methods, the vector is determined purely from the geometry of the shape of the surface in the vicinity of v. In image-based, the vector is considered to be the gradient of the given image at v; that is, the direction of the vector is the same as the direction in which image intensity changes most rapidly at v. Given the normal vector N at v, the shading assigned to p is determined usually as $[f_d(v, N, L) + f_s(v, N, L, V)] f_D(v)$. Here f_d is the *diffuse component* of reflection, f_s is the *specular component*, f_D is a component that depends on the distance of v from the viewing plane, and L and V are unit vectors indicating the direction of the incident light and the viewing rays. The diffuse component is independent of the viewing direction, but depends only on L (as a cosine of the angle between L and N). It captures the scattering property of the surface. The specular component captures surface shininess. It is maximum in the direction of ideal reflection R whose angle with N is equal to the angle between L and N. This reflection dies off as a cosine function on either side of R. By weighting the three components in different ways, different shading effects can be created.

Image-based volume rendering – In image-based surface rendering, a hard object is implicitly created and rendered on the fly from the given image. In image-based volume rendering [19], a fuzzy object is implicitly created and rendered on the fly from the given image. Clearly, surface rendering becomes a particular case of volume rendering. The central idea in volume rendering is to assign an opacity to every voxel in the image that takes on any value in the range 0% to 100%. The opacity value is determined based on the objectness value at the voxel and how prominently we wish to portray this particular grade of objectness in the rendition. This opacity assignment is specified interactively via an opacity function, such as the trapezoidal function mentioned earlier. Here, the value of the function now indicates percentage opacity. Every voxel is now considered to *transmit*, *emit*, and *reflect* light. Our goal is to determine the amount of light reaching every pixel in the viewing plane. The amount of transmission depends on the opacity of the voxel. Its emission depends on its objectness, and hence on opacity. The greater the objectness, the greater is the emission. Its reflection depends on the strength of the surface. The greater the strength, the greater is the reflection. Just as in surface rendering, there are three basic steps: projection, hidden-part

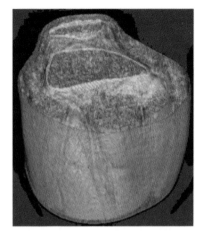

Figure 12.9. A rendition of bone and soft tissue which are segmented by using fuzzy thresholding of the CT scene of a subject's knee.

removal, shading or compositing. The principles underlying *projection* are identical to those described under surface rendering.

Hidden-part removal is much more complicated than in surface rendering. In ray casting, a common method is to discard all voxels along the ray from the viewing plane beyond a point at which the "cumulative opacity" is above a high threshold (say 90%) [25]. In voxel projection, in addition to a similar idea, a voxel can be discarded if the voxels surrounding it in the direction of the viewing ray have "high" opacity. The *shading* operation, more appropriately called *compositing*, is more complicated than for surface rendering. It has to take into account all three components – transmission, reflection, and emission. We may start from the voxel furthest from the viewing plane along each ray and work toward the front, calculating for each voxel its output light. The net light output by the voxel closest to the viewing plane is assigned to the pixel associated with the ray. Instead of this back-to-front strategy, calculations can be done from front to back, which is actually shown to be faster than the former.

As with surface rendering, voxel projection methods for volume rendering are substantially faster than ray casting. Figure 12.9 shows a CT knee dataset rendered by using this method, wherein two types of tissues – bone and soft tissue – have been identified, each with a separate trapezoidal function.

Object-based methods

In these methods of visualization, objects (hard or fuzzy) are explicitly defined first and then rendered.

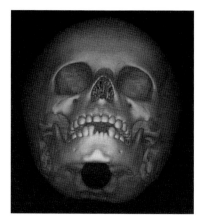

Figure 12.10. An object-based surface rendition of the skull of a child by using triangles to represent the surface.

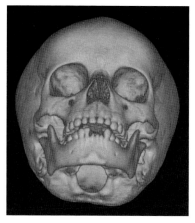

Figure 12.11. An object-based volume rendition of the data of Figure 12.10. A fuzzy object representation was first obtained by using fuzzy thresholding.

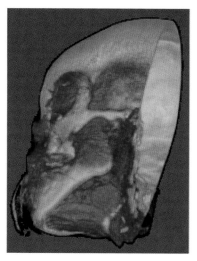

Figure 12.12. Object-based volume rendering of bone and soft tissues. Bone and soft-tissue structures (muscles) were detected as separate 3D fuzzy connected objects from a craniofacial 3D CT image. Skin is effectively peeled off because of its weak connectedness to muscles.

In difficult segmentation situations, or when segmentation is time-consuming or when it has too many parameters, it is not practical to do direct image-based rendering. The intermediate step of completing object definition then becomes necessary. Depending on whether the object definition method is hard or fuzzy, we have object-based surface and volume rendering methods, respectively.

Object-based surface rendering – These methods take as input hard object descriptions and create renditions. The methods of projection, hidden-part removal, and shading are similar to those described under image-based surface rendering. The only difference here is that a variety of surface description methods have been investigated by using voxels, voxel faces [26], triangles [12], and other surface patches. Therefore, the projection methods that are appropriate for the specific surface elements have been developed. Figure 12.2b shows a rendition of a child's skull based on voxels, while the same object is rendered by using triangles in Figure 12.10. Object-based surface rendering of large surfaces consisting of 10 million voxels/triangles can be done at the rate of about 10–20 frames per second on modern PCs (2 GHz Pentium) entirely in software, which is about 10–30 times faster than rendering the same surfaces in hardware rendering engines.

Object-based volume rendering – These methods take as input fuzzy object descriptions, which are in the form of a set of voxels wherein each voxel has an objectness value and a number of other parameters, such as gradient magnitude, associated with it. Since the object description is more compact than the original image, and since additional information to speed up computation can be stored as part of the object description, volume rendering based on fuzzy object descriptions can be done at interactive speeds on modern PCs entirely in software. Figure 12.11 shows a fuzzy object rendition of the dataset in Figure 12.10. Figure 12.12 shows a rendition of craniofacial bone and soft tissue both of which have been defined separately by using the fuzzy connected methods described earlier. If we used a direct image-based volume rendering method, then the skin would become inseparable from other soft tissues and would always obscure the rendition of muscles and neurovascular structures.

227

Several erroneous statements relating to visualization appear in the literature, with the following being the most frequent areas of confusion:

(1) *Surface rendering equated to thresholding.* Clearly, thresholding is only one (actually the simplest) of the many available hard region- and boundary-based segmentation methods, the output of any of which can be surface rendered.

(2) *Volume rendering not requiring segmentation.* The phrase "volume rendering" is very general and is used in different senses. This is clarified below. In whatever sense it is taken, it is not right to suggest that volume rendering does not require segmentation. The only useful volume rendering/visualization technique that does not require segmentation of any sort is maximum intensity projection. The opacity assignment schemes described under image-based visualization are clearly fuzzy segmentation strategies, and they face the same problems that any segmentation method encounters. Note how unconvincing it is to say that opacity functions such as the trapezoidal function do not represent segmentation, when its particular manifestation when $t_1 = t_2$ and $t_3 = t_4$, which corresponds to thresholding, is indeed segmentation.

(3) *The meaning of volume rendering.* The meaning conveyed by the phrase "volume rendering" varies quite a bit in the literature. Frequently, it is used to refer to any image-based rendering techniques, hard as well as fuzzy. It is also used to refer to object-based rendering techniques. In the general sense, clearly the slice mode of visualization is also captured within this phrase. It is better to reserve this term to refer only to fuzzy object rendering, whether it is done via image-based or object-based methods, but not to hard object-rendering methods.

Among the challenges of visualization is the fact that the pre-processing operations and subsequently the visualization operations can be applied in many different sequences to get to the desired end result. For example, the sequence filtering → interpolation → segmentation → rendering may produce significantly different renditions from those produced by interpolation → segmentation → filtering → rendering. Considering the different methods for each operation and the parameters associated with each operation, there is a large number of ways of producing the desired end results. A systematic study is needed to understand what combination of operations is best for a given application. Usually, whatever fixed combination is provided by the CAVA system is taken to be the best for the application. Because of these variations, objective comparison of visualization methods becomes a daunting task. A further challenge is to achieve realistic tissue display including color, texture, and surface properties.

Manipulation

The main purpose of these operations, *given* an object system, is to *create* another object system by altering the individual objects or their relationship in the system. The main motivation for these operations is to simulate surgical procedures based on patient-specific image data, and to develop aids for interventional and therapy procedures. Compared to pre-processing and visualization, work on manipulation is quite meager. Operations to *cut*, *separate*, *add*, *subtract*, *move*, *mirror*, *stretch*, *compress*, *bend* objects and their components have been developed. The idea here is that the user directly interacts with an object-based surface or volume rendition of the object system to execute these operations. Clearly, for the operations to be practically useful, they should be executable at interactive speeds.

Analysis

The main purpose of these operations, *given* a set of images $I_1, …, I_m$ or an object system $S_1, …, S_n$ pertaining to a body region under study, is to *generate* a quantitative description of the morphology, architecture, and function of the object system in the body region. The goal of many CAVA applications is analysis of an object system. Although visualization is used as a visual aid, that in itself is not always the end goal. As such, many of the current application-driven works are in analysis. As in other operations, we may classify them into two groups: *image-based* and *object-based*. In image-based methods, the quantitative description is based directly on image intensities. Examples of measures include ROI statistics, density, activity, kinetics, perfusion, and flow. Object structural information derived from another modality is often used to guide the selection of regions for these measurements. In object-based methods, the quantitative description is obtained from the objects based on their morphology, their architecture, how they change with time, or on the relationship between and among objects in the system – and how that changes. Examples of measures include distance, length, curvature, area, volume, kinematics, and mechanics.

In summary, there appears to be a dichotomy that is pervasive in all CAVA operations, namely that these operations may be image-based or object-based. The challenges encountered in most CAVA operations are attributable to the difficulties encountered in image segmentation, since object information is vital for filtering, interpolation, registration, detection, realistic rendering, manipulation, and analysis. Currently most of the efforts in CAVA technology are focused on segmentation, registration, and analysis. Future research in image segmentation is likely to explore more hybrid strategies to investigate how best to combine prior object models and the information that can be best extracted from the given image.

References

1. Udupa JK, Herman GT, eds. *3D Imaging in Medicine*, 2nd edn. Boca Raton, FL: CRC Press, 2000.

2. Raya SP, Udupa JK. Shape-based interpolation of multidimensional objects. *IEEE Trans Med Imag* 1990; **9**: 32–42.

3. Grevera GJ, Udupa JK. Shape-based interpolation of multidimensional grey-level images. *IEEE Trans Med Imag* 1996; **15**: 882–92.

4. Goshtasby A, Turner DA, Ackerman LV. Matching tomographic slices for interpolation. *IEEE Trans Med Imag* 1992; **11**: 507–6.

5. Gerig G, Kübler O, Kikinis R, Jolesz FA. Nonlinear anisotropic filtering of MRI data. *IEEE Trans Med Imag* 1992; **11**: 221–32.

6. Sonka M, Hlavac V, Boyle R. *Image Processing, Analysis, and Machine Vision*, 2nd edn. Pacific Grove, CA: Brooks/Cole, 1999.

7. Gong L, Kulikowski C. Comparison of image analysis processes through object-centered hierarchical planning. *IEEE Trans PAMI* 1995; **17**: 997–1008.

8. Christensen GE, Rabbitt R, Miller MI. 3-D brain mapping using a deformable neuroanatomy. *Phys Med Biol* 1994; **39**: 609–18.

9. Cootes TF, Taylor CJ, Cooper DH, Graham J. Active shape models: their training and application. *Comput Vision Imag Und* 1995; **61**: 38–59.

10. Doyle, W. Operations useful for similarity-invariant pattern recognition, *J ACM* 1962; **9**: 259–67.

11. Udupa JK, Srihari S, Herman GT. Boundary detection in multidimensions. *IEEE Trans PAMI* 1982; **4**: 41–50.

12. Lorensen W, Cline H. Marching cubes: a high resolution 3D surface construction algorithm. *Comput Graph* 1989; **23**: 185–94.

13. Levoy M. Display of surfaces from volume data. *IEEE Comput Graph Appl* 1988; **8**: 29–37.

14. Herman GT, Liu HK. Dynamic boundary surface detection. *Comput Graph Image Proc* 1978; **7**: 130–8.

15. Kass M, Witkin A, Terzopoulous D. Snakes: active contour models. *Int J Comput Vision* 1987; **1**: 321–31.

16. Cohen I, Cohen LD, Ayache N. Using deformable surfaces to segment 3-D images and infer differential structures. *CVGIP Image Understand* 1992; **56**: 242–63.

17. Falcao A, Udupa JK, Samarasekera S, *et al.* User-steered image segmentation paradigms: live wire and live lane. *Graph Mod Imag Proc* 1998; **60**: 233–60.

18. Duda RO, Hart PE, Stork DG. *Pattern Classification*. New York, NY: Wiley, 2001.

19. Drebin R, Carpenter L, Hanrahan P. Volume rendering. *Comput Graph* 1988; **22**: 65–74.

20. Udupa J K, Odhner D, Samarasekera S, *et al.* 3DVIEWNIX: an open transportable, multidimensional, multimodality, multiparametric imaging software system. *SPIE Proc* 1994; **2164**: 58–73.

21. Udupa JK, Saha PK. Fuzzy connectedness in image segmentation. *Proce IEEE* 2003; **91**: 1649–99.

22. Chu S, Yuille A. Region competition: unifying snakes, region growing and Bayes/MDL for multi-band image segmentation. *IEEE Trans PAMI* 1996; **18**: 884–900.

23. Napel S, Marks MP, Rubin GD, *et al.* CT angiography with spiral CT and maximum intensity projection. *Radiology* 1992; **185**: 607–10.

24. Goldwasser S, Reynolds R. Real-time display and manipulation of 3-D medical objects: the voxel machine architecture. *Comput Vision Graph Imag Proc* 1987; **39**: 1–27.

25. Levoy M. Display of surfaces from volume data. *ACM Trans Graph* 1990; **9**: 245–71.

26. Herman GT, Udupa JK. Display of 3-D information in 3-D digital images: computational foundations and medical application. *IEEE Comput Graph Appl* 1983; **3**: 39–46.

Chapter 13

Registration and atlas building

James C. Gee

Spurred by the advent of *in vivo* imaging methods, computational anatomy, in particular the development of digital atlases, has emerged over the last decade as a major discipline in biomedical science [1], engaging diverse fields such as computer science, mathematics, signal processing, and statistics. This new field is greatly advancing medical research, basic biological science, and clinical practice. An atlas may be used as an instance of anatomy upon which teaching or surgical planning is based, a reference frame for understanding the normal and pathological variation of anatomy, a coordinate system for functional localization studies, and as a probabilistic space into which functional or structural features are mapped. Within the context of bioinformatics, the atlas serves as the mechanism through which novel sources of spatially indexed or image-based information may be linked with other databases in order that new relationships may be derived. In this chapter, we introduce the technology involved in constructing digital atlases, most notably image registration, and highlight some of the most promising applications in biomedicine, with particular focus on contemporary brain mapping research.

Brain mapping

One of the greatest challenges facing modern science has been the task of relating the functions of the mind to the structures of the brain. Success in this endeavor was long recognized as a prerequisite for both basic understanding and progress towards treatments for a range of neurological and psychiatric disorders. The development of *in vivo* structural and functional neuroimaging – primarily via magnetic resonance imaging (MRI) – suddenly promises to bring such results to reality. However, the adoption of this new and powerful tool into brain studies has highlighted the need for a reference neuroanatomic template. Such a resource is critical for several reasons:

- All brains are to a certain degree different in structure from one another. If comparisons are to be made, it is necessary to have a common anatomic substrate as a reference. Individual brains can then either be compared with, or spatially normalized into, this reference so that group comparisons can be made.

- Studies involving functional neuroimaging are performed either to determine which areas of the brain are involved with implementing a particular cognitive function or to investigate the possible neural bases for deficits in that function displayed by a target population. The results of the studies are sets of three-dimensional (3D) coordinates depicting areas of neural activation in the brain of an individual subject in response to specific tasks or conditions. By referring to a common reference it can be determined which specific structure or neural region was responsible for that activation.

Because the spatial nature of the information extracted from neuroimaging data is a distinguishing feature when compared with other phenotypic measures, a natural means of encoding this information is to establish a referential or template coordinate system with which the image-based measures can be indexed. Once available, these databases or atlases may incorporate any kind of data that is anatomically labeled – the labels allow the data to be mapped to the atlas, with the localization precision depending on the specificity of the label. In this way, diverse sources of neuroscientific information may be integrated and logically organized. Moreover, by organizing the data with respect to a coordinate frame, the latter provides an anatomy-driven mechanism with which

Introduction to the Science of Medical Imaging, ed. R. Nick Bryan. Published by CAMBRIDGE University Press. © Cambridge University Press 2010.

multivariate – for example, genotype–phenotype – associations may be made.

Brain atlas construction

Methodology

The construction of referential coordinate systems of neuroanatomy and the atlases they spawn applies to the brain the same cartographic principles used in map-making. Essentially, a pictorial representation of the brain is required (typically obtained via histology or MRI), over which a coordinate parameterization must then be specified, enabling one to locate positions in the picture and finally label these according to standard anatomical nomenclature. Just as one is able to look up, for instance, a particular city in a world atlas, an analogous resource for the brain would permit neuroanatomical features to be similarly identified. Furthermore, in the same way that geographic information systems are the computerized extension of textbook atlases, digital brain atlases offer the promise of versatile new means for encoding and manipulating neuroanatomically referenced information.

In traditional approaches, a single individual is chosen to serve as the canonical model, to which a Cartesian coordinate system is referenced and used to locate anatomy. The Talairach coordinate system, widely used in brain mapping, sets its origin at the anterior commissure, and orients its axes with respect to the line connecting this anatomic landmark with the posterior commissure [3]. Computerized versions of the Talairach textbook atlas have extended the original, sparse annotation to cover the entire brain, so that every coordinate is anatomically labeled. The coordinate systems can also be specialized to particular brain structures, where, not surprisingly, the cortical mantle has received special attention. Drawing again the analogy to geographic map-making, the development of map projection methods for unfolding the cortex has found important application in functional imaging studies of the brain [4].

Clearly, the underlying imagery on which an atlas is based determines to a great extent the level or kind of detail that can be documented. All brain atlases necessarily reflect the limitations of the acquisition technologies of their time; however, the current state of the art (an example of which is shown in Figure 13.1) is producing volumetric data with spatial resolution that exceeds our ability to annotate in a timely manner.

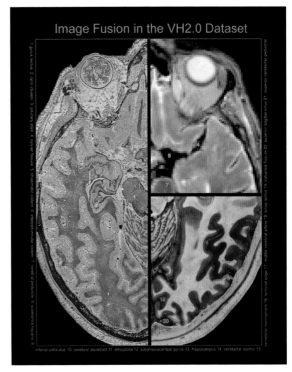

Figure 13.1. Detailed anatomy from the Visible Human Project merges information from x-ray computed tomography, MRI, cryosections, and histological sections to produce anatomical images able to resolve fine structures as small as 25 microns in size [2].

Challenges

Unlike the problem of mapping the world, brain atlases gain their full power when representative populations of individuals are characterized for their construction, raising issues about how best to summarize group data on neuroanatomy, and how to relate these to new instances of individuals.

Atlases based on the brain of a single individual, even one who is healthy and normal, will, by definition, represent a biased sample of neuroanatomy. Ideally, the geometry and signal appearance of a group of individuals can be rigorously combined to define the underlying anatomic template, from which a population-specific coordinate system is derived. One strategy is to choose the anatomic configuration nearest to the centroid of a population distribution. Mappings to these templates reflecting average morphology will require minimal distortion, as the subjects will deviate least from such a template. Performance of algorithms based on manipulating canonical information should also improve when using an average model. Average shapes are gained by estimating the average of these transformations, which

231

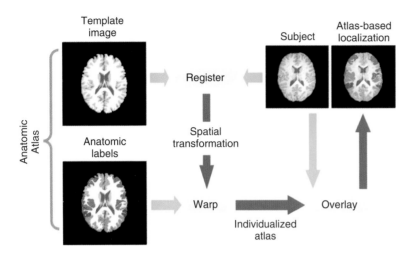

Figure 13.2. Anatomic localization via atlas warping. Relying on the knowledge that different instances of the same anatomy share a common topological scheme, the problem of localizing anatomic structures in a subject image can be reduced to that of determining the spatial correspondence between the anatomy depicted in the image and a template, or atlas, representation of the same anatomy. Using this mapping, information encoded in the atlas – such as anatomic labels and structural boundaries – is transferred to the subject image. The transformed atlas labels automatically localize their corresponding structures in the images. Moreover, the inverse mapping allows subject data from a population to be standardized to a common coordinate frame, opening the way to a powerful alternative for performing group statistics.

relates a given member of the population to the remainder of the data. There is growing recognition that the Euclidean spaces traditionally used to represent brain shape limit our ability to quantify the ways in which neuroanatomy can vary in nature, over time, or as a consequence of disease or intervention; instead, new statistics for manifold-valued data are required [4], and its development is emerging as a major research focus in the field.

Once available, a digital atlas of the brain (unlike its hard-copy variants) can be computationally re-shaped to accommodate the anatomic variability of new individuals. The individualized brain templates that are produced in this way facilitate anatomic localization as well as transfer of information associated with the atlas, such as, for example, maps of cytoarchitecture, biochemistry, and gene expression, as well as functional and vascular anatomy. The shape of the atlas is adapted using spatial transformations to warp the template into correspondence with the anatomy of an individual (Figure 13.2). The challenge of registering brain image volumes has become a major research focus in medical image analysis.

The ability to relate atlas data to a new subject's brain images also operates in reverse, enabling population data to be spatially normalized to the template and subsequently compared across individuals, with subject-specific anatomic differences removed. The algorithmic techniques key to the development of deformable brain atlases are the same tools with which population-specific templates can be constructed [5].

Emerging modalities such as diffusion tensor MRI provide an additional opportunity for computing

anatomically and functionally meaningful mappings between subjects, as shown in Figure 13.3. The processing of these unique data types with their special characteristics, as well as their combination with complementary information from other modalities to support multivariate analysis, continually introduces new challenges to the field. Special populations with significantly altered neuroanatomic appearance also present challenges to the current state of the art, which is limited in its ability to accommodate changes in both signal intensity and non-topology-preserving variations in shape.

Enabling technology: image registration

The technology integral to all of the developments above is image registration [8]. Given a pair of images, the object of image registration or matching is to find a spatial transformation or geometric mapping f: $\Omega_1 \rightarrow \Omega_2$ that brings the features of one image $I_1(x)$ into alignment with those of the second image $I_2(x)$, where Ω_1 and Ω_2 are the respective spatial domains of images I_1 and I_2:

$$I_1(x) = I_2(f(x)) \qquad (13.1)$$

For an arbitrary location x in one image, this mapping specifies its corresponding position $f(x)$ in the second image. Such mappings are required in solutions to a variety of general problems in image analysis, an example of which is shown in Figure 13.4a. For example, to infer the motion or measure the shape change of objects over sequential image acquisitions, one must

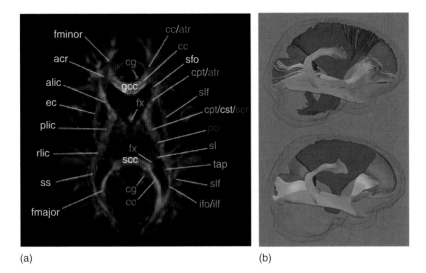

Figure 13.3. Diffusion tensor imaging-based white-matter atlas: (a) with annotations [6] and (b) with tracts depicted in three dimensions [7]. (Reproduced with permission from Mori *et al.*, 2005 [6], and Yushkevich *et al.*, *NeuroImage* 2008; **41**: 448–61 [7].)

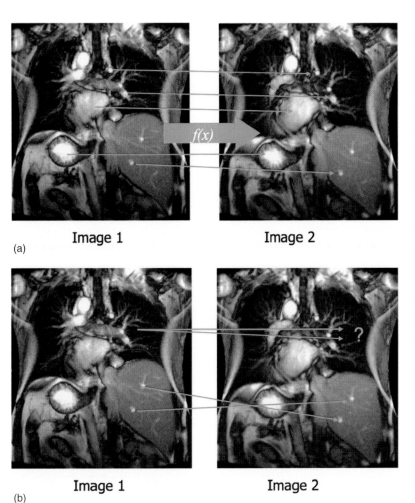

Figure 13.4. The image registration problem. Given a pair of images as shown in (a), the registration problem is to find *f* such that *Image₁* (x) = *Image₂* $(f(x))$, where the spatial transformation *f* specifies for each point *x* in *Image₁* its corresponding location *f(x)* in *Image₂*. In the majority of applications, mappings are sought between images that arise from distinct but topologically similar sources, so the equality or correspondence constraint in the preceding definition does not strictly apply; the success of image registration therefore depends both on the degree to which two anatomies actually bear topological resemblance and on the level of localization accuracy required by the analysis. Another challenge with the correspondence constraint is that its optimization may not yield a unique solution, as illustrated in (b). Depending on the way in which the image "equality" or similarity is evaluated, there may be multiple candidate mappings for some *x* that are all equally plausible. To disambiguate among these possibilities, an additional constraint is typically imposed that restricts the family of admissible mappings from which the solution is drawn. This constraint may be implemented by specifying the transformation type (for example, rigid, affine, polynomial, elastic, etc.) and/or requiring a certain degree of smoothness in the solution mapping (by, for example, penalizing some measure of deformation induced by the mapping). Such a constraint would eliminate the candidate solution shown in (b), in which a fold is introduced in the transformation of *Image₁*.

determine the correspondence between the features in each consecutive pair of images; images of the same anatomy observed by different modalities usually are first fused into the same coordinate space to facilitate their interpretation.

Its application in diverse problem settings has resulted in numerous implementations of the registration operation, each specialized to the type of data or the information that is being sought in the problem. In most instances, the optimal mapping f is obtained by maximizing some "similarity" metric that evaluates the "goodness of match" induced by f between the registered images. Many approaches to measuring image similarity have been proposed, including a strategy as simple as subtracting the registered images and examining the residual intensity difference at each image voxel:

$$\Sigma_\Omega [I_1(x) - I_2(f(x))]^2 \qquad (13.2)$$

which is the basis of so-called optical flow methods. Instead of looking at individual voxel values, it may be more effective to compare signal patterns within a small neighborhood of voxels. These region-based patterns would potentially provide more salient image information with which to identify corresponding positions between different images. For example, aspects of local image geometry can be characterized by computing the gradient of the original images, as shown in Figure 13.5. Another class of metrics that rely on ensemble groups of voxel values examines the probabilistic relationships between image signals in similar anatomic regions. In this way, images acquired even from different modalities may be compared by studying their statistical "correlation" via, for example, the normalized cross-correlation:

$$\Sigma_\Omega \langle F/|F|, G/|G| \rangle \qquad (13.3)$$

where $F = \Sigma\ I_1 - I_1^{mean}$ and $G = \Sigma\ I_2 - I_2^{mean}$ are computed over a fixed neighborhood centered at the relevant points in I_1 and I_2, respectively, or by the application of various information-theoretic measures. The different metrics can be combined to further detail the various aspects of the images that together best characterize the most likely correspondence mapping. Ideally, an image signature can be found for uniquely associating pairs of voxels in the different images.

It is important to note that the metrics above apply not just to medical imagery, and this lack of domain specificity can lead to images being aligned without the correct match between the underlying anatomies represented in the images. This potentially significant limitation stems from our inability in most instances to precisely quantify what we mean by "anatomic correspondence." As a consequence, image similarity is typically applied as a surrogate measure.

Once a similarity metric is specified, its optimization will in general be an ill-posed problem in that many solutions are possible. Because the image features on which registration is based are often sparsely distributed – for example, within the white matter or cerebrospinal fluid spaces in brain MR images – the optimization problem is inherently underconstrained. As illustrated in Figure 13.4b, ambiguity may arise as a result of multiple candidate voxels with identical similarity scores. This is resolved by additionally requiring that the registration mapping be "smooth," and then choosing as the solution the smoothest mapping, which typically translates to the transformation that induces the least amount of deformation on the transformed image.

The smoothness constraint can be imposed implicitly via choice of parameterization of admissible transformations or explicitly – through regularization – by specifying an additional "deformation" term to be optimized along with the similarity measure; for example:

$$\Sigma_\Omega \langle u, u \rangle \qquad (13.4)$$

where $u(x) = f(x) - x$ is the displacement at x. In other words, additional consideration must be made in image registration regarding the plausible characteristics that the solution mappings should exhibit. The dimensionality of the transformation parameterization will dictate whether explicit regularization is necessary. In order to account for fine variation in the local shape details of the brain, for example, many applications solve for transformations with as many degrees of freedom as voxels in the image data. Additional attention is required in many of these cases to ensure that anatomic topology is preserved by the computed mappings.

Estimation of the registration solution is complicated both by the potentially very large number of transformation unknowns and by the highly non-linear nature of the similarity measures, which are often non-linear functions of image inputs that are, in turn, non-linear signal functions of location. Iterative techniques must therefore be used to search for the solution, and their development remains an important area of research in the field [9].

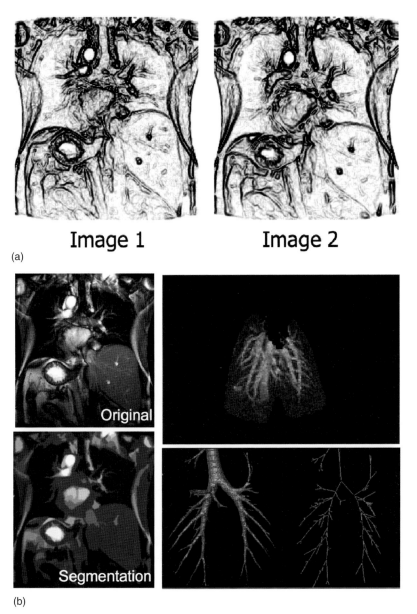

Figure 13.5. Evaluating image similarity and anatomic correspondence. An explicit assumption in image registration is that corresponding features may be identified in the images to be aligned, and registration of these features will yield the desired mappings. By definition, each particular form of correspondence has associated with it a metric for quantifying the degree of similarity between two feature instances. In (a), instead of comparing the intensity value between pairs of potentially corresponding voxels, a neighborhood of voxel values is considered by examining the gradient magnitude value between voxel pairs. Such a region-based measure may provide a more discriminatory image signature or feature for a voxel, with which candidate-matching voxels in the target image may be more reliably found. Ideally, the features directly support the alignment of anatomy, and strategies toward this end, as shown in (b), include first segmenting or classifying the images into general corresponding anatomic regions and then registering these segmentations, or specializing the alignment to particular structural features, such as the airway tree or vasculature in lung imagery.

Another way the registration problem has been popularly conceptualized is to imagine the images to be modeled as idealized, say elastic, continua [5,9]. Registration then mimics the process of physically reshaping one image until its appearance matches that of the second image. The external forces are derived from a potential energy that acts as the similarity measure. The amount of elastic deformation as a result is given by the internal strain energy. The equilibrium configurations, which locally minimize the total potential energy (deformation – similarity), represent solutions to the corresponding registration problem. In addition to its intuitive appeal, the continuum mechanical viewpoint allows rigorous treatment of the deformation associated with registration mapping and opens new modeling possibilities through the range of different materials for which mathematical idealizations have been developed. By re-expressing the registration problem as one of statics, a ready collection of well-established techniques, including the finite element method, can be brought to bear on its numerical solution.

The analysis of image registration in terms of mechanical systems is not the most general, and further insights can be gained with a probabilistic formulation [5]. For computational anatomy, the probabilistic approach will figure importantly in addressing the challenges outlined previously to develop a knowledge representation scheme that encompasses predictive and explanatory studies of both normal and pathological conditions.

New discoveries

The availability of powerful image registration methods capable of registering fine details from different image volumes has opened new avenues of research and discovery in biomedical science and clinical applications. As already noted, data from different modalities can be fused or integrated to facilitate their interpretation, as shown in Figure 13.6, and registration enables changes over time to be detected and quantified in serial or longitudinal studies by examining the displacement of material points between the different time instances at which the serial images were acquired. Figure 13.7

shows one of the first MRI-based regional maps of pulmonary ventilation–perfusion ratio by applying multimodality registration methods to align dynamically acquired ventilation data to blood flow maps from perfusion imaging.

Note that the spatial transformations that connect between images inform directly in quantitative form how the anatomy changes in geometry over the images. By way of illustration, Figure 13.8 plots the paths that points within a circle travel as they are transformed into their corresponding positions in the larger square, to which the smaller circle is registered. The differences in size and shape are both visually captured by the field of vectors which, importantly, represents a mathematical quantity that precisely encodes the geometric difference between the registered objects. As a consequence, image registration provides a remarkable new tool capable of extracting and quantifying morphologic information from image data. For example, by registering an image volume into its mirrored version, Figure 13.9 demonstrates a novel

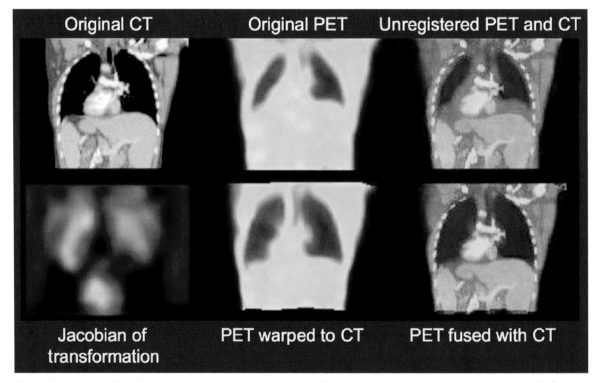

Figure 13.6. Fusing multimodality studies via image registration. The map of the transformation Jacobian visualizes the amount of deformation that was required to warp the PET image into alignment with the subject's corresponding CT image. For an application such as that shown here, a natural requirement is that the domain topology of an image is maintained after its transformation. These diffeomorphic mappings allow information to be carried in either direction, so the example in this case could have just as easily shown the CT image warped into correspondence with the PET image. The particular choice of mapping direction in a given instance will depend on the application, as well as on the resolution and quality of the images involved.

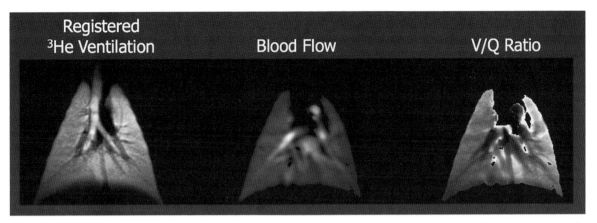

Figure 13.7. MR ventilation–perfusion ratio mapping in a porcine model. Voxel-wise V/Q ratio values were obtained by treating as images the parametric maps of blood flow numerically generated from breath-hold-acquired data and registering these to dynamic ventilation images.

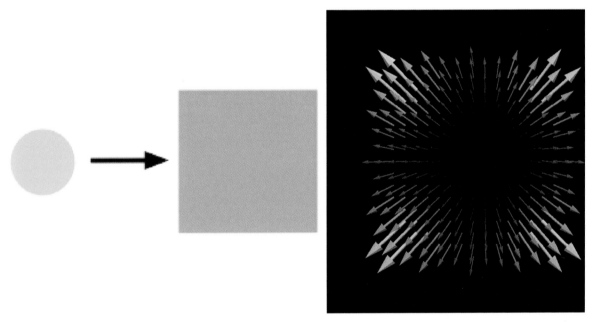

Figure 13.8. Correspondence mappings quantify shape and size differences. The vector field (right) visualizes the paths that points within the circle travel as they are transformed into their corresponding positions in the square (left). The displacement vectors specify for each point in the circle its location in the target domain of the square. Note how the size difference between the objects is captured by the way in which the vectors are directed away from the circle's center, filling out the circle to fit the larger square. Careful examination will also reveal how the mapping adjusts for the shape difference between the circle and square. The mappings encode these qualitative impressions as rigorous mathematical quantities that are the basis for registration's application as a powerful tool for quantitatively extracting morphological information from image data.

approach for detailed characterization of left–right asymmetries of imaged anatomy. Determining the transformations between average configurations of different groups then allows us to compare shape distributions across groups, which is useful for localizing significant differences between these groups to parameterize morphological variations across health and disease [5].

The moving lung presents a different kind of anatomical variation that can nevertheless be characterized in the same way as in the preceding examples. In particular, pulmonary motion between consecutive phases is given directly by the spatial transformation that brings the images into register. This ability to quantify lung deformation, as demonstrated in

237

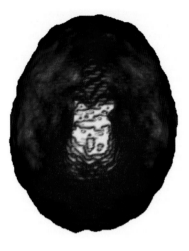 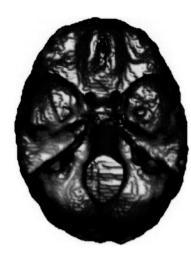

Figure 13.9. CT characterization of left–right asymmetries of fossil endocasts that potentially inform our understanding of evolutionary changes in the brain. Endocasts of hominid fossil crania often have features suggestive of modern human endocasts. For example, the region over Broca's area is sometimes reported to be enlarged, just as in modern humans. By morphing left endocast hemispheres into their right hemispheres and evaluating the corresponding Jacobian maps, as exemplified in this figure, image registration provides for the first time a technique for quantifying this impression.

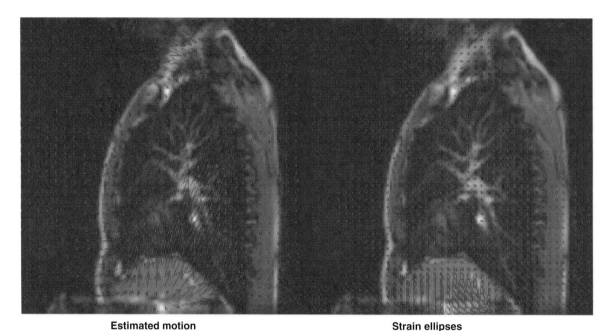

Estimated motion **Strain ellipses**

Figure 13.10. *In vivo* assessment of regional lung motion. From the registration mapping, representing pulmonary motion, between different respiratory phases, one can directly derive a quantitative description of tissue deformation (strain) or volume change (ventilation).

Figure 13.10, represents a novel opportunity to determine those mechanical characteristics which may predict the severity of disease and the extent of recovery in the afflicted lung.

Brain atlases, made possible by registration technology, provide the foundation on which modern neuroinformatics infrastructure is built, their importance evidenced by a series of large-scale initiatives, including the National Institutes of Health Human Brain Project and MRI Study of Normal Brain Development, designed to advance neuroscience research through

the development of public brain databases. Our understanding of the genetic bases for health and disease is also being advanced by the use of atlas technology. A prominent example is the Allen Brain Atlas, a highly detailed, cellular-resolution, genome-wide map of gene expression in the mouse brain [10], as illustrated in Figure 13.11. Discovering which genes are active in different regions of the brain is a first step toward understanding functional differences between neurons on the cellular and molecular level, and potentially what percentage of the human genome is involved in

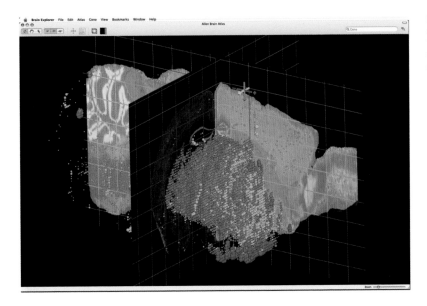

Figure 13.11. Allen Brain Atlas: expression profile, colored by expression intensity, of *Pde10* gene in three dimensions, shown with coronal and sagittal planes of anatomic reference atlas. (Reproduced with permission.)

building and operating the human brain. With a goal to comprehensively define the unique molecular properties of brain cells that may underlie neural functions such as learning, memory, emotions, and cognition, the Allen Brain Atlas program is positioned to facilitate the construction of other types of maps, including those based upon proteomics and imaging.

Conclusions

The atlases made possible by the developments described above promise to implement a flexible means to store and access diverse bioscientific information, enable model-based methodologies to extract the latter, and facilitate novel multivariate correlative studies, thus opening hitherto unexplored avenues of research in biomedical science. Atlases are therefore a key element of a comprehensive informatics platform for biomedical and clinical research and an essential tool in imaging-based studies of structural and functional correlates in health and disease.

References

1. Chicurel M. Databasing the brain. *Nature* 2000; **406**: 822–5.

2. Ratiu P, Talos IF. *Cross-Sectional Atlas of The Brain.* Cambridge, MA: Harvard University Press, 2005.

3. Talairach J, Tournoux P. *Co-planar Stereotaxic Atlas of the Human Brain: 3-Dimensional Proportional System. An Approach to Cerebral Imaging.* New York, NY: Thieme, 1988.

4. Thompson PM, Miller MI, Ratnanather JT, Poldrack RA, Nichols TE. Mathematics in brain imaging. *NeuroImage* 2004; **23** (Suppl 1).

5. Gee JC. On matching brain volumes. *Pattern Recognit* 1999; **32**: 99–111.

6. Mori S, Wakana S, van Zijl PCM, Nagae-Poetscher LM. *MRI Atlas of Human White Matter.* Amsterdam: Elsevier, 2005.

7. Yushkevich P, Zhang H, Simon T, Gee JC. Structure-specific statistical mapping of white matter tracts. *NeuroImage* 2008; **41**: 448–61.

8. Yoo TS. *Insight into Images: Principles and Practice for Segmentation, Registration, and Image Analysis.* Wellesley, MA: A. K. Peters, 2004.

9. Modersitzki J. *Numerical Methods for Image Registration.* Oxford: Oxford University Press, 2004.

10. Ng L, Pathak SD, Kuan C, *et al.* Neuroinformatics for genome-wide 3D gene expression mapping in the mouse brain. *IEEE/ACM Trans Comput Biol Bioinform* 2007; **4**: 382–93.

Christos Davatzikos and Ragini Verma

The widespread use of medical imaging as a means for diagnosis and monitoring of diseases, as well as for offering prognostic indicators, has enabled the collection of large imaging databases from healthy and diseased populations. Although earlier advanced imaging studies typically involved a few dozen subjects each, many current clinical research studies involve hundreds, even thousands of participants, often with multiple scans each. This has created a significant demand for quantitative and highly automated methods for population-based image analysis.

In order to be able to integrate images from different individuals, modalities, and time points, the concept of a *statistical atlas* (Figure 14.1) has been introduced and used extensively in the medical image analysis literature, especially in the fields of computational anatomy and statistical parametric mapping of functional brain images [1]. An atlas reflects the spatiotemporal characteristics of certain types of images for specific populations. For example, a statistical atlas of the typical regional distribution of gray and white matter (GM, WM) in the brain can be constructed by spatially normalizing a number of brain images of healthy individuals into a common stereotaxic space, and measuring the mean and standard deviation of the amount of GM and WM in each brain region (Figure 14.2). This atlas can also be more specific, for example, as to age, gender, and other characteristics of the underlying population. Similarly, a statistical atlas of cardiac structure and function can provide the average myocardial wall thickness at different locations, its change over time within the cardiac cycle, and its statistical variation over a number of healthy individuals or of patients with specific cardiac pathology. Finally, an atlas of the spatial distribution of prostate cancer [2] can be constructed from a number of patients undergoing prostatectomy, in order to guide biopsy

procedures aiming to sample prostate regions that tend to present a higher incidence of prostate cancer (e.g., Figure 14.3).

A statistical atlas is analogous to the knowledge acquired by a radiologist during clinical training, in that it learns patterns from a large number of scans, and represents anatomical or functional variability in a group of individuals. The two most common ways in which atlases are used are the following:

(1) To compare two groups of individuals, for example a group of patients with a specific disease and a group of healthy controls, or groups of subjects divided on the basis of age, gender, or some other physical characteristic. Conventional approaches have used standard linear statistics [3]. However, an increasingly common use of multiparametric or multimodality images calls for more sophisticated statistical image analysis methods that determine often non-linear relationships among different scans, and therefore lead to the identification of subtle imaging phenotypes. Some of these approaches and challenges are discussed below.

(2) To compare an individual with a group of individuals. For example, one might want to evaluate whether a patient with cognitive impairment presents the spatial pattern of brain-tissue atrophy that is common to Alzheimer's disease patients. The individual's scans can then be compared with the statistical atlas of AD patients. High-dimensional pattern classification methods are finding their way into the imaging literature more and more frequently, providing a new class of imaging-based diagnostic tools. Some of the work in this direction follows.

Introduction to the Science of Medical Imaging, ed. R. Nick Bryan. Published by Cambridge University Press. © Cambridge University Press 2010.

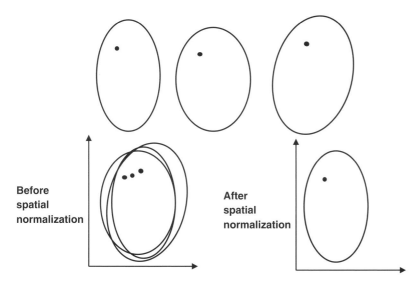

Figure 14.1. Schematic diagram showing the principle of a statistical atlas. Different anatomies are combined together into the same spatial coordinate frame, in a way that accounts for inter-individual morphological variability. If an area of interest, denoted here by a dot, is to be studied, it will be spatially co-registered across individuals, if the proper spatial alignment (registration) is applied. One can then investigate structural or functional characteristics at that specific (and any other) spatial location.

Before spatial normalization

After spatial normalization

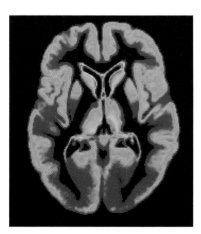

Figure 14.2. A statistical atlas of the spatial distribution of gray matter in a population of elderly healthy individuals. Hot colors indicate brain regions with the highest frequency/volume of gray matter in the population. A new individual's spatial distribution of gray matter can be contrasted against this atlas, in order to identify regions of potentially abnormal brain atrophy.

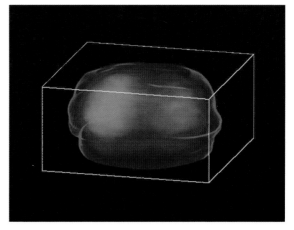

Figure 14.3. A statistical atlas of the spatial distribution of prostate cancer obtained from co-registered prostatectomy specimens. Brighter green indicates areas of higher cancer incidence. This atlas can potentially be used to guide biopsy procedures aiming to obtain tissue from regions more likely to host cancer.

Multiparametric statistics and group analysis

A fundamental process in constructing a statistical atlas is that of *registration*, i.e., the process of bringing scans from different sessions and different individuals into a common spatial coordinate system of a template, where they can directly be compared with each other and integrated into a statistical atlas. This process is shown schematically in Figure 14.1, and it is described in Chapter 13. These spatially normalized images can now be incorporated into a statistical atlas for group analysis, as will be discussed next. The method adopted for group-based analysis depends completely on the type of data (scalar or high-dimensional) used for representing the subjects.

Statistical analysis of scalar maps

Traditionally, in the standard framework of voxel- and deformation-based analysis, scalar images, such as tissue density maps [4] or Jacobian determinants [5], are used for group analysis. In diffusion tensor images (DTI), one of the several scalar maps of fractional anisotropy or diffusivity may be used to represent each of the subjects. Such scalar maps are then smoothed by a Gaussian filter: (1) to Gaussianize

241

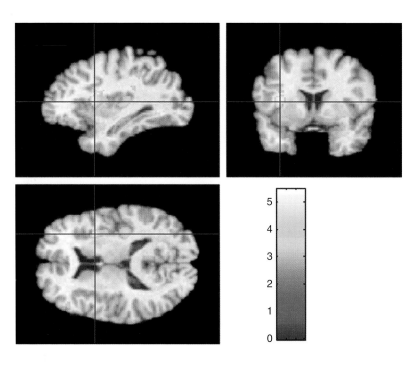

Figure 14.4. Regions of volumetric difference between schizophrenia patients and healthy controls using voxel-wise application of linear statistics. The color scale represents the *t*-statistic.

the data, so that linear statistics are more applicable, (2) to smooth out the noise, or (3) to analyze the image context around each voxel, since structural changes are unlikely to be localized at a single voxel, but are rather more likely to encompass entire regions. *Voxel-wise* statistical tests, such as the general linear model, are then applied to the spatially normalized and smoothed data. The output is a voxel-wise map which identifies regions of significant difference based on some user-defined threshold. Statistical parametric mapping or SPM has been a tool widely used for this purpose. Using MRI data, Figure 14.4 shows an example of voxel-based statistical analysis performed on a group of patients with schizophrenia versus a group of healthy controls. Figure 14.5 shows the regions of change in an aging brain over a period of four years. Similar analyses have been performed on anisotropy and diffusivity maps computed from DTI data. These regions can be further analyzed with respect to the clinical correlates to determine the biological underpinnings of the group changes. This is a very popular and widely accepted form of analysis.

In addition to the application of voxel-wise statistical tests, analysis can also be performed on a *region-wise* basis, using regions of interest (ROIs) that have been defined on a template or average atlas of subjects that has been created using the process of spatial normalization. Figure 14.6 shows regions identified in the template. By the process of

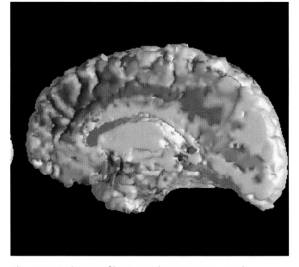

Figure 14.5. Pattern of brain atrophy in an aging population created using 107 individuals followed over four years (color scale).

spatial normalization, each of these regions can be warped to each of the subjects (or vice versa), and group-based analysis may be performed using region-based values of scalar quantities that characterize the effect of pathology on these regions. For example, tissue atrophy during the course of aging or as a manifestation of disease could be evaluated percentage-wise in each of the regions that have been outlined in the atlas of ROIs.

Statistical analysis of multi-parametric and multimodal data

While the general linear model has been used effectively for the statistical analysis of scalar map representation of subjects, with the increasing use of multiparametric or multimodality images, the general linear model (GLM) with Gaussian smoothing does not suffice. Firstly, the simple spatial filtering and subsequent linear statistics are not a valid approach for the multiparametric data such as tensors and multimodality data. This is because the high-dimensional data, which has non-linear behavior at each voxel due to its inherent structure as well as the changes induced by pathology, are typically distributed along submanifolds of the embedding space. A manifold is a generalization of a surface to higher dimensions; it reflects non-linear correlations in the data, which restrict the values that a collection of measurements can have. In tensors, this embedding space could be of R^6, if single voxel data are to be considered. In multimodality data, the dimension of the embedding space will be the number of modalities combined to represent the data. Figure 14.7 demonstrates this concept for the

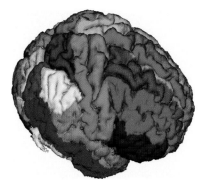

Figure 14.6. An atlas of anatomic ROIs can be warped to the template and vice versa to perform region-based analysis.

case of tensors, but instead of ellipses any high-dimensional structure could be used to emulate the voxel-wise structure of multimodality data. The curved surface running through the tensors is a manifold. In general, a manifold can be thought of as an abstract geometric space in which every point has a neighborhood that resembles a Euclidean space, but the global structure may be more complicated. Figure 14.7a shows such a structure, where each of the triangles is a plane in Euclidean space. Thus lines in two dimensions, spheres in three dimensions, including a globe, and surfaces in higher dimensions are all examples of a manifold. Along with the concept of a manifold comes an important idea of distance along the manifold, which is crucial for us. In Figure 14.7b the red line is the distance along the manifold. Intuitively, this can be compared with the distance between two cities such as New York and Philadelphia: the distance measured along the curved surface of the earth is the distance along the manifold (equivalent to the red line), as compared to the crow's flight distance (equivalent to the green line). In addition, non-linearity may arise due to changes introduced by the pathology. The filtering and subsequent statistics need to be performed on the underlying manifold on which the data lie. In addition to the underlying structure of the data, another reason for the lack of feasibility of the GLM for these data is that the shape and size of a region of interest, such as a region of growth or abnormal morphological characteristics, is not known in advance. The way in which a disease process is likely to affect the local tissue structure of the brain is highly unlikely to follow a Gaussian spatial profile of a certain predefined size. Thus the two main challenges that we need to address in order to form statistical atlases of these higher-dimensional data and subsequent group analysis are: (1) determining the true underlying structure of the data in the form of

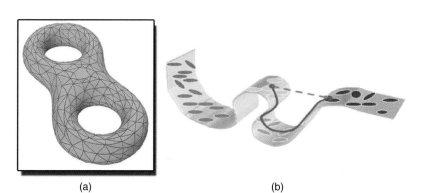

(a) (b)

Figure 14.7. (a) Example of a manifold with complex global structure and local Euclidean structure of triangles. (b) Manifold structure of tensors. The gray surface represents the non-linear manifold fitted through the tensors or any high-dimensional structure represented as ellipses. The green dotted line represents the Euclidean distance between tensors treated as elements of R^6 and the red line represents the geodesic distance along the manifold that will be used for all tensor manipulations.

a non-linear manifold and (2) estimating the statistical distribution of the data on that manifold.

In order to address these two issues, more sophisticated image analysis methods need to be developed that determine the often non-linear relationships among different scans and therefore lead to the identification of subtle imaging phenotypes. In relation to tensors, methods based upon Riemannian symmetric spaces [6] rely upon the assumption that the tensors around a given voxel from various subjects belong to a principal geodesic (sub)manifold and that these tensors obey a normal distribution on that submanifold. The basic principle of these methods is sound, namely that statistical analysis of high-dimensional data must be restricted to an appropriate manifold. However, there is no guarantee that the representations of the tensors on this submanifold will have normal distribution. More importantly, restricting the analysis on the manifold of positive definite symmetric tensors is of little help in hypothesis-testing studies, since the tensors measured at a given voxel or neighborhood, from a particular set of brains, typically lie on a much more restricted submanifold of the space of symmetric positive definite matrices. For example, if all voxels in a neighborhood around the voxel under consideration belong to a particular fiber tract, then the tract geometry will itself impose an additional non-linear structure on the subspace of the tensors at those voxels from all subjects. In addition, non-linear changes introduced by pathology are not accounted for when considering the full tensor space. Some of these issues were alleviated by the development of a manifold-based statistical analysis framework which focuses on approximating/learning the local structure of the manifold along which tensor/higher-dimensional measurements from various individuals are distributed. The learned features belonged to a low-dimensional linear manifold parameterizing the higher-dimensional tensor manifold and were subsequently used for group-wise statistical analysis. The filtering and subsequent statistical analyses were then performed along the manifold, rather than in the embedding space.

We now explain this in greater detail in the context of multiparametric data as represented by tensors. This analysis can be extended to multimodality data. The two frameworks that are discussed below are from the perspective of whether: (1) the manifold is explicitly determined and (2) the data distribution is determined by implicitly incorporating the underlying structure of the data.

Statistical analysis on the estimated manifolds

Suppose the problem is to investigate and determine whether or not two groups (e.g., schizophrenia patients and controls) display morphological differences on a voxel-wise basis, using diffusion tensor imaging (DTI) data available for these subjects. Having spatially normalized this data, we will analyze group differences voxel by voxel. At a particular voxel, we form a dataset by collecting tensors from that location from all subjects. For purposes of smoothing the data locally, tensor measurements from all voxels in a surrounding neighborhood are collected, as well as from all subjects of our study. This collection of tensors generally does not follow a Gaussian distribution in R^6, but rather lies on a submanifold of R^6. We have applied various manifold learning methods that aim to learn the structure of this manifold. We initially applied Isomap [7], a method that first builds a graph from these tensor samples and subsequently uses graph-searching methods to calculate geodesics along the submanifold, and finally applied multidimensional scaling on these geodesics, in order to flatten the submanifold. Standard multivariate statistical tests such as Hotelling's T-square test, can then be applied on the flattened submanifold, determined at each voxel. Mathematical details of the method can be found in [8].

Determining the statistical distribution on high-dimensional data

In the above manifold learning approach, the underlying structure is explicitly determined. This approach is quite effective if a sufficient number of samples are available, so that the submanifold is properly sampled. While this can be obtained by using neighborhood tensors from around the voxel under consideration, thereby indirectly imposing spatial smoothness, some practical applications do not offer a sufficiently large number of samples. Hence the results of undersampling the submanifold can be quite unpredictable. While the issue can be somewhat alleviated by using neighborhood samples from all subjects to determine the underlying structure at a point, there are no methods for determining the correctness of the underlying manifold. Also, it increases the dimensionality of measurement at each voxel, thereby changing the embedding space. Second, Isomap or any other manifold learning technique flattens a submanifold, but it

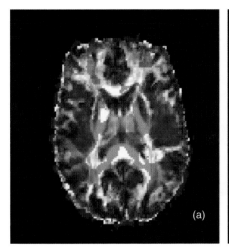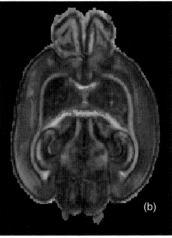

Figure 14.8. Regions of significant differences between (a) schizophrenia patients and controls and (b) young and old mice obtained using statistical analysis of multiparametric data. The colored regions are areas exceeding a statistical threshold of group difference.

does not Gaussianize or otherwise estimate the statistical distribution of the data on the flattened manifold. Therefore, standard statistical tests may still be inappropriate for use on the flattened submanifold.

Thus in the process of collecting samples voxel-wise for statistical analysis, it can be observed that this dataset has unknown statistical distribution on some non-linear manifold. Therefore, it is particularly important to analyze the underlying structure in each such dataset and to use this structure to estimate features that can identify group differences. It is not enough to non-linearly approximate the probability density from a number of samples; one must also obtain a representation that will enhance group separation. In order to overcome these limitations, kernel-based principal component analysis (kPCA) and kernel-based Fischer discriminant analysis (kFDA) methods have been developed. These methods effectively estimate the non-linear distribution of tensors or other higher-dimensional data on the underlying manifold as well as their statistical separation, without the need to construct the manifold from a large number of samples. kFDA focuses on finding non-linear projections of the tensorial data which can optimally discriminate between the two groups. The common idea behind kernel-based techniques is to transform the samples into a higher-dimensional reproducible kernel Hilbert space (RKHS), which can be used for statistical analysis and for density estimation. For the tensorial datasets, such an analysis also linearizes the tensors, thereby simplifying further group analysis by allowing the use of linear tests for statistical inference. Having obtained the kernel-based features, standard statistical tests, such as the Hotelling's T-square test can be applied.

Using either manifold learning or kernel-based techniques, p-value maps may be obtained using Hotelling's T-square statistic in a parametric analysis (with underlying distributional assumptions regarding normality of the kernel projections) or in a non-parametric manner (via permutation tests and without any distributional assumptions). Regions with significant differences between the two groups are identified from the parametric or non-parametric p-value maps by controlling the false discovery rate (FDR) using a suitable p-value threshold. Testing for multiple comparisons is an essential last step in such an analysis in order to validate the regions that have been found to be different. It is possible to directly obtain thresholded p-value maps using a more complex form of the permutation test by controlling the family-wise error rate due to multiple comparisons [9]. However, we prefer to use FDR-based multiple comparisons correction after the non-parametric p-value map is fully computed, because this facilitates easy comparison with the parametric p-value map. Figure 14.8a identifies regions of difference between schizophrenia patients and controls using kernel-based methods. Figure 14.8b shows the kernel-based framework applied to mouse images (the two groups being the young and the old) at a much higher level of significance. These regions survive multiple comparisons testing using the FDR.

Forming group averages

An important aspect of statistical atlases is the ability to obtain average maps that are representative of a particular group property. This has been achieved by simple linear averaging when scalar maps are used for statistical analysis, as all the maps have already been spatially normalized to a template. This problem is slightly more challenging in the case of higher-dimensional data. This is then handled using manifold learning. On the lines of the framework described above under *Statistical analysis on the estimated manifolds*, a manifold is fitted to the data at each voxel (accumulated within a spatial neighborhood and across subjects) and the average is computed on the manifold [8].

In the above discussion involving manifold learning and kernel-based methods, although the data at each voxel were tensors, the frameworks can easily lend themselves to higher-dimensional data as is derived from multimodality data. The difference would be the manifold learned and the nature of the embedding space.

Individual patient analysis and high-dimensional pattern classification

Although informative from a biological point of view, group analyses such as those described in the previous sections are not meant to provide diagnostic tools for individuals. This is because two groups can have highly overlapping values of a structural or functional variable, e.g., the volume of a structure, but with a sufficiently large sample size a group analysis will identify significant group differences, even of the smallest magnitude, if they are present. For example, Figure 14.9 shows the joint histogram of the volume of the hippocampus and the volume of the entorhinal cortex (ERC) in a group of healthy elderly individuals and a group with mild cognitive impairment (MCI). Statistically significant group differences exist between these two sets of measurements. However, if we are given a new individual's volumes of the hippocampus

and the ERC, we will not be able to correctly classify this individual, because of the overlap between the two joint histograms.

In order to address this issue, high-dimensional pattern classification methods have been pursued with increasing frequency in the recent literature. A pattern is formed by a collection of image-derived measurements, typically obtained from a number of different anatomical regions. Figure 14.10 shows a schematic representation of a pattern analysis and recognition system that can be used in detecting and quantifying patterns of structure or function. A statistical atlas is of fundamental importance in these

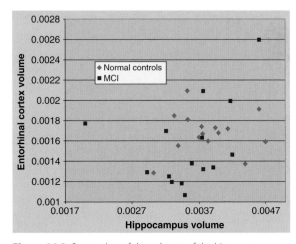

Figure 14.9. Scatterplots of the volumes of the hippocampus (horizontal) and entorhinal cortex (vertical), of healthy elderly and MCI individuals, after dividing each measurement by the respective total intracranial volume. Although a statistical test reveals significant group differences, the volumetric measurements are of relatively modest diagnostic value, due to the overlap of the two distributions. Given an individual's volumetric measurements of these two structures, we cannot classify him/her.

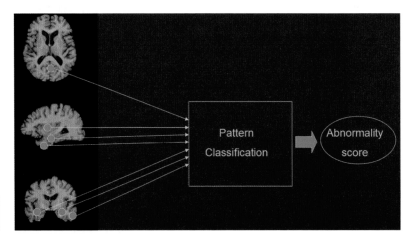

Figure 14.10. A schematic diagram demonstrating the concept of a pattern classification system. Imaging information is extracted from a number of spatial (or spatiotemporal) locations, and is integrated by a pattern classification system that outputs a score that is positive or negative. Positive value indicates the presence of a pattern of interest, perhaps the spatial pattern of brain atrophy seen in Alzheimer's patients or the spatiotemporal pattern of cardiac deformation. Selecting the best way to sample a spatial pattern is an important topic of active research in machine learning and medical image analysis.

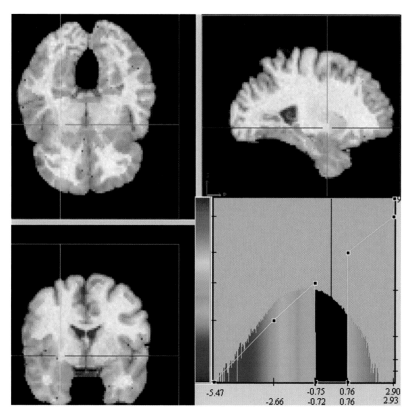

Figure 14.11. An individual is compared against a statistical atlas of normal elderly individuals, in order to determine whether the pattern of brain atrophy is typical of a normal elderly person or not. The figure displays a z-score map, i.e., a voxel-by-voxel evaluation of the individual's gray matter volume against the statistical atlas. A pattern of frontotemporal atrophy indicates Alzheimer's-like pathology.

methods, since it represents the range of variation of the features that are used to construct the pattern. A simple example is illustrated in Figure 14.11, which displays the z-score map of an Alzheimer's patient's regional distribution of gray matter tissue in the brain. Pattern recognition methods are trained to recognize such spatiotemporal patterns of structure and function.

One of the motivating factors behind these developments is the complex and spatiotemporally distributed nature of the changes that many diseases cause, particularly in the brain and the heart. For example, in Alzheimer's disease, the anatomical structures that carry most discriminative power are likely to depend on the stage of the disease as the disease progressively spreads throughout various brain regions – and also on age and other demographic and genetic factors, since disease is to be distinguished from complex and progressively changing background normal variations in anatomy and function that may depend on demographic and/or genetic background. Moreover, in addition to causing brain atrophy, i.e., volumetic changes, Alzheimer's disease might cause changes in the signal characteristics of an image. For example,

tissue demyelination, deposition of minerals, or other macro- or microstructural changes caused by disease can affect the MR signal intensity. Vascular disease also causes well-known MR signal changes, for example in the white matter of the brain (e.g., increasing T2 signal). It is thus becoming clear that, in order to achieve the desirable diagnostic power, multiple modalities and multiple anatomical regions must be considered jointly in a (possibly non-linear) multivariate classification fashion. Moreover, regions that are relatively less affected by disease should also be considered along with regions that are known to be affected (which in the case of Alzheimer's disease might include primarily temporal lobe structures, in relatively early disease stages), since differential atrophy or image intensity changes between these regions are likely to further amplify diagnostic accuracy and discrimination from a background of normal variation. Certain cardiac diseases also have subtle and spatiotemporally complex patterns of structural and functional change. For example, arrhythmogenic right ventricular disease involves spatial patterns of structural and physiological change that are not always easy to distinguish from normal inter-individual

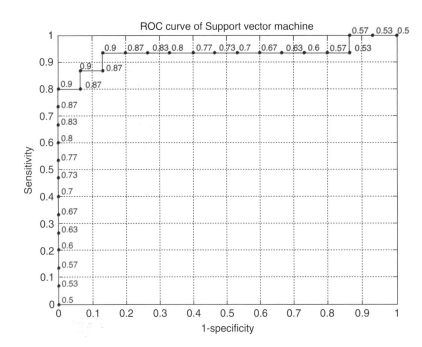

Figure 14.12. ROC curve of the MCI versus normal classification problem of Figure 14.9. High classification rates are achieved, using high-dimensional pattern classification.

variability. Finally, patterns of the spatial distribution of prostate cancer can potentially be used to develop optimized biopsy protocols that maximize cancer detection [2].

A fundamental challenge faced by high-dimensional pattern classification methods in medical imaging is the curse of dimensionality, i.e., the fact that imaging measurements have vastly larger dimensionality than the number of samples available in the typical study. Extraction, selection, and reduction of all spatiotemporal information included in a medical scan to a small number of features that optimally distinguishes between two or more groups is an open problem. Some approaches have employed global dimensionality reduction methods, such as principal or independent component analysis, before feeding the reduced features into a pattern classifier.

More localized approaches have been developed. Spatiotemporal patterns of regional brain atrophy are examined by hierarchically decomposing an image into images of different scales, each of which captures structural and/or functional characteristics of interest at a different degree of spatial resolution. The most important parameters are then selected and used in conjunction with a non-linear pattern classification technique to form a hypersurface, the high-dimensional analog to a surface, which is constructed in a way so that it optimally separates two groups of interest, for example normal controls and patients

with a particular disease. Effectively, that approach defines a non-linear combination of a large number of image-derived measurements from the entire anatomy of interest, each taken at a different scale that typically depends on the size of the respective anatomical structure and the size of the region that is most affected by the disease. This non-linear combination of volumetric measurements is the best way, according to the respective optimality criteria, to distinguish between two groups, and therefore to perform diagnosis via classification of a new scan into patients or normal controls. Figure 14.12 shows the ROC curve obtained by a high-dimensional non-linear classification system applied to the same population of healthy controls and MCI patients described in Figure 14.9. Very good diagnostic accuracy can be achieved using high-dimensional pattern classification, in contrast to the discrimination capability of ROI-based measurements, as in Figure 14.9.

In summary, the availability of large numbers of medical image datasets has necessitated the development and validation of image analysis tools that capture the range of variation of image-derived structural and functional characteristics of populations of patients and healthy subjects. A new generation of techniques for statistical analysis and pattern classification has appeared in the literature over the past decade, aiming not only to help identify anatomical and functional differences across different groups, but also to classify individual scans against baseline statistical atlases of normal and diseased populations. These new tools are gradually being adopted in clinical studies.

References

1. Csernansky JG, Wang L, Joshi SC, Ratnanather JT, Miller MI. Computational anatomy and neuropsychiatric disease: probabilistic assessment of variation and statistical inference of group difference, hemispheric asymmetry, and time-dependent change. *NeuroImage* 2004; **23**: 56–68.

2. Zhan Y, Shen D, Zeng J, *et al.* Targeted prostate biopsy using statistical image analysis. *IEEE Trans Med Imaging* 2007; **26**: 779–88.

3. Friston KJ, Holmes AP, Worsley K, *et al.* Statistical parametric maps in functional imaging: a general linear approach. *Hum Brain Mapp* 1995; **2**: 189–210.

4. Ashburner J, and Friston KJ. Voxel-based morphometry: the methods. *NeuroImage* 2000; **11**: 805–21.

5. Davatzikos C, Vaillant M, Resnick S, *et al.* A computerized approach for morphological analysis of the corpus callosum. *J Comput Assist Tomogr* 1996; **20**: 88–97.

6. Fletcher PT, Joshi S. Principal geodesic analysis on symmetric spaces: statistics of diffusion tensors. In: Sonka M, Kakadiasis IA, Kybic J, eds. *Computer Vision and Mathematical Methods in Medical and Biomedical Image Analysis.* Heidelberg: Springer, 2004: 87–98.

7. Tenenbaum JB, de Silva V, Langford JC. A global geometric framework for nonlinear dimensionality reduction. *Science* 2000; **290**: 2319–23.

8. Verma R, Khurd P, Davatzikos C. On analyzing diffusion tensor images by identifying manifold structure using isomaps. *IEEE Trans Med Imaging* 2007; **26**: 772–8.

9. Nichols TE, Holmes AP. Nonparametric permutation tests for functional neuroimaging: a primer with examples. *Hum Brain Mapp* 2002; **15**: 1–25.

Biomedical applications
Morphological imaging

R. Nick Bryan

Introduction

From a simplistic, yet practical perspective, the goal of biomedical science is to identify and cure disease. Imaging plays a critical role in the former, which is a prerequisite for the latter. One can frame disease from an imaging perspective, as we did with nature in Chapter 1. Nature, or the universe, is defined as

$$U = (m, E)(x, y, z)(t) \qquad (15.1)$$

An image of a part of nature is a function of measurements of these physical parameters:

$$I = f(m, E)(x, y, z)(t) \qquad (15.2)$$

In the case of medicine, the parts of nature in which we are most interested are our patients and their diseases. Patients can be overly simplified as abnormal (diseased) subjects from a total population of normal (N) and diseased (D) subjects. This division into normal and diseased is applicable not only to populations of individuals but to tissues within an individual, e.g., cancerous versus normal breast tissue. Following from Equations 15.1 and 15.2, we might define disease then as:

$$D = (m, E)(x, y, z)(t) \qquad D \neq N \qquad (15.3)$$

and an image of disease as:

$$D = f(m, E)(x, y, z)(t) \qquad D \neq N \qquad (15.4)$$

What we strive for in biomedical imaging is to identify abnormal subjects or diseased tissue by making signal measurements as a function of location and time. Useful images distinguish between, or in imaging lingo show contrast between, normal and diseased tissue. For practical purposes, it does not matter which of these parameters, m, E, x, y, z, or t, are

abnormal and, as long as they distinguish between normal and abnormal biological states, they may be useful medically.

Biomedical science has long been subdivided into three major branches: morphology, physiology, and molecular (biochemistry). This section of the book will expand on imaging applications in each of these fields. It should be understood that the definitions of these fields are arbitrary and more historic than contemporary. Interestingly, however, these biological fields have their analogous components in the above formalizations of nature, image, and disease.

Morphological imaging

Morphology is the study of the form or structure of something, anything. It is the branch of biology that deals with the form and structure of organisms without consideration of function. Morphology relates to the size, shape, and structure of an organism and its parts. In medicine, morphology has generally been subdivided into macroscopic anatomy and microscopic histology. Morphology primarily relates to the spatial domain of biology: the x, y, z aspects of a patient or sample. Morphological imaging will be the focus of most of this chapter, but first let us briefly introduce physiological and molecular imaging, which will be more extensively addressed in Chapters 16 and 17, respectively.

Physiological imaging

Physiology is the study of the functions of living organisms and their parts. It involves the scientific investigation of an organism's vital functions, including growth and development, the absorption and processing of nutrients, the synthesis and distribution of proteins and other organic molecules, and the functioning of different tissues, organs, and other anatomic

Introduction to the Science of Medical Imaging, ed. R. Nick Bryan. Published by Cambridge University Press. © Cambridge University Press 2010.

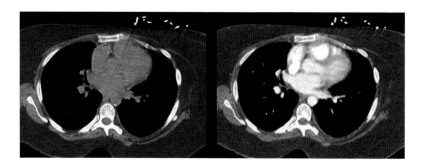

Figure 15.1. Pre- and post-contrast CT abdomen: morphological, physiological.

structures. The dynamism implicit in this definition incorporates the concept of change, specifically change over time. Time, t, is the critical domain of physiology. Hence physiological imaging often involves imaging at multiple time points.

The image signal of interest varies as a function of time. A single image of a blood vessel such as the aorta on an x-ray CT scan provides morphological, but no dynamic or physiological, information. In fact, such morphological images may not distinguish between the live and dead state. However, a series of x-ray CT scans after a bolus injection of radiographic contrast agent is dynamic, showing a change in radiodensity over time due to the flow of blood through the vessel (Figure 15.1). Physiological images show evidence of life. While it is true that most physiological imaging requires multiple time-dependent images, some do not. In these cases, the detected signal itself contains dynamic information. An example is Doppler ultrasound (US) imaging. The detected signal incorporates a frequency shift that relates to the velocity of blood flow. FDG-PET images are dependent on the functional ability of cells to metabolize glucose.

Morphological imaging tends to focus on relatively permanent, well-defined structures, objects, or diseases – such as organs, foreign bodies, or tumors. Both the normal and the diseased objects we define or distinguish morphologically have a relatively fixed physicality. This is not true for most of the physiological phenomena we image, which tend to be transient patterns as demonstrated by fMRI of brain function or dynamic processes such as cardiac ejection fraction. Since time is so critical to physiological imaging, temporal sampling rate can be a limiting factor. By the Nyquist principle, to distinguish a temporally dynamic event, one has to sample (in our case image) at twice the frequency of the fastest changing component of the process. Consider an image of the heart made with x-ray CT. A reasonable, high-resolution image might consist of $512 \times 512 \times 512$ isotropic $8\,\text{mm}^3$ voxels (2 mm cubes) and take 10 seconds to make. However, since the living human heart beats at approximately 1 Hz, cardiac motion would be averaged over many voxels and the physiological information would be blurred beyond recognition. There would be no dynamic information, even if one made multiple images. If one wants to capture the heart chambers during the systolic and diastolic phases of the cardiac cycle, one has to image at half the duration of systole (the fastest component of the cardiac cycle), approximately every 50 ms. Recalling that image SNR decreases as the square root of imaging time, a 50 ms CT image, with the same scanning parameters and spatial resolution, would have 14 times less SNR. While temporal resolution may be a limiting factor in physiological imaging of fast events, this is not the case for slow events such as tumor growth.

Molecular imaging

Biochemistry has evolved into molecular biology, which is the study of biology at the chemical, molecular level. Contemporary molecular biology involves the biochemistry of cells and is closely linked to cell biology. It includes the study of the structure and activity of macromolecules essential to life, in particular nucleic acids and proteins involved in cell signaling, survival, replication, and transmission of genetic information. This biological field perhaps relates mostly to the m,E aspects of our definition of nature. Molecular imaging is highly dependent on signal sensitivity to the very low concentrations of the many important biological molecules such as enzymes and other regulatory molecules. This is a bit of a forced classification, as these molecules are critically dependent on the spatial structure of their atomic components and the temporal expression of their activity. However, from a biomedical imaging perspective, it is the need to measure extremely small molecular signals that defines this field. Like morphological and physiological imaging, molecular imaging is driven and simultaneously constrained by sensitivity and specificity, in this case to chemical signals. The desire to detect signals from a specific protein having picomolar tissue concentration from a cellular mix of over 100 000 different proteins is an enormous challenge at best; doing this non-invasively and *in vivo* remains at the edge of possibility.

One can put this molecular sensitivity and specificity in perspective by looking at molecular imaging as done by common medical imaging devices. The x-ray CT signal is a function of linear attenuation coefficient, μ, of which electron density may be a significant component (see Chapter 5). All tissue electrons contribute to the signal regardless of whether the electrons are from molecules in calcium in bone, amino acids in proteins, lipids in fatty tissue, or water in cells. Hence there is a relatively large signal due to the large numbers of electrons in all molecules; the signal, however, is very non-specific. In practice, conventional x-ray easily differentiates the extremely low electron density of gases (air in the lungs) and the very high electron densities of metals such as calcified bone, whereas it is barely able to distinguish watery from fatty soft tissues because of their relatively similar number of electrons (Figure 15.2). The MRI signal is primarily due to the protons in water molecules and hence is actually relatively specific from a molecular viewpoint. It is also moderately sensitive, since protons have a relatively high gyromagnetic ratio and water accounts for approximately 80% of the mass of most biological tissues. However, most biological tissues have about the same water content and the number of water molecules in a tissue is not a particularly distinguishing feature. As noted in Chapter 7, MRI contrast is not primarily a function of water concentration (or proton density, p), but a function of the biophysical characteristics of the water, particularly T_1 and T_2. Hence MRI might be generalized as having moderate molecular sensitivity and specificity. On the other hand, the signal from FDG-PET is related to trapped intracellular deoxyglucose, one specific molecule that has tissue concentrations in the micromolar range. This is what one imagines as molecular imaging in contemporary biomedicine. However, it is easy to appreciate the technological challenges that must be met to move from imaging 80 molar water to micromolar glucose – seven orders of magnitude difference in concentration. Recall the basic formula from Chapter 2:

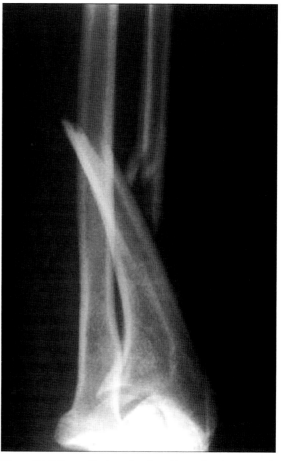

Figure 15.2. X-ray of fracture of radius with excellent bone contrast but poor soft-tissue contrast.

$$\frac{S}{N} \propto V\sqrt{t} \qquad (15.5)$$

Consider making a $128 \times 128 \times 128$ 3D MR image of a kidney with isotropic 1 mm^3 voxels. Using a conventional proton-density-weighted pulse sequence, this is easily accomplished in five minutes; recall that the proton density signal is primarily due to water concentration – 80 molar. Now consider making the same image, but now measuring signal only from 5 μ molar glucose. One could do this, but to have comparable signal-to-noise and spatial resolution in the image, one would have to scan for 1.6×10^7 minutes – more than a year! Needless to say, physiological imaging, observing changes in glucose concentration over time, is a moot point not only from a feasibility perspective, but from a biological perspective in that there is little biological interest in glucose dynamics at this time scale. One

Table 15.1. Spatial dimensions

Factor (m³)	Multiple	Value
10^{-45}	—	Volume of an *electron* ($\sim$9.4 $\times$ 10^{-44} m³)
10^{-42}	—	Volume of a *proton* ($\sim$1.5 $\times$ 10^{-41} m³)
10^{-33}	—	Volume of a *hydrogen atom* (6.54 $\times$ 10^{-32} m³)
10^{-21}	1 attoliter	Volume of a typical *virus* (5 attoliters, a million million times a hydrogen atom)
10^{-18}	1 femtoliter	Volume of a *human red blood cell* (90 femtoliters, 9 $\times$ 10^{-17} m³)
10^{-12}	1 nanoliter	Individual *calcification* in breast cancer A medium grain of sand (0.5 mm diameter, 1.5 milligrams, 62 nanoliters, almost 500 small sand grains)
10^{-6}	1 milliliter (1 cubic centimeter)	Volume of *gallbladder bile* 20 milliliters 1 teaspoon = 3.55–5.00 milliliters (about 1000 large sand grains)
10^{-3}	1 liter (1 cubic decimeter)	Volume of *human brain* 1.5 liters
10^{-1}	100 liters	Volume of average *human body* 70 liters

could decrease the spatial resolution by a similar factor, resulting in an image with perhaps one voxel, i.e., no spatial resolution within the kidney, again an image of little biomedical interest. Concentration sensitivity is one of the two basic challenges to molecular imaging, the other being how to image not a few, but thousands of different molecules. The previous chapters on nuclear and optical imaging, and the following chapter on molecular imaging, present a few of the many important biomedical techniques and applications in this field.

Morphological imaging

Spatial resolution

Since morphological imaging focuses on spatial attributes, spatial resolution is obviously important but can be a limiting factor as well. The potential spatial range of biomedical imaging extends from large animals such as humans (measured in meters) through animal organs such as mouse kidneys (measured in millimeters) to small blood vessels such as arterioles (measured in hundreds of microns), to single cells (less than 10 microns), down to intracellular molecular complexes measured in nanometers (Table 15.1). There are at least 10 orders of magnitude difference in size from the smallest to the largest biological structures of potential interest. However, for practical purposes, *in vivo* clinical imaging extends three orders of magnitude from meters to millimeters, while *in vivo* experimental imaging offers an additional 2–3 orders of magnitude of spatial resolution, down to tens of microns. At present, non-invasive *in vivo* imaging is not possible beyond these spatial dimensions.

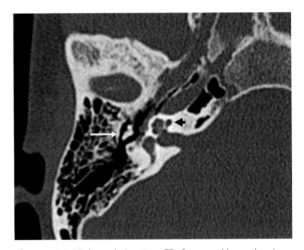

Figure 15.3. High-resolution x-ray CT of temporal bone showing cochlea (black arrow) and ossicles (white arrow). Voxel size 0.5 mm isotropic; scan time 30 seconds.

According to the Nyquist principle, to resolve a small structure such as the turns of the cochlea and ossicles of the temporal bone, which are approximately 1 mm in diameter, an image should have 0.5 mm spatial resolution. This requisite spatial resolution is not just voxel resolution, which requires 0.5 mm in plane voxel dimensions, but overall image resolution. This can be achieved with x-ray CT but this is near the clinical limit of this technology (Figure 15.3). In fact, 1 mm³ is about the spatial-resolution limit of any clinical imaging technique. This limitation is due to a variety of factors, some relating to the specific imaging technology while others are patient-related. Technological limitations are often due to inadequate signal sensitivity, while patient-related factors include practical imaging times (less than one hour) and motion. One reason the temporal-bone semicircular canals can be imaged by CT is that the scan can be performed within 30 seconds and patient head motion can usually be constrained for this time period. On the other hand, CT images of structures in the chest and abdomen rarely have comparable spatial resolution because of cardiac, vascular, and breathing motions.

Some of the clinical limitations to imaging at higher spatial resolution do not apply to other biomedical imaging opportunities. Mice can be anesthetized, rigidly fixed by a specimen holder, and scanned over hours in order to obtain high-spatial-resolution images. *In vivo* CT images of bone in mice may have spatial resolution of a few hundred microns, while *ex vivo* CT images may have spatial resolution of 50 microns and resolve complex trabecular anatomy (Figure 15.4). However, in order to maintain adequate SNR for such small voxels, scan time has to increase proportionally. Imaging 100-micron-diameter mouse semicircular canals takes hours, not seconds.

It is critical to remember that images are a function of signal, space, and time, and that image acquisition is interdependent on all three. Given the same imaging device, images of greater spatial resolution either require longer data-acquisition (scan) times or have lower SNR. However, different instruments may have greater signal, spatial, or temporal resolving powers, and in practice one always attempts to use the instrument that provides the most critical information at least cost and damage or risk to the sample, ALARA.

Morphological analysis

As previously noted, morphology involves spatial information, and morphological analysis uniquely requires imaging, the only measurement tool that explicitly incorporates spatial information. Given an image with morphological information, how does one apply it to a biomedical question? First an observer must extract the image encoded information using various image analysis tools as presented in Chapters 11, 12, 13, and 14. Most frequently, an observer identifies "objects" or distinct components within an image and then either classifies the object and/or assesses specific morphologic features of the object. Although human observers have tended to use qualitative feature descriptors such as smooth, irregular, lobulated, etc., the spatial inadequacies of language have been and remain a scientific limitation. One of the great ongoing changes in biomedical imaging is the evolution to quantitative analysis, including quantitative spatial analysis.

Morphological analysis starts with the detection of an object, generally an organ, tissue, or pathological lesion. All subsequent analytical steps are dependent upon this initial step, generally termed segmentation. Image objects have previously been defined as a non-random collection of signals (see Chapter 3). To detect an object within an image, observers (human or computer) search an image for spatially non-random signals. Computers approach this task statistically; humans presumably do the same, though in still incompletely understood ways. Once an object has been "officially" detected by passing some threshold of non-randomness, further analysis proceeds. A common task is to classify an object, usually performed by some type of "pattern matching." In biomedicine, the beginning "pattern" is that of normal; in the case of morphology, normal anatomy. Radiologists observe hundreds of normal chest films and build an internal reference pattern against which they test all new studies (Figure 15.5). This process requires a training set upon which to build the pattern and a learning process that is at least partially conscious. However, once the pattern is built, the matching process may be very automatic and at least partially unconscious, particularly the positive match. It takes an experienced

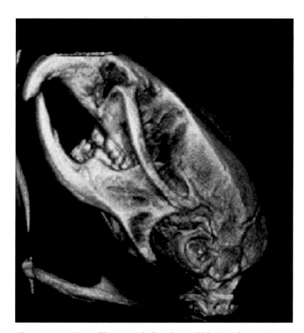

Figure 15.4. X-ray CT mouse skull and mandible. Voxel size 0.25 mm isotropic; scan time 32 minutes.

255

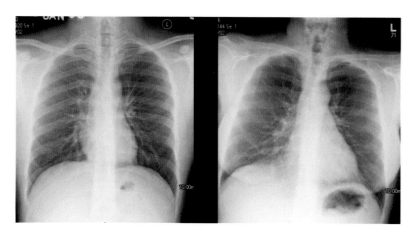

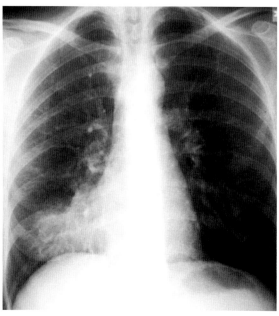

Figure 15.6. Pattern matching of distinctive, triangular radiodensity of right-middle-lobe pneumonia on chest x-ray. Courtesy of Detroit Receiving Hospital, www.med.wayne.edu/diagradiology/TF/Chest/CH09.html.

radiologist less than five seconds to make most normal/abnormal decisions. If a "not-normal" decision is made, then the matching process starts all over again. The observer searches his/her library of known abnormal patterns for a match. Perhaps the radiologist observes the lesion in Figure 15.6, and, having seen 10 right-middle-lobe pneumonias and built a pattern thereon, makes a diagnostic match. Such a diagnosis is made primarily on morphological, i.e., spatial, characteristics of a lesion. Comparable computer image analysis methods have now been developed, as described in Chapters 13 and 14. Large numbers of normal images are co-registered to a standard template in order to

create a statistical atlas, the computer's "normal pattern," against which new test cases are statistically compared.

While human pattern matching can be automatic and mysteriously intuitive, there are specific morphological features of objects that presumably play a role in this process – morphological features that can and are often used in more deliberate analysis and are requisite for computer analysis. The basic morphologic descriptors are quite simple – *number*, *size*, *shape*, *position*. We shall not belabor number, which is just a count of objects, but its practical importance should not be underestimated. In clinical imaging, multiple similar objects often suggest an entirely different diagnosis than only one of the same object. For instance, multiple lesions in the liver are suggestive of metastatic cancer while a single, similar-appearing lesion is more suggestive of a benign condition (Figure 15.7).

The basic geometric descriptors – *number*, *size*, *shape*, *position* – may be used in describing any kind of object, including abnormal organs and tissues. "The lateral ventricles are abnormally *large*; an *irregular, lobulated* mass; a *triangular* density in the right upper lobe" are phrases frequently seen in radiological reports that use simple morphological descriptors (Figure 15.8). While literally thousands of morphological descriptive words are used in describing biomedical images, most are relatively crude and ambiguous, such as large/small, pea-sized, lobulated, ovoid, etc. A useful biomedical lexicon probably needs no more than five or six descriptive terms for any particular morphological feature, and there are probably no more than a few dozen useful morphological features. The new RadLex radiological lexicon is being developed to define and standardize medical imaging terminology [1]. It contains approximately 200 terms called "morphologic" (Table 15.2).

Table 15.2. RadLex morphological characteristics

aerated	discoid	hyperinflated	obstructed	retractile	smooth
amorphous	distorted	impinged	occluded	ruptured	tethered
aphthous	emphysematous	indented	patent	scarred	thickened
atrophic	eroded	invaginated	patulous	sclerosing	thinned
bilobed	fatty	lacunar	plaque-like	septated	thinned
blunted	fibrous	lipid	pleomorphic	serpentine	tortuous
bulky	flattened	long	puckered	serpiginous	truncated
compressed	fungating	mixed	punctate	shallow	tubular
conglomerate	fusiform	multilocular	reconstructed	sharp	ulcerated
consolidated	hydrated	narrowed	reticular	short	unilocular
					varicoid

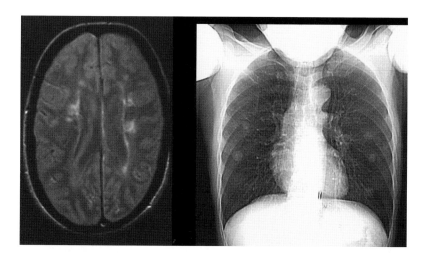

Figure 15.7. Number: multiple lesions reflecting "multiple sclerosis" of the brain and metastasis to the lung.

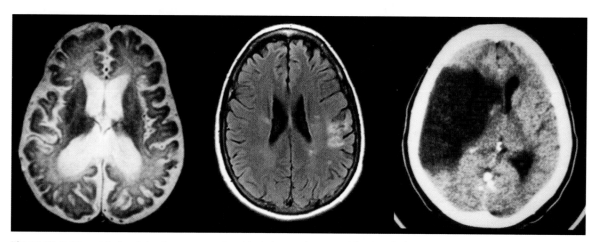

Figure 15.8. Geometric descriptors from cross-sectional brain images: *large* ventricles; *irregular* hyperintensity; *triangular* radiolucency.

Because of the relatively tight relationship between structure and function, size is not just a descriptor but a predictor (Table 15.3). For whole organs and defined structures, larger than/smaller than, whether expressed qualitatively or quantitatively, suggests certain types of pathological conditions. An abnormally small structure suggests underdevelopment, a destructive insult such as an infarct, or a degenerative process. A large

257

organ suggests a congenital anomaly, hypertrophy, or pathological swelling (edema). In terms of pathological lesions, big is usually worse than small. For example,

a 5 mm nodule in the lung is probably benign and can be conservatively managed (watched). A 15 mm nodule is much more likely to be cancer and needs intervention (Figure 15.9).

Qualitative size descriptors are rapidly being replaced by quantitative measurements, from linear dimensions to 3D volumes. Linear measurements such as the RECIST (Response Evaluation Criteria in Solid Tumors; maximum diameter) and WHO (maximum orthogonal diameters) for tumor size can be easily performed by human observers without extensive training (see Chapter 16). Sequential tumor size measurements are now standard for evaluating tumor progression. More complex structures and lesions, such as white-matter ischemic lesions of the brain, do not lend themselves to such simple measurements. The size or spatial extent of diffuse, poorly defined lesions has until recently been described subjectively or with crude ordinal grading systems such as the

Table 15.3. RadLex size modifiers

asymmetric size	giant
collapsed	inflated
constricted	intermediate
contracted	large
decreased in height	over-inflated
deflated	prominent
dilated	shrunken
distended	small
ectatic	symmetric size
engorged	too small to characterize
enlarged	widened
expanded	

(a)

(b)

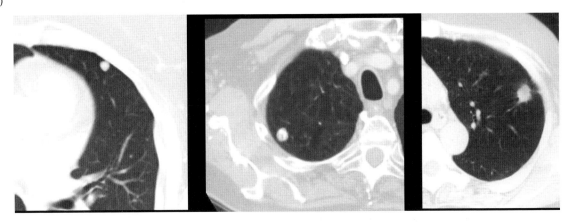

Nodule size (mm)*	Low-risk patient†	High-risk patient‡
≤	No follow-up needed§	Follow-up CT at 12 mo; if unchanged, no further follow-up
>4–6	Follow-up CT at 12 mo; if unchanged, no further follow-up	Initial follow-up CT at 6–12 mo then at 18–24 mo if no change
>6–8	Initial follow-up CT at 6–12 mo then at 18–24 mo if no change	Initial follow-up CT at 3–6 mo then at 9–12 and 24 mo if no change
>8	Follow-up CT at around 3, 9, and 24 mo, dynamic contrast-enhanced CT, PET, and/or biopsy	Same as for low-risk patient

* Average of length and width; † Minimal or absent history of smoking and of other known risk factors; ‡ History of smoking or of other known risk factors; § The risk of malignancy in this category (<1%) is substantially less than that in a baseline CT scan of an asymptomatic smoker.

Figure 15.9. Size: diagnosis and management of pulmonary nodules based on size. Smaller to larger, benign to malignant. MacMahon H, Austin JH, Gamsu G, et al. Guidelines for management of small pulmonary nodules detected on CT scans: a statement from the Fleischner Society. *Radiology* 2005; **237**: 395–400. Used with permission.

Cardiovascular Health Study (CHS) grading system (Figure 15.10). More rigorous quantitation requires more complex volumetric analysis. However, volumetric analysis requires segmentation of an entire structure, which for humans is not only tedious but often poorly reproducible. More efficient automated computer segmentation software as described in Chapters 13 and 14 will be critical for these more complex spatial analyses.

Shape is a more complex morphological feature, though with one of the more limited RadLex lexicons –

just 16 terms (Table 15.4). Yet shape is the most distinctive feature of most objects, biological or non-biological [2]. Gross shape distinguishes coffee cups from cars. Subtle shape differences easily distinguish thousands of different coffee cups from each other (Figure 15.11). While there is enormous potential for using shape discrimination in biomedical imaging, in practice it is applied at only the crudest level. Perhaps the RadLex lexicon reveals the underlying problem. These few words are remarkably inadequate in reliably conveying spatial information about biological objects. Only the simplest of these shape descriptors are of scientific value, the others being poorly defined, imprecise, and irreproducible. This is a prime example of the visual system's and imaging's superiority over all other human sensory and communication systems in conveying spatial information. From a scientific perspective, a thousand-word description of an image is still inadequate. Fortunately, digital image analysis now offers increasing capabilities for quantitative shape analysis, bringing numbers into morphological analysis and thus increasing its scientific power (at least according to Kelvin's admonition about numbers and science). With the use of anatomic templates

Table 15.4. RadLex Shape

asymmetrically shaped	pedunculated
beaded	plate-like
curved	polypoid
irregularly shaped	round
linear	spoke-wheel
lobular	straightened
nodular	symmetrically shaped
ovoid	wedge-shaped

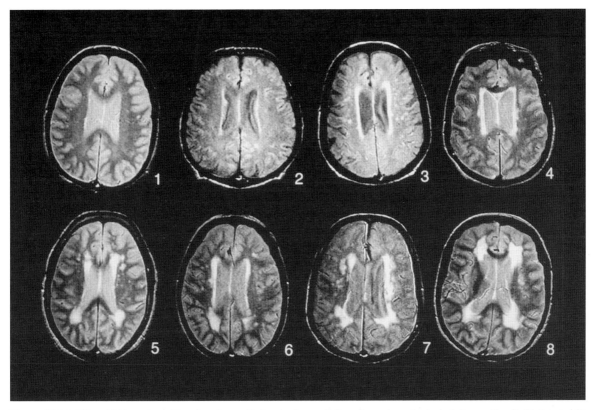

Figure 15.10. Diffuse MRI hyperintensities of small-vessel ischemic disease. CHS grading system of extent of disease. Manolio TA, Kronmal RA, Burke GL, *et al.* Magnetic resonance abnormalities and cardiovascular disease in older adults. *Stroke* 1994; **25**: 318–27.

embedded within well-defined geometric systems that allow global as well as local quantitative spatial analysis, morphological tasks previously impossible can now be performed (see Chapter 14).

While many shape features can be of biological importance, one is worth specific comment – *margin* (Table 15.5). The edges of structures, especially pathological lesions, reveal much about their biological aggressiveness and destructiveness. A smooth, well-defined lesion margin is much more likely to be associated with a benign, slowly growing condition than an irregular, poorly defined lesion, which is more likely to reflect a malignant condition such as cancer (Figure 15.12). Perhaps this is a biological reflection of entropy. High entropy reflects disorganized, more randomly arranged tissue while low entropy reflects

well-organized, normal, or benign tissues [3]. As with other morphological descriptors, specific numbers are replacing vague words. Edges or margins of structures or lesions can be detected and quantified by computer algorithms using such parameters as diffusivity, gradients, and even entropy, which can be a numerical spatial descriptor (see Appendix 3) (Figure 15.13).

Position is somewhat an exception in terms of number of useful words. The position of a structure or lesion may be qualitatively described in image space (object in the upper right side of image) using a limited lexicon, or much more precisely described in object space using anatomic terms (lesion in the anterior nucleus of the thalamus). Anatomy provides the traditional spatial labeling for biological organisms. There are thousands of anatomic terms, some describing structures only a few millimeters in size. Cartography has supplemented geographic names and qualitative descriptors with a quantitative framework, Cartesian latitude and longitude. Biomedical imaging is increasingly using similar quantitative spatial systems, such as the Cartesian-based Talairach coordinate system for stereotactic neuroanatomy and, more recently, fMRI (Figure 15.14).

Table 15.5. RadLex margin characteristics

circumscribed margin	poorly defined margin
irregular margin	smooth margin
lobulated margin	spiculated margin
obscured margin	

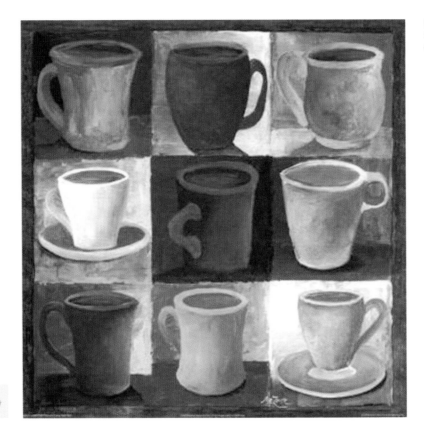

Figure 15.11. Coffee cups distinguished by shape. Mary Beth Zeitz, www.marybethzeitz.com. Used with permission.

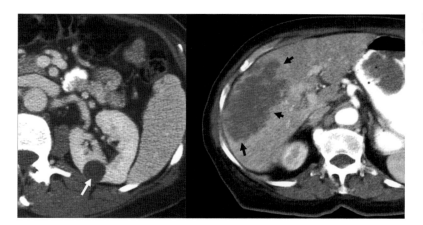

Figure 15.12. Shape: round, benign renal cyst (white arrow); irregular liver cancer (black arrows).

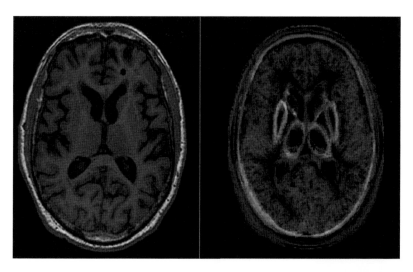

Figure 15.13. Edges of putamen and thalamus accentuated by "entropy" analysis. Courtesy of E. Herskovits.

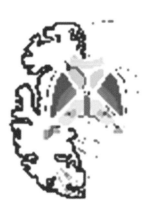
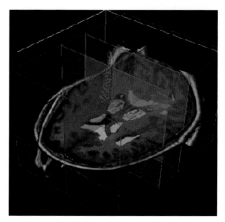

Figure 15.14. Talairach Cartesian coordinate system for stereotactic neurosurgery. Derived from interactive software in Nowinski WL, Thirunavuukarasuu A, Bryan RN. *The Cerefy Atlas of Brain Anatomy*, Vs. 1.0. Thieme, New York; Stuttgart, 2002. (CD format.)

It should be noted that morphological features are relatively independent of imaging modality. The number, size, shape, and position of the lateral ventricles of an individual are the same on CT, MR, or US scans (Figure 15.15).

Morphology and signal

The previous discussion of morphological imaging focused on the spatial components of an image, but an image is a composite of signal, space, and time – and

Table 15.6 Hemorrhage in MRI of the brain

	Age	T_1-weighted	T_2-weighted
Hyperacute	Hours old, mainly oxyhemoglobin with surrounding edema	Hypointense	Hyperintense
Acute	Days old, mainly deoxyhemoglobin with surrounding edema	Hypointense	Hypointense, surrounded by hyperintense margin
Subacute	Weeks old, mainly methemoglobin	Hyperintense	Hypointense, early subacute with predominantly intracellular methemoglobin. Hyperintense, late subacute with predominantly extracelluluar methemoglobin
Chronic	Years old, hemosiderin slit or hemosiderin margin surrounding fluid cavity	Hypointense	Hypointense slit, or hypointense margin surrounding hyperintense fluid cavity

Reproduced with permission from Culebras et al., Stroke 1997; **28**: 1480-47 [4].

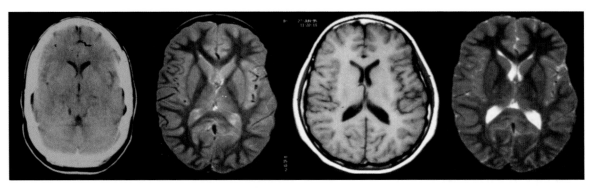

Figure 15.15. Spatial independence, signal dependence on imaging modality. The size, shape, and position of the lateral ventricles is the same on CT and PD, T_1 and T_2 MRI, while CSF signal intensity varies by modality.

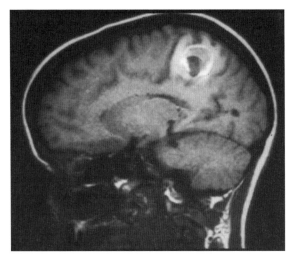

Figure 15.16. MRI signal specificity of subacute brain hematoma due to methemaglobin.

even for morphological imaging, signal cannot be ignored. For morphological analysis, a biomedical object – organ, structure, lesion – must be identifiable in an image before its morphological features can be appreciated. This implies that an object must have signal that distinguishes it from surrounding objects. In the case of imaging, an object must have sufficient difference in signal contrast to distinguish it from its surroundings. Therefore, at a minimum, morphological analysis requires enough signal-based object contrast to detect a lesion. Object signal, as specifically reflected by image contrast, determines the sensitivity of an imaging study. Object contrast must also be sufficient to allow definition of any morphological feature to be evaluated. Object contrast may be described categorically (a radiodense lesion in the lung), ordinally (decreased/iso/increased lesion brightness on brain MRI), or numerically (HUs on CT scans).

In addition to the critical role that signal plays in test sensitivity, it also plays a role in specificity as it is an additional descriptor to be used for lesion classification. In contrast to morphological features, the signal features of an object are completely

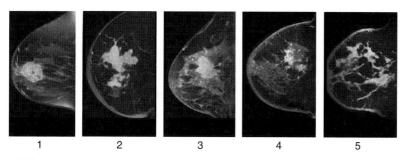

Figure 15.17. Contrast-enhanced MRI of increasing grades of breast tumor malignancy. Verbal and quantitative texture (Gabor filter) descriptors. Courtesy of C. Davatzikos.

1. Unicentric mass; well marginated
2. Multilobulated mass; well marginated
3. Area enhancement, irregular margins; nodular
4. Area enhancement, irregular margins without nodularity
5. Septal spread

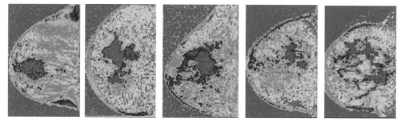

Gabor filter features

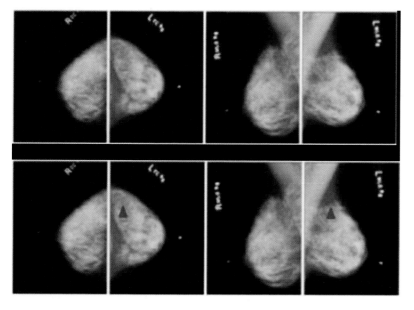

Figure 15.18. Digital mammogram images with and without suspicious regions marked by CAD system. Courtesy of Hologic, www.hologic.com/breast-screening/imagechecker/.

dependent on the imaging modality. The imaging modality determines what is bright or dark on an image. Cerebrospinal fluid is dark on CT, T_1 MR, and US images while bright on T_2 MR images and of intermediate brightness on so-called FLAIR-

MR images (Figure 15.15). Hemorrhagic blood is associated with a sequence of degradation molecules as it ages, and these molecules have different MRI signal characteristics. These signals are used to classify brain hematomas into acute, subacute, or chronic (Table 15.6, Figure 15.16). These distinctive signal descriptors are independent of spatial features. The T_1 bright signal of a subacute hematoma is specifically related to the molecule methemaglobin. More refined and detailed signal analysis quickly takes us to physiological and molecular imaging, as presented in the following chapters.

Perhaps the most complex morphological feature of a structure is *texture*. Texture is a measure of the overall spatial organization and signal variability in an object. Simply stated, texture relates to the uniformity of signal spatial distribution. Many of the "morphological" descriptors, verbal and numerical, relate to texture. *Amorphous*, *mixed*, *multilocular*, *pleomorphic*, *reticulated*, etc. verbally describe textural aspects of a tissue. Quantitative measures of texture include skewness, coarseness, contrast, energy, entropy, uniformity, fractile dimensions (Figure 15.17). While, once again, words seem wanting in describing image data, it must be admitted that the biomedical significance of these newer quantitative measures of texture remains an open question. However, in breast imaging computer-assisted diagnosis (CAD) has become a routine diagnostic tool for diagnosing breast cancer,

though still used as a supplementary tool by the mammographer (Figure 15.18).

In conclusion, biomedical imaging applications relate to all of the traditional biological subdivisions of morphology, physiology, and biochemistry. Morphological imaging focuses on the geometric, spatial attributes of image objects but requires adequate signal contrast for object detection and feature extraction. Spatial and signal features in combination determine specificity.

References

1. Langlotz CP. RadLex: a new method for indexing online http://radlex.org/viewer educational materials. *Radiographics* 2006; **26**: 1595–7.

2. Pizlo Z. *3D Shape: its Unique Place in Visual Perception.* Cambridge, MA: MIT Press, 2008.

3. Gatenby RA, Frieden BR. Information theory in living systems, methods, applications, and challenges. *Bull Math Biol* 2007; **69**: 635–57.

4. Culebras A, Kase CS, Masdeu JC, *et al.* Practice guidelines for the use of imaging in transient ischemic attacks and acute stroke: a report of the Stroke Council, American Heart Association. *Stroke* 1997; **28**: 1480–97.

Chapter 16

Physiological imaging

Mitchell D. Schnall

Biomedical images represent spatial maps of signals collected from the interaction of energy with the body at a specific time. The signals themselves represent a property of the tissue. There are two strategies to infer functional status of tissue and whole organisms from biomedical images. The first relies on the signals from which the image is collected to target properties that directly relate to function. A common example of this approach is the use of FDG-PET to measure glucose uptake, providing a direct window into tissue glucose metabolism. A single image collected after the injection of radiolabled FDG provides a spatial distribution of the rate of glucose uptake. As the functional signals often target events that occur in cells at a molecular level, this approach to functional imaging is often referred to as molecular imaging. In molecular imaging the key information is included in the spatial distribution of a signal at a single time point.

A second approach to inferring tissue function from biomedical images relies on the evolution of the image as a function of time. With this approach, images from a single time point do not contain functional information. However, tracking a tissue property over time allows information regarding function to be extracted. The time axis contains the critical information in this approach to imaging tissue function. We will define the measurement of tissue function by detecting time changes in images as *physiological imaging*. There is a large array of physiological imaging methods, including the tracking of a morphological tissue property such as the size of a tumor or the change in a tissue property in response to a physiological stimulus, such as detecting the blood oxygen level-dependent (BOLD) response to neurological stimulus. In addition, physiological imaging can track properties over a wide range of time scales, from years (detecting atrophy associated with neurodegenerative disease) to fractions of a second (detecting mechanical properties of

contracting myocardium). In this section we will illustrate the various approaches to physiological imaging in more detail.

Detecting changes in special dimensions over a long time scale

Tumor response assessment

Perhaps the most often-practiced application of physiological imaging is the assessment of the response of cancer to treatment. This is among the few imaging assessments that serves as a surrogate marker for clinical outcome in approving cancer treatments [1]. Traditionally, tumors were assessed by clinical examination, which included an estimate of the tumor size through palpation. This approach has obvious limitations. The emergence of cross-sectional imaging has provided a more objective means to assess tumor size, and is not limited by accessibility to palpation. The basic approach is simple. Patients are imaged prior to starting therapy and then at fixed intervals after treatment has been initiated. The intervals are defined based on the expected time course of growth and response of a specific tumor type (a crude application of the Nyquist sampling theorem), but are typically of the order of weeks to months. Tumor size is measured at each time point. Tumor growth is defined as disease progression, tumor shrinkage is defined as a therapeutic response, and no change in tumor size is defined as stable disease. Figure 16.1 illustrates CT scans demonstrating a 31% increase in the longest diameter of a tumor. By RECIST criteria, this change in tumor size would be defined as disease progression, providing functional evidence of disease status.

Although appearing trivially simple, the assessment of tumor response through changes in size remains a controversial process. There are multiple issues that

Introduction to the Science of Medical Imaging, ed. R. Nick Bryan. Published by Cambridge University Press. © Cambridge University Press 2010.

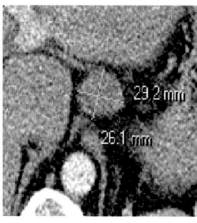
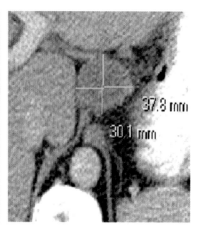

Pre-treatment   Post-treatment

Figure 16.1. CT images before and after chemotherapy demonstrate an increase in the longest diameter of a tumor focus from 2.9 to 3.8 cm. This increase is over 30% of the longest diameter and would be classified as tumor progression by RECIST criteria.

must be addressed in establishing a method to address tumor size. The first issue is exactly how you assign a measurement variable to the tumor. There are multiple possibilities, including linear dimensions (diameters), area of the cross-section through the center of the tumor, and tumor volume. There are two sets of standards that are generally adopted to assess tumor size: RECIST (Response Evaluation Criteria in Solid Tumors) and WHO (World Health Organization), both of which are based on linear dimensions. Linear measurement was adopted as a metric for several reasons. It parallels the classic assessment of size through palpation. It is also easily disseminated, and does not require special software tools or laborious manual tumor outlining to generate area or volume measurements. There is a distinct difference between the WHO and RECIST criteria, however. The RECIST assessment of a single tumor is based on measuring a single longest diameter. The WHO assessment is based on measurement of the longest and orthogonal diameters. There remains controversy regarding the added value of the WHO bi-dimensional measurement relative to the RECIST single diameter measurement.

Treatment effect is a patient-level assessment requiring a set of rules for assessing the patient's entire disease burden and assigning a patient-level category of response. This required a standard for accommodating multiple lesions. The current RECIST standard requires the assessment in a single patient of up to 10 lesions and up to five lesions in each organ system. The patient-level RECIST measurement includes the summation of the longest diameter for each "target lesion" for a given patient. A decrease in this index by 20% is defined as a positive treatment response, while an increase by more than 30% is defined as disease progression.

Looking ahead, there is intense research in the development and implementation of volumetric approaches to assess tumor size. Manual definition of tumor margins to enable volumetric assessment is burdensome and only practical in small selected research studies. Computer automated segmentation is actively being developed. Although apparently simple, this development is complicated by the fact that medical images are not exact representations of anatomic details, but are close approximations. This means that the borders of structures on medical images are not perfectly defined, i.e., they do not have a finite transition width. The sharp images that we view are a result of display cutoffs applied to the image data. Applying different display cutoffs can actually shrink or expand the apparent lesion size, as shown in Figure 16.2. The details of the shape of the border transition for an object in a medical image is a complex function of the physics of the imaging modality, the specifics of a particular embodiment of imaging acquisition technology, and the particular reconstruction algorithm applied. Although computers can be trained to detect and consistently apply cutoffs to define tumor edges for a given border transition function, maintaining the same consistency across the variability of technologies is challenging. This remains an area of active research, and it will likely affect the way tumor size is assessed in the future.

Measuring brain structural changes associated with aging

Normal anatomic structures have complex shapes and often require a more complex approach to assess changes over time than a single anatomic dimension,

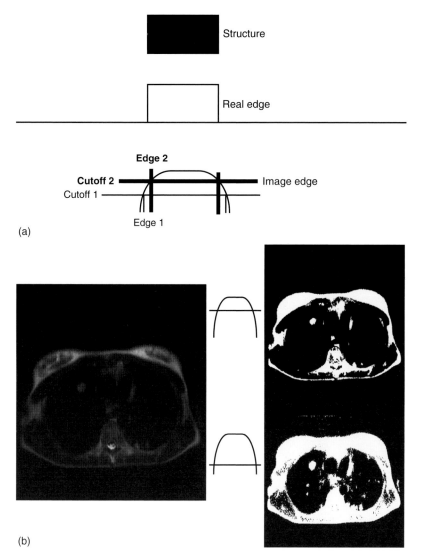

Figure 16.2. (a) The image representation of a rectangular object would result in indistinct object edges, resulting in different perceived sizes based on different image display cutoffs. (b) Displays from the same image of lung metastasis using different display cutoffs change the apparent lesion size.

area, or volume. An example of an important application of complex morphological analysis is the detection of changes in the brain associated with aging. Although it would be possible to measure specific linear or volume measurements of selected brain structures, such as the lateral ventricles, such an analysis would limit the detection of changes to only those that were pre-selected. More complex analytic approaches allow exploration of the entire brain for age-related changes.

One class of image analysis approaches maps the image of a subject onto a specific template and characterizes the subject's brain based on the differences between the subject and an anatomic template (Chapters 13 and 14). An example of such an approach

is the RAVENS method described by Davatzikos et al. [2]. The RAVENS method is based on initially segmenting the brain tissue into white matter, gray matter, and CSF, based on MRI signal intensity. The segmented brain is then registered using a complex elastic mapping to a selected standard anatomic atlas. During the registration step, the signal intensity of each pixel is encoded with the pixel volume change associated with the registration. The result is a representation of the gray matter, white matter, and CSF components of an individual's brain, mapped to a template with the intensity of each pixel representing the local change in volume between the subject and the template (Figure 16.3). By representing the local (pixel-level) changes in volume by intensity, statistical

267

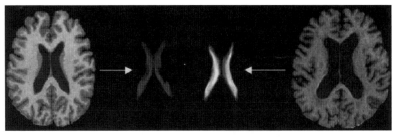

Figure 16.3. MR images from two different subjects with different degrees of ventricular atrophy and their respective CSF RAVENS maps. Although the ventricles of the RAVENS maps have the same shape after elastic normalization, their brightness differs, reflecting the fact that relatively more CSF was forced to fit the same template for the brain with larger ventricles (shown on the right). Voxel-wise comparisons of RAVENS maps can be performed using voxel-wise statistical tests. (Reproduced with permission from Davatzikos *et al., NeuroImage* 2001; **14**: 1361–9 [2].)

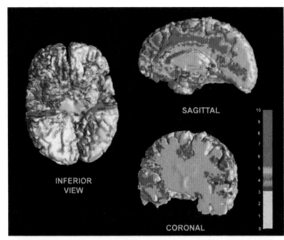

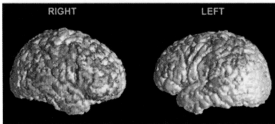

Figure 16.4. Longitudinal magnetic resonance imaging studies of older adults: a shrinking brain. (Reproduced with permission from Resnick *et al., J Neurosci* 2003; **23**: 3295–301 [3].)

approaches can be applied to determine significant changes in pixel intensity (and thus volume) between populations across all pixel locations within the template. The result is the identification of all locations in the brain in which the morphology of the brain differs between the populations.

This approach has been applied to identify the pattern of brain atrophy associated with normal aging. Resnick *et al.* studied 92 adults at baseline, two years, and four years with MRI [3]. They applied

the RAVENS approach to measure local volume changes over the follow-up period, presumed to be related to atrophy. Figure 16.4 demonstrates a map of gray-matter loss. Similar methods have been used to identify morphological changes associated with Alzheimer's dementia and psychiatric conditions such as schizophrenia.

Tracking cardiac motion

Tracking the motion of the heart wall under normal and stress conditions is important to assessing cardiac function. The predominant technology used clinically to evaluate cardiac motion is ultrasound. The ability to rapidly acquire images in real time provides cine loops of cross-sections through the heart moving in real time. Newer four-dimensional ultrasound techniques allow complete three-dimensional datasets of the moving heart to be acquired. Although ultrasound represents an ideal technique to rapidly assess gross regional cardiac contractility, it has limitations. The need to find an acoustic window through which the image can be collected results in occasional difficulty in assessing part of the heart wall. This is particularly the case in assessing the right ventricle. In addition, ultrasound imaging provides imaging of the heart shape as a function of time, but does not provide data to allow an element of myocardium to be tracked as a function of time through the cardiac cycle. Thus ultrasound will not allow the detection of any shear motion along the plane of the myocardium.

MRI has emerged as a powerful technique to assess cardiac function by tracking cardiac motion. Several technology barriers had to be overcome to develop MRI into a viable method to track cardiac motion. The formation of an MR image typically requires the acquisition of over 100 individual lines of data, each representing a view of the anatomy in k-space. Even with repetition times (T_R) as short as 5 ms, this would produce an image every half-second, which is incompatible with the time scale of cardiac motion. In order to overcome this limitation, investigators have developed methods to acquire a fraction (or segment) of the image in a single cardiac cycle, while accumulating the full image over multiple cycles. As an example, consider the acquisition of a single cross-section of the heart in the short axis over a 256×128 matrix. This would typically be performed by acquiring 128 phase encode steps (lines in k-space), each of which would be collected as an echo with 256 points. If the image were broken into segments of 8 phase encode steps, each segment could be acquired in 40 ms (assuming a 5 ms T_R). If the heart rate were 60 beats per minute, 25 temporal frames could be acquired during each cardiac cycle. This would provide ample time resolution to track the motion of the myocardium over a cardiac cycle. However, in order to collect the entire data set of 128 lines of k-space needed to reconstruct each image, 16 different segments would need to be collected in each of 16 different heart beats. Respiratory motion can be eliminated so long as patients can hold their breath for 16 heart beats. Gating the acquisition to the cardiac contraction through the simultaneous collection of the EKG signal allows consistent timing of the segments for each cardiac cycle. This scheme works well if the heart rate (time scale of the cardiac contraction) is consistent beat-to-beat. In the setting of cardiac disease, there are often ectopic beats with variable timing. In order to overcome this problem, the development of methods to reject beats that vary in time beyond a set threshold have been developed. The strategy of gated acquisition in segments has proven effective in providing maps of cardiac motion with MRI.

The method described so far will not only suffer from the limitation of mapping the shape of the heart as a function of time, but will also be unable to detect motion in the plane of the myocardium. In order to overcome this limitation, investigators have developed a method to magnetically tag the myocardium in order to track it over time. The application of a radiofrequency (RF) pulse in the setting of a gradient disturbs the magnetization in a slice of anatomy. This principle allows a slice of anatomy to be "tagged" by destroying the magnetization in the slice, resulting in a dark line in the image [4]. A labeling grid can be developed by applying a series of saturation pulses in a rectilinear

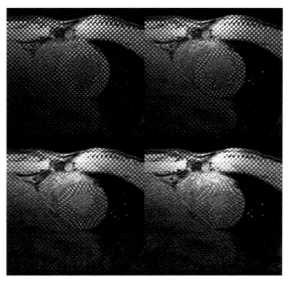

Figure 16.5. Sequential SPAMM (spatial modulation of magnetization) images of the heart acquired in the short axis (time sequence from top left to bottom right) during cardiac systole. Note the contraction of the left ventricle. Also note the decay of the contrast of the labeled grid due to the T_1 relaxation of the myocardium.

grid covering the heart. This labeling is performed immediately before the first temporal frame is collected for each heart beat. The labels established by saturating spins will disappear over time due to T_1 relaxation. Since T_1 relaxation is of the order of a second, the labels will persist for approximately one beat if the heart rate is not too slow. Each intersection of two orthogonal saturation bands represents a point in the myocardium that can be tracked over time. An example of a time sequence of tagged images is illustrated in Figure 16.5. The individual frames from a gated tagged cine MRI image acquisition can be used to develop a map of the vector displacements of each tag intersection as a function of time by calculating the difference in the location of the tag intersections between each temporal frame. These data can be used to assess the motion of myocardium anywhere in the acquisition plane. There are several software approaches to automatically detect the labeling grid in the image, track it over time, and develop stress and strain maps across the myocardium. The example of cardiac motion tagging illustrates how the development of multiple image acquisition and analysis technologies operating in concert can provide powerful maps of important functional parameters based on changing anatomy as a function of time. This approach continues to evolve through the development of faster imaging approaches, improvement of gating technology, the development of 3D approaches, and the use of higher field strength magnets.

Changing signal as a function of time: dynamic contrast-enhanced MRI

Monitoring the change in signal, rather than spatial position, as a function of time can also provide powerful techniques to measure physiology. Of all imaging modalities, MRI appears to dominate this approach to measuring physiology. This is likely because of the richness of the dependence of the MRI signal intensity on acquisition technique and molecular milieu, and the ability of changes in signal to provide a window into physiology.

Among the most important physiological parameters to assess in multiple disease states is blood flow. This has become particularly important in assessing tumors, given the recent successes in targeting angiogenesis as a strategy to treat cancer. Dynamic contrast imaging has become a popular method for assessing tumor blood flow and tracking changes in blood flow in response to anti-angiogenesis therapy. The technique is based on observing the change in signal as a function of time after the injection of an exogenous contrast agent. In principal this can be performed with any imaging modality. Methods based on CT, MRI, ultrasound, and PET have been described. Concerns related to radiation exposure of multiple sequential CT acquisitions have limited the use of CT. The lack of widespread availability of ultrasound contrast agents has limited the use of ultrasound. Although the use of labeled water with ^{15}O and sequential PET acquisitions had been the standard for estimating perfusion by imaging, this technology is difficult to disseminate due to the short half-life of ^{15}O. Of all modalities, MRI has generated the greatest interest as a modality to estimate blood flow through a dynamic contrast-enhanced technique. This is based on the inherent safety profile of the contrast, the sensitivity of MRI to detect contrast-related signal changes, and the ability to perform repeated studies without radiation exposure.

The approach to dynamic contrast-enhanced MRI (DCE-MRI) is based on acquiring a time series of T_1-weighted images during the intravenous injection of a bolus of low-molecular-weight gadolinium (Gd)-based contrast. The low-molecular-weight Gd diffuses relatively freely out of the tissue capillaries into the extracellular space except in the brain, where it is restricted to the intravascular space by the blood–brain barrier. The pharmacokinetics of the contrast is most often modeled using a two-compartment model initially popularized by Tofts et al. [5] that is applied as the *general kinetic model*. The general kinetic model describes the concentration of contrast in the tissue as a function of time according to Equation 16.1:

$$C_T(t) = K_{trans} * C_a(t) \exp(K_{trans}/V_e * t) \quad (16.1)$$

The quantities measured by the MRI imaging sequence include the contrast concentration as a function of time ($C_T(t)$) and the concentration of contrast in arterial supply to the tissue of interest immediately after the contrast injection ($C_a(t)$: arterial input function or AIF). The resultant parameter extracted from fitting the model includes the extracellular tissue volume (V_e) and the exchange constant between the intravascular and extracellular space (K_{trans}). K_{trans} is often used as a surrogate for tissue perfusion.

There are multiple technical considerations that must be addressed to make measurements of the tissue Gd concentration and AIF after an injection of contrast. The first important consideration is that the relationship between Gd and the MRI signal intensity is complex. Gd is detected indirectly by its influence on the T_1 relaxation rate of water. Gd has the effect of changing the water T_1 such that $1/T1_{Gd} = 1/T1 + R$ [Gd]. The ratio of the NMR signal intensity acquired after Gd administration to that acquired prior to Gd administration is:

$$Signal\ ratio = (1 - \exp^{-T_R/T_1})(1 - \cos(\alpha)$$
$$\exp^{-(T_R/T_1 + R[Gd])})/(1 - \cos(\alpha)\exp^{-T_R/T_1})$$
$$(1 - \exp^{-(T_R/T_1 + R[Gd])})$$

$$(16.2)$$

Thus, in order to estimate the concentration of Gd after the injection of the contrast, several measured quantities are necessary: the ratio of the post- to pre-contrast signal intensity (measured), the pre-contrast T_1 relaxation time, T_R and α (constants determined by the pulse sequence), and R (relaxivity of Gd). Therefore, in order to accurately fit the generalized kinetic model, one must have a map of the pre-contrast tissue T_1 times that can be registered to the pre- and post-contrast image sets. The ideal approach is to actually collect a set of images with varied flip

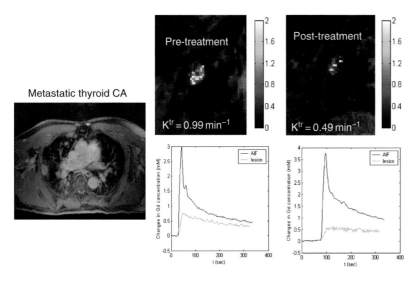

Metastatic thyroid CA

Pre-treatment $K^{tr} = 0.99\ min^{-1}$

Post-treatment $K^{tr} = 0.49\ min^{-1}$

Figure 16.6. Dynamic contrast-enhanced MRI. Left: axial MRI image demonstrating a metastatic thyroid carcinoma in the right chest wall. Right: Pre- and post-treatment DCE-MRI exams. Top: K_{trans} maps. Bottom: arterial and lesion signal intensity as a function of time after contrast injection. Note the response to sorafenib treatment.

angle that allows direct calculations of the tissue T_1. Unfortunately, this adds time to the examination. Alternatively, T_1 can be estimated based on historical data. A T_1 map can be combined with a map of the ratio of post-contrast to pre-contrast images and pulse sequence parameters to estimate the tissue Gd concentration as a function of time.

The AIF offers additional challenges. The contrast bolus is typically administered over a time scale of approximately 10 seconds. This results in rapidly increasing signal intensity within the arterial system that requires very high temporal resolution to sample accurately. Although individual image planes can be acquired with the required 1–2 second time resolution, this would preclude the DCE-MRI examination to study an entire tumor volume. Several approaches have been proposed to address this challenge. A small test dose of Gd can be injected prior to the DCE-MRI image acquisition and could be used to measure the AIF. The high concentration of contrast within the arterial system allows the AIF to be measured with one-tenth of the dose used for the DCE-MRI study. This allows the DCE to be performed after the AIF measurement without contaminating the tissue with Gd. A second approach involves estimating the AIF from models that can be fitted with lower time-resolution data. This is often done on a population and not an individual exam basis. Obviously this represents a compromise to measuring the AIF directly.

The final result of a DCE-MRI study is an estimate of K_{trans}. This can either be generated on a specific region of interest by collecting the full set of signal intensity data from a prescribed region of interest within the tumor. This approach is often used when there is motion between the time series of images. If the anatomy is stationary, and all images can be directly superimposed, K_{trans} maps of the entire tumor can be generated. An example of a K_{trans} map through a metastatic tumor to the right lung before and after anti-angiogenic therapy is illustrated in Figure 16.6. K_{trans} is used to predict and monitor tumor treatment with anti-angiogenic therapy.

Change in signal in response to applied energy: arterial spin-labeled perfusion

DCE-MRI relies on detecting changes in signal intensity related to an exogenous contrast agent that is injected intravenously. However, it is possible to essentially create an internal contrast agent by labeling the arterial blood through spin-inversion. Imagine that a plane perpendicular to the direction of flow of a blood vessel is exposed to RF energy that selectively inverts the water protons passing through the plane. The labeled arterial spins flow into the tissue of interest, exchange across the capillary membrane, and mix with the tissue water, resulting in cancellation of some of the positive spins in the tissue water. The net effect is a decrease in the MRI signal that can be acquired from the tissue water protons. The magnitude of the signal decrease is related to the rate of flow of the inverted water protons into the tissue of interest [6]. The

271

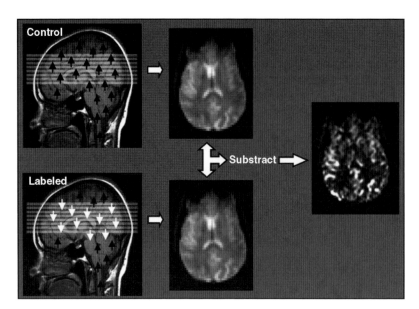

Figure 16.7. Arterial blood is labeled or tagged and, after a delay, moves into the imaging plane or volume, during which time there is T_1 decay of the label. Snapshot images are acquired in labeled and control conditions and subtracted, yielding a difference image with intensity proportional to cerebral blood flow (CBF). (Reproduced with permission from Wolf and Detre, *Neurotherapeutics* 2007; **4**: 346–59 [7].)

technique is illustrated in Figure 16.7. In the original description of the arterial spin-label (ASL) technique, the use of a continuous inversion of the inflowing arterial spins using a spin-lock pulse was described. Under these conditions the blood flow (*f*) can be calculated to be:

$$f = (\lambda / T1_{\text{apparent}})(M_{\text{control}} - M_{\text{steady state}})/2M_{\text{control}}$$

(16.3)

Where λ is the blood–brain partition coefficient, $T1_{\text{apparent}}$ is time for the brain magnetization to approach steady state after inversion is applied (close to the blood T_1), $M_{\text{steady state}}$ represents the brain magnetization in the setting of continuous inversion, and M_{control} represents the brain magnetization in the absence of labeling.

This approach has the obvious appeal of avoiding the need for injecting contrast. It also labels the actual blood water, which is freely diffusible across the capillary membrane and allows for an accurate estimate of actual tissue perfusion. In addition, since the label is placed via spin-inversion, it disappears with T_1 relaxation, allowing repeated measures to be performed in one examination time frame.

However, the arterial spin-label (ASL) technique presents new challenges. This includes establishing the label in the arterial supply. The use of continuous labeling as described in the original publication of ASL is not practical in many settings due to specific absorption rate (SAR) limitations. Several creative

pulse techniques have been developed to balance the RF exposure and the extent of inversion. In addition, since the net effect on the MRI signal related to arterial inversion is small, care has to be taken to adjust for the small direct effect that the labeling pulses have on the imaging volume. This is typically achieved by applying an identical pulse along a plane parallel to the labeling plane on the opposite side of the imaging volume from the labeling plane. Finally, since this technique requires detecting a difference between two images to detect flow, motion between the acquisitions will effect the measurement.

Change in signal in response to physiological stimulus: blood oxygen level determination

Perhaps the most widely used physiological imaging method is blood oxygen level-dependent (BOLD) MRI. BOLD-MRI relies on detecting MRI signal changes related to changes in the magnetic properties of the iron bound to hemoglobin, which is related to changes in the blood oxygen tension. The iron in oxygenated hemoglobin is less magnetic than the iron in deoxyhemoglobin. If a physiological perturbation is applied to a tissue that affects the level of oxygen extraction, the magnetism of the venous blood changes, resulting in a change in the MRI signal. The MRI signal change is related to changes in the dephasing of the tissue protons by changes in the local magnetic field

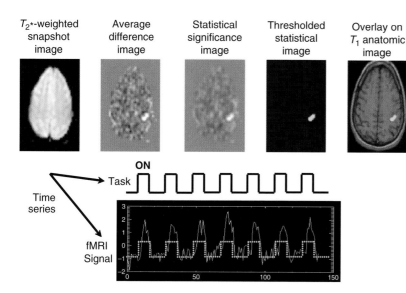

| T_2*-weighted snapshot image | Average difference image | Statistical significance image | Thresholded statistical image | Overlay on T_1 anatomic image |

Figure 16.8. Typical BOLD experiment. Top row demonstrates the base T_2* image, the averaged difference signal between the base image in the stimulus and non-stimulus condition, the statistical-difference image between the stimulus and non-stimulus conditions and the statistical-difference image after applying a threshold demonstrating the functional area. This can be overlaid on a T_1-weighted anatomic image (top right). Bottom of figure includes the stimulation pattern and the actual signal intensity from the MRI image in the functional regions as a function of time, related to the stimulation patterns. Courtesy of John Detre.

Time series

ON
Task

fMRI Signal

associated with the hemoglobin in the blood stream. This effect is best measured with T_2* imaging.

The most common application of BOLD imaging is to detect brain activity [8]. The brain has a very high metabolic rate and associated high oxygen consumption. It also has sensitive regulation of blood flow, increasing flow with increased energy demand to ensure adequate levels of metabolites are available. Thus, in response to activation, there is an increased blood flow to the activated brain tissue, typically beyond that needed to supply metabolic oxygen. This so-called luxury perfusion results in an increase in the level of blood oxygen in the venous blood in activated tissue. Thus, on a T_2*-weighted image there is a small signal difference detected between the activated and unactivated state. Detecting the signal difference provides a unique window into brain activity.

The signal change related to the BOLD effect is quite small. The difference between single measurements performed in the activated and unactivated states typically cannot be detected by simple inspection. The usual method for detecting the BOLD effect is to repeatedly toggle on and off the physiological stimulus, resulting in alternating periods of stimulated and basal state. The images are analyzed to detect pixels that have a statistical correlation with the stimulus input. An example of a BOLD measurement is demonstrated in Figure 16.8. The detection of functional brain activation with BOLD has had a major impact on cognitive neuroscience. Creative approaches to presenting complex auditory, visual, and tactile stimuli in the setting of an MRI scanner have been developed. This has allowed the investigation of brain activation patterns associated with complex stimuli in normal volunteers and patients afflicted with neurologic and psychiatric illness, providing insight into normal and pathologic brain function.

Conclusions

Although anatomic images are often considered static representations of structural information, their time evolution provides a rich opportunity to probe biological function. Changes in anatomic structure in response to evolving biological processes including tumor growth and brain atrophy can be used to quantify these important events. This is particularly useful to measure the effects of therapeutic interventions. Methods for quantifying structure can be as simple as measuring a linear dimension or as complex as developing three-dimensional maps of local volumetric change.

Changes in anatomic images can also be induced by extrinsic stimuli. Labeling structures in MRI images with saturation bands allows the detection of anatomic motion on short time scales such as cardiac motion. Changes in signal induced by contrast injection or arterial blood saturation can provide measures of perfusion, an important parameter to describe tissue viability. Finally, signal changes in response to external stimuli such as the detection of the BOLD effect can provide a powerful method to detect neuronal activity in the living brain. A common thread that joins the techniques described above is the requirement to integrate the image acquisition technique to the image analysis method. Physiologic imaging represents a systems problem that requires consideration of the entire imaging system in order to generate viable approaches to assaying biological function.

References

1. Therasse P, Arbuck SG, Eisenhauer EA, *et al.* New guidelines to evaluate the response to treatment in solid tumors. *J Natl Cancer Inst* 2000; **92**: 205–16.

2. Davatzikos C, Genc A, Xu D, Resnick SM. Voxel-based morphometry using the RAVENS maps: methods and validation using simulated longitudinal atrophy. *NeuroImage* 2001; **14**: 1361–9.

3. Resnick SM, Pham DL, Kraut MA, Zonderman AB, Davatzikos C. Longitudinal magnetic resonance imaging studies of older adults: a shrinking brain. *J Neurosci* 2003; **23**: 3295–301.

4. Axel L, Dougherty L. MR imaging of motion with spatial modulation of magnetization. *Radiology* 1989; **171**: 841–5.

5. Tofts PS, Kermode AG. Measurement of the blood–brain barrier permeability and leakage space using dynamic MR imaging. 1. Fundamental concepts. *Magn Reson Med* 1991; **17**: 357–67.

6. Detre JA, Leigh JS, Williams DS, Koretsky AP. Perfusion imaging. *Magn Reson Med* 1992; **23**: 37–45.

7. Wolf RL, Detre JA. Clinical neuroimaging using arterial spin-labeled perfusion magnetic resonance imaging. *Neurotherapeutics* 2007; **4**: 346–59.

8. Ogawa S, Lee TM, Kay AR, Tank DW. Brain magnetic resonance imaging with contrast dependent on blood oxygenation. *Proc Natl Acad Sci USA* 1990; **87**: 9868–72.

Molecular imaging

Jerry S. Glickson

Molecular imaging is the characterization, visualization, and measurement of biological processes in space and over time at the molecular and cellular level in humans and other living systems. There are two types of molecular imaging probes: naturally occurring *intrinsic probes*, consisting of molecules that can be visualized in the host or in isolated tissues by appropriate imaging techniques, and *extrinsic probes*, usually synthetic, which are introduced into the host to facilitate detection by a specific imaging technique.

A very important subclass of extrinsic probes is *nanoparticles*, consisting of large molecules or particles to which extrinsic imaging probes are attached for diagnosis of specific lesions or diseases. Ideally, these nanoparticles are selectively targeted to specific cells via antibodies or receptor-targeting components of the nanoparticle (e.g., the receptor-binding sequence of a lipoprotein or of a protein like transferrin). These nanoparticles may also deliver therapeutic agents, thereby facilitating a seamless transition between diagnosis and therapy. Such versatile probes, called theranostic agents, lie at the heart of the individualized diagnosis and therapy that is the goal of much current medical research.

Table 17.1 lists the various targets of molecular imaging. Except for the drugs, these targets are all intrinsic to the body. Some can be imaged directly and hence are considered intrinsic probes, but others require the addition of an extrinsic probe that binds to the target molecule and thereby makes it detectable by a molecular imaging technique. For example, serum albumin is not readily detected by any of the imaging techniques, but indocyanine green (ICG) is a near-infrared (NIR) extrinsic probe approved by the US Food and Drug Administration (FDA) for human use that binds tightly to albumin and makes it readily detectable by optical imaging. Gadolinium complexes that bind tightly to serum albumin facilitating its detection by T_1-weighted dynamic contrast-enhanced MRI have also been prepared.

Molecular beacons are molecular switches that can exist in a fluorescent state or in a state in which fluorescence is quenched by fluorescence energy transfer (FRET) to a proximal quencher (which could be the same fluorophore if the fluorophore exhibits self-quenching), or it can be a separate entity in the beacon. When the fluorophore is separated from the quencher, fluorescence is restored, and the molecular beacon is activated. Utilization of near-infrared (NIR) fluorophores permits *in vivo* detection of these molecular beacons since the penetration depth of NIR light can be several centimeters, depending on the wavelength and the intensity of the light source. For example, antisense peptide nucleic acids or nucleotides have been prepared that hybridize with a specific mRNA and in the process activate a fluorophore and thereby indicate transcription of a specific gene [1]. The method can also be used to detect any molecule that is cleaved by a specific enzyme. For example, Tung *et al.* [2] used a graft copolymer of poly-L-lysine with peptide substrates of cathepsin D attached to the lysine side-chain amino groups. Each peptide was linked to a cy-5 NIR fluorophore at its amino terminus. In the intact graft copolymer, self-quenching efficiently eliminated fluorescence, but cleavage of the small peptides by cathepsin D liberated free and highly fluorescent cy-5, indicating the presence of this proteinase. A simpler approach using specific peptides with fluorophores on one end and quenchers on the other was recently introduced by Stefflova *et al.* to detect apoptosis by the activity of caspase 3 [3]. Analogous methods have been used to detect specific phospholipases and glycosidases. The fluorophore could also be a photodynamic therapy agent that not only detects a specific mRNA or enzyme but uses it as a trigger to generate cytotoxic singlet oxygen in the presence of near-infrared

Introduction to the Science of Medical Imaging, ed. R. Nick Bryan. Published by Cambridge University Press. © Cambridge University Press 2010.

Table 17.1. Targets of molecular imaging

Target	Concentration range	Imaging modality
Nucleic Acids		
mRNA	picomolar	Optical NIR (molecular beacons)
DNA	picomolar	PET (^{11}C- ^{18}F-labeled drugs), bioluminescence
Proteins		
Serum albumin	micromolar	MRI (Gd complex) NIR (ICG complex)
Hemoglobin	micromolar	NIR
Myoglobin	nanomolar	NIR, ^{1}H MRS
Amyloid β	nanomolar	PET, SPECT
AKT	femtomolar	Bioluminescence–split luciferase
P53	femtomolar	Bioluminescence
Cartilage (GAGs)	micromolar	^{23}Na and ^{1}H (GdDTPA) MRI
Polysaccharides		
Glycogen	millimolar	^{1}H MRS magnetization transfer MRI
Receptors		
Lipoproteins	nanomolar	Optical NIR, MRI (Gd, FeO), PET, SPECT
Folate	nanomolar	NIR, MRI (FeO)
Her2nu	nanomolar	MRI (Gd)
Neurotransmitters/ neuroreceptors	nanomolar	PET
Insulin-like receptor 1 (IGF-1)	Nanomolar	PET, NIR
Integrins	nanomolar	PET, SPECT, NIR
Metabolites		
ATP	5 mM	^{31}P MRS
ADP	<1 mM	^{31}P MRS
AMP	~1 mM	^{31}P MRS
Pi (pH)	millimolar	^{31}P MRS
Phosphocreatine	millimolar	^{31}P MRS
Phosphocholine (PC)	millimolar	^{31}P MRS
Phosphoethanolamine (PE)	millimolar	^{31}P MRS
Glycero-PC	millimolar	^{31}P MRS
Glycero-PE	millimolar	^{31}P MRS
Lactate	millimolar	^{1}H MRS, ^{13}C MRS
Choline	millimolar	^{1}H MRS
Citrate	millimolar	^{1}H MRS
Amino acids	millimolar	^{1}H MRS
N-acetylaspartate	millimolar	^{1}H MRS
Glucose	millimolar	^{1}H MRS, ^{13}C MRS
Oxygen	<1 Tor – 150 Tor	^{15}O PET, ^{19}F MRI, phosphorescence, hyperpolarized ^{3}He MRS

Table 17.1. (cont.)

Target	Concentration range	Imaging modality
Drugs		
^{18}FDG	nanomolar	^{18}F PET
5-fluorouracil	millimolar	^{19}F MRS, ^{18}F PET
Temozolomide	millimolar	^{13}C MRS, ^{11}C PET
Doxorubicin	nanomolar	Optical
Gancyclovir	nanomolar	^{18}F PET
Steroids (estrogens, androgens)	nanomolar	^{18}F PET
Opioids	nanomolar	^{18}F PET
Hypoxia Probes		
(EF5, ATSM, misonidazole, etc.)	nanomolar	^{18}F PET
HIF1α-GFP activation	femtomolar	Optical
Apoptosis Probes		
Caspase 3	nanomolar	NIR beacon
Annexin V	nanomolar	^{99m}Tc-SPECT, ^{1}H MRS (FeO)
Perfusion		
^{99m}Tc-sestemibi	nanomolar	SPECT
Gd-DTPA	micromolar	^{1}H MRI
Potassium Analogs (membrane integrity)		
^{201}Thallium, ^{87}Rb	nanomolar	SPECT

radiation [3]. Thus, extrinsic probes could be both diagnostic and therapeutic.

Marker genes are genetic probes that detect specific promoters, such as HIF1α that is activated under hypoxic conditions, or expression of specific genes such as those introduced by gene therapy. Examples of marker genes are thymidine kinase, which can be detected by PET with fialuridine (FIAU) or other PET probes, creatine kinase and arginine kinase for MRS detection, luciferase for bioluminescence detection, or fluorescent proteins emitting different colors or wavelengths of light in the NIR for optical detection. The Tsien laboratory has introduced a novel molecular switch consisting of a split luciferase molecule that is bioluminescent when the two pieces are permitted to come together in a conformation similar to the conformation of the intact luciferase. Conformational changes, calcium levels, and protein–protein interactions can be detected *in vivo* by attaching the half-luciferase fragments to different regions of proteins or different proteins [4]. Rehemtullah and colleagues [5] have designed a molecular beacon consisting of a split luciferase molecule attached to the signaling protein AKT. Using an ingenious construct that separates the two halves of the luciferase protein when AKT is phosphorylated, these authors have designed a molecular switch that can signal phosphorylation of this key signaling protein. However, a key limitation of the bioluminescence and fluorescent protein probes is that they cannot be applied to human subjects in the clinic; they can, however, be used in mice to evaluate the activity of drugs that target the signaling pathway or activate specific promoters, or they can be used to study inter-protein interactions. Development of optical probes that can perform similar functions in humans is one of the key challenges to molecular imagers.

In terms of the basic definition in Chapter 1, Equation 1.15 indicates that the radiologically detected signal is basically a five-dimensional vector quantity dependent on mass or energy, which are relativistically interconvertible, spatial coordinates, and the time required to detect the signal:

$$S = f(m, E)(x, y, z)(t) \qquad x, y, z < \infty \qquad (17.1)$$

Table 17.2 summarizes the ranges of these vector coordinates defining the signals detected by various

Table 17.2. Ranges of molecular imaging coordinates ($S = f(m,E; x,y,z; t)$)

Modality	Concentration	Frequency, wavelength or energy	Spatial resolution volume/linear	Temporal resolution
MRS				
^{1}H	0.0001–100 M	63–500 MHz	0.012–2 ml/2.3–12.6 mm @ 4.7T	6–30 min
^{1}H/Dy liposomes	$\sim 10^{-6}$ M	300 MHZ	$\sim$0.15 mm @ 7T	$\sim$30 min
^{1}H/magnetite	$\sim 10^{-6}$ M	63–500 MHz	0.15 mm @ 7 T	2 hr
^{31}P	0.001–0.010 M	25.9–202 MHz	0.5–27 ml/ 5–30 mm	$\sim$30 min
^{13}C	0.003–0.026 M	15.7–123 MHz	0.5–27 ml/ 5–30 mm	5–60 min
Hyperpolarized ^{13}C	10^{-8}–0.001 M	15.7–123 MHz	$\sim 10^{-5}$–1 ml/ $\sim$1 mm	1.5 min
^{19}F	0.0001–0.100 M	59–459 MHz	0.015–2 ml/ $\sim$2–13 mm	$\sim$30 min
MRI				
^{1}H	$\sim$100 M 10 mM Gd	63–500 MHz	$\sim$0.001 ml/ $\sim$0.5 mm	2–3 min
PET				
^{18}F	10^{-11}–10^{-12} M	High-energy γ-rays	0.001–10 ml/ 1–5 mm	10 sec to min
SPECT				
^{99m}Tc	$\sim 10^{-10}$ – 10^{-11} M	Low-energy γ-rays	1–5 mm	min
CT	1 mM iodine	x-rays	0.050 mm	min
Optical				
NIR	$\sim 10^{-9}$ M	$\lambda = 650$–900 nm	$\sim$0.001 ml/ 2–3 mm	<1 min–10 min
Bioluminescence	10^{-15}–10^{-17} M	<560 nm	$\sim$1 cm	sec to min
Ultrasound	1 bubble	High-frequency sound	0.050–0.500 mm	sec to min

molecular imaging modalities. In terms of rank order of concentration sensitivity, bioluminescence is the most sensitive imaging modality, detecting to about 0.01 femtomolar (10^{-17} M) concentrations. PET and near-infrared (NIR) imaging can detect into the picomolar (10^{-12} M) range, whereas SPECT is slightly less sensitive ($\sim 10^{-11}$). The sensitivity of ultrasound is not well defined, but the method is capable of detecting a single bubble in the blood stream. MRI is capable of monitoring micromolar and tens of micromolar concentrations with magnetite and gadolinium contrast agents, respectively, and MRS generally monitors between a tenth and tens of millimolar levels of metabolites (ATP, P_i, lactate, glucose, etc.). On the other hand, MRI has the highest spatial resolution ($\sim$1 µL and $\sim$0.5 nm in 2–3 minutes at 4.7 T and $\sim$50 nm in 60 minutes at 9.4 T). Overall, the MR methods, with their high resolution and sensitivity to chemical structure and dynamics, are probably the most versatile methods, but they have distinct limitations with respect to concentration sensitivity (being the least sensitive of all the imaging techniques) and their inability to detect large rigid macromolecules like

DNA or various globular proteins, although macromolecules like glycogen which undergo rapid internal rotation can be completely "NMR visible."

Each of the modalities has unique advantages for specific applications. Thus, NIR and bioluminescence optical imaging offer the advantages of low cost, portability, and extremely high sensitivity, but at the cost of poor spatial resolution at depths below a few millimeters below the surface, which makes these methods difficult or impossible to implement in many clinical settings. Cell surface receptors such as LDL, insulin, and folate receptors typically occur at a concentration of about 1000 copies per cell, which translates to about 10^{15}/L (assuming 10^9 cells/mL); dividing by Avogadro's number, this is equivalent to about 1.6×10^{-9} M, which make receptors ideal for PET detection with tomographic resolution. This is why PET imaging is routinely used to image neuroreceptors and neurotransmitters in the brains of animals and humans. None of the other imaging modalities are suitable for this purpose. However, recycling of cellular receptors facilitates the accumulation of much higher intracellular concentrations of molecular probes over the course of time, thus enabling the application of much less sensitive techniques like MRI for detection of cells carrying appropriate receptors [6]. MRI can detect single cells loaded *ex vivo* with large iron oxide particles in living mice [7].

We are ultimately interested in defining concentrations of metabolites in space and time in living tissues. The tissues may be specific organs or parts thereof (brain, heart, liver, kidneys). They may be part of the vasculature, lymphatics, CNS, neuronal system, hematological system, immune system, skeletal system, etc., or they may be portions of diseased tissues such as tumor, infarcts, etc. If spatial resolution permits, the signal may be subdivided on the basis of its spatial coordinates, but in many instances an entire organ or simulated organ (such as a tumor simulated by attaching isolated tumor cells to microcarrier beads or to gel threads in a perfusion chamber) may constitute the sample. Suspensions of multicellular spheroids of aggregated tumor cells have served as models of the natural heterogeneity of tumors. Bioreactors constructed from thin dialysis tubes embedded in a cylindrical perfusion chamber have also been used to study high concentrations of normal and malignant cells. The variation of metabolite concentrations over this isolated organ is often investigated as a function of time without delineating the spatial dependence of the signal. The intent is eventually to delineate the complete spatial dependence of the signal in the *in vivo* organ or tissue in the host, but preliminary studies are first performed in the isolated perfused organ or tissue. In other instances, the organ might be modified by introducing a perturbation of the flow of perfusate in part of it (e.g., by ligating specific arteries of the heart) or by varying the global flow of perfusate. In this case, imaging may delineate the spatial and temporal dependence of the signals.

We also need to include the concept of composite or average organs or tissues, for which a signal may be averaged over the same organ or tissue in a number of animals or humans. For example, a number of matched animals or patients may be examined to determine the average metabolic characteristics of specific organs or tissues in the normal animal, and these characteristics may then be compared with those of a diseased cohort. Alternatively, a diseased organ or tissue (isolated or *in vivo*) might be examined as a function of time in cohorts of animals or humans who are therapeutically treated with some agent, and these organs or tissues can be compared with corresponding organs in sham-treated or placebo-treated controls. Average values of the molecular imaging parameters might be compared in the treated and control cohorts to determine if a statistically significant difference can be detected. Alternatively, patients or animals may serve as their own controls by comparing their characteristics as a function of time with pretreatment values.

Molecular imaging has been applied to disease diagnosis, staging, monitoring therapy, and the evaluation of metabolic pathways. This chapter will examine a number of examples of these types of molecular imaging applications. We will emphasize the use of nanoparticles as delivery systems for diagnostic and therapeutic (i.e., theranostic) agents, and also the use of MRS and MRI in monitoring therapeutic response of cancer. Finally we will demonstrate how ^{13}C MRS kinetic measurements can quantitatively delineate metabolic flux through glycolytic and oxidative pathways of cellular energy production in hearts and tumor cells.

Lipoprotein theranostic agents

Lipoproteins provide a versatile natural platform for delivery of diagnostic and therapeutic agents to cell surface receptors. Nanoparticles are large natural or synthetic macromolecular structures that are used for delivery of large payloads of diagnostic and/or therapeutic agents for the detection and treatment of a broad range of diseases. Some of these agents are targeted to pathological tissues by specific cell-surface receptor-binding moieties, antibodies, or antibody fragments, whereas others non-specifically accumulate in tumor or other tissues that typically exhibit leaky vasculature, through which these particles readily extravasate. Examples of nanoparticles include synthetic polymers, liposomes, polymerosomes, emulsions, and receptor-binding proteins.

Lipoproteins constitute a versatile nanoparticular platform that includes a large family of macromolecular particles varying in size from ~10 nm (HDL) to over a micron (chylomicrons). The key advantages of these nanoparticles is that they occur naturally in humans and other mammals and hence are non-immunogenic, and that they are readily amenable to incorporation of optical, MRI, PET, and SPECT contrast agents as well as a variety of chemotherapeutic, photodynamic therapy (PDT), and radiotherapeutic agents. The archetypical lipoprotein, low-density lipoprotein (LDL, commonly referred to as "bad cholesterol")

279

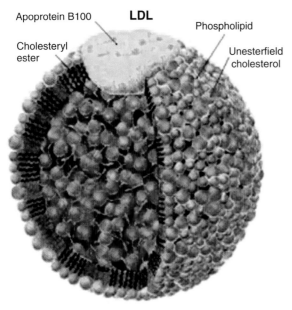

Apoprotein B100   **LDL**

Cholesteryl ester

Phospholipid

Unesterfield cholesterol

Figure 17.1. Cartoon depicting probable structure of LDL. The particle consists of a phospholipid monolayer shell containing free cholesterol and cholesterol esters surrounding a lipid core containing triglycerides and cholesterol esters. Each particle contains one copy of the apoprotein ApoB100, one of the largest proteins known (~550 kDa). Modeling suggests that APoB100 contains a globular N-terminal domain followed by a sequence of alternating amphipathic α-helices and β-sheets. Since the helices are too short to span the phospholipid monolayer, they are probably adsorbed on the monolayer with their hydrophobic faces on the outer surface of the monolayer. The β-sheets are similar to those on the primordial lipoprotein vitellogenin and are probably adsorbed directly to the lipid core. The dimensions of ApoB100 would permit it to form a belt spanning the entire surface of LDL. ApoB100 contains a highly cationic sequence, Arg-Leu-Thr-Arg-Lys-Arg-Leu-Lys, which is believed to bind to a complementary anionic sequence at the cell surface receptor.

served as the starting point for development of this platform. This ~22 nm diameter nanoparticle is depicted in Figure 17.1.

LDL binds to cell surface receptors (LDLR) in the liver, adrenals, and ovaries. Since a number of tumors overexpress LDLRs, LDL has been used as a vehicle for delivery of a number of antineoplastic agents. Brown and Goldstein [8] have delineated the mechanism by which LDL binds to cell surface receptors, undergoes endocytosis, and is degraded in lysosomes, so that the receptor is recycled to the cell surface. This provides a very efficient mechanism for delivery of drugs or diagnostic agents to cells expressing LDLRs. PET and SPECT agents have been covalently attached to ApoB100 to permit monitoring LDLRs by nuclear medicine imaging techniques. Commercial visible and

NIR fluorophores that intercalate in the phospholipid monolayer of LDL are available for both *ex vivo* and *in vivo* tracking of cells overexpressing these receptors (DiI and DiR, Invitrogen, Carlsbad, CA, USA). Cholesterol ester conjugates of NIR dyes have also been synthesized and permitted to intercalate into the phospholipid monolayer on the surface of human LDL [9]. These probes enabled NIR monitoring of the accumulation of these dyes in xenografts of melanoma B16 and HepG2 tumors that overexpress LDLRs [9]. Bis-stearyl-Gd-chelates have also been inserted into the LDL phospholipid monolayer and detected in a human hepatoma xenograft in a nude mouse by MRI (Figure 17.2) [10].

However, the presence of LDLRs in normal tissues diminishes the tumor specificity of LDL-delivered contrast agents and drugs. Zheng *et al.* [11] have therefore developed a method for redirecting LDL to receptors that are more specific to neoplastic tissues, such as the folate receptor which is overexpressed in a number of malignancies including ovarian and breast cancer. ApoB100 contains 357 lysine side-chain amino groups, of which 225 are exposed and 132 buried. Among the exposed lysines, there are 53 active lysine amino groups (pK$_a$ 8.9) with the rest exhibiting normal pK$_a$s (10.5) and normal reactivity [11]. The presence of clusters of cationic amino acids in the backbone sequence could account for all or some of these acidic amino side-chains. Because the receptor-binding site contains a sequence rich in lysines, alkylation of this side-chain quickly eliminates the ability of LDL to bind to LDLR, whereas attachment of folate redirects the particle to folate receptors which internalize and degrade LDL in much the same way as LDLR does. The same scheme could be used to redirect lipoproteins (including HDL and others to various receptors). Zheng *et al.* [11] attached folate groups to 170 or 47.6% of the lysine side-chains of LDL, which totally abolished binding to LDLR (see below). To enable confocal microscopy, surface loading of the commercial visible dye DiI (Invitrogen, Carlsbad, CA, USA) to the folate-conjugated LDL was performed. The molar ratio of the DiI:LDL:FA (folic acid) was 55:1:~150–200; the diameter of the particle measured by electron microscopy was 26.1 ± 3.0 nm, which is slightly larger than native LDL (see above). Specificity for folate receptors was demonstrated by comparative confocal microscopy of various cell types that expressed folate or LDL receptors.

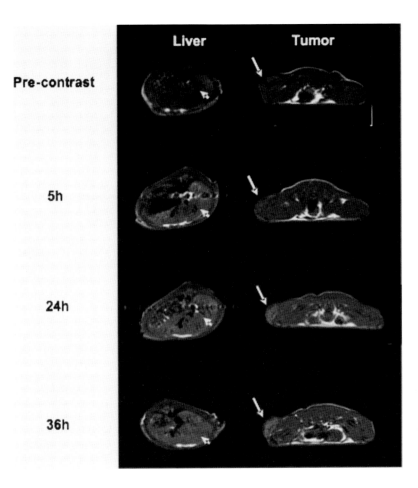

Figure 17.2. Comparison of T_1-weighted MRI of nude mouse with subcutaneous HepG2 tumor before injection of GdDTPA-SA-LDL (180:1; 0.04 mmol/kg) (top images), five hours after injection (liver 55% enhancement, tumor 9%), 24 hours after injection (liver 25% enhancement, tumor 25%), and 36 hours after injection (liver ~25% enhancement, tumor 25%). (Reproduced with permission from Corbin et al., Neoplasia 2006; **8**: 488–98 [10].)

Preliminary *in vivo* tumor localization studies were performed on mice with a subcutaneous HT1080 (FR⁻) tumor on one thigh and a KB (FR⁺) tumor on the other thigh [12]. At $t = 0$, 0.77 µM LDL-FA surface loaded with the NIRF DiR (Ex 748 nm, Em 780 nm) was injected intravenously into the tail vein; the molar ratio was DiR : LDL : FA = 8 : 1 : 105. Xenogen images (Ex 710–760 nm, Em 810–875 nm) measured at various times post-injection are shown in Figure 17.3. Five minutes after injection, the dye was distributed throughout the animal and in both tumors. At two hours post-injection, the dye had cleared from the FR⁻ HT1080 tumor but was retained in the FR⁺ KB tumor. However, the bulk of the dye remained outside of the tumor, particularly in the liver. At 24 hours, fluorescent intensity had increased substantially in the KB tumor and almost disappeared from the abdomen. The study demonstrates that the LDL particle can diffuse through leaky blood vessels into both tumors but is retained and accumulates in the tumor that contains the FRs. There also appears to be slow transfer of the nanoparticles between binding sites in the abdomen and in the tumor. The mechanism underlying this transfer requires further study. However, the data demonstrate that redirection of the particle to the folate receptor has taken place.

Corbin *et al.* [13] have utilized the same principle to redirect HDL to folate receptors (Figure 17.4). Studies are now in progress to develop folate-targeted LDL or HDL to ovarian tumors together with paclitaxel and carboplatin (A. Prantner, A. Popov, G. Coukos, N. Scholler, and J. D. Glickson, unpublished). A method has also been developed to encapsulate iron oxide into the lipid core of HDL-like particles targeted to folate receptors that can be used for early detection of tumors by T_2-weighted MRI (I. W. Chen, R. Zhou, H. Choi, and J. D. Glickson, unpublished). The lipoprotein delivery system could provide a method for *in situ* labeling of cells with iron oxide, and hence could provide an extremely sensitive method for early detection of cancers such as ovarian cancer that often go undetected until they reach an advanced state.

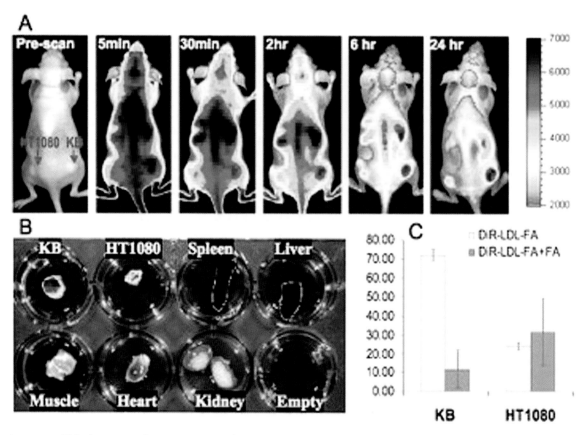

Figure 17.3. (A) Real-time *in vivo* fluorescence images of KB/HT1080 dual tumor mice with IV injection of DiR-LDL-FA (5.8 µM); (B) fluorescence images of tissues and tumors excised at 24 hours post-injection; (C) fluorescence readings of tumor extracts from *in vivo* FA inhibition assay. (Reproduced with permission from Chen *et al., J Am Chem Soc* 2007; **129**: 5798–9 [12].)

Prediction and early detection of therapeutic response

Availability of rapid, reliable, and non-invasive methods for predicting and detecting therapeutic response to anti-cancer therapy would facilitate both the rational design and optimization of treatment protocols to meet the needs of the individual cancer patient. Optimization of individualized treatment protocols would spare non-responsive patients unnecessary toxicity and cost and permit them to explore more effective alternative therapeutic options at an earlier stage of their disease. The central hypothesis of molecular imagers working in this critical field is that there exist biomarkers of therapeutic response that predict or detect response to treatment of an individual tumor and can be detected by non-invasive or minimally invasive methods before treatment is initiated or soon after it has been initiated. While the mechanistic basis on which such response prediction or early detection is based is still not well

defined, two molecular imaging methods have proven useful for such applications – MRS detection of phospholipid metabolites [14], lactate [15], and citrate [16], and PET imaging of the glucose analog fluoro-2'-deoxyglucose (FDG) [17] or nitroimidazole indicators of tumor hypoxia [18].

We will restrict ourselves in this chapter to discussion of MRS studies of non-Hodgkin's lymphoma (NHL), which has been the focus of research at various institutions collaborating in an NCI-sponsored cooperative program. Following an NCI workshop in 1992, a multi-institutional program was funded by the NIH to explore the potential utility of ^{31}P MRS for prediction and early detection of therapeutic response in four types of human cancer: NHL, squamous cell carcinoma of the head and neck, soft-tissue sarcoma, and locally advanced breast cancer. These malignant diseases were chosen because they lent themselves to ^{31}P MRS measurements and because they exhibited an approximately 50:50 probability of local therapeutic

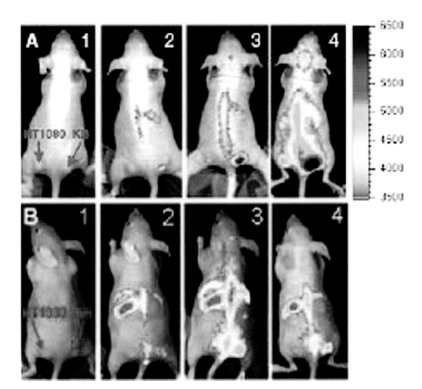

Figure 17.4. (A) *In vivo* fluorescent imaging of dual tumor (KB/HT 1080)-bearing mouse before and at several time points following intravenous injection of (DiR-BOA)-HDL-FA (15 μM). (B) *In vivo* inhibition study was performed with 30-fold excess free folic acid (FA). The numbers refer to the imaging times: (1) pre-contrast, (2) 1 h, (3) 5 h, (4) 24 h. (Reproduced with permission from Corbin *et al.*, *J Biomed Nanotechnol* 2007; **3**: 367–76 [13].)

response. Due to limited patient accrual, the program eventually focused exclusively on NHL. The clinical exploratory trial, which has currently accrued over 100 patients, includes Columbia University, Memorial Sloan-Kettering, University of Pennsylvania, Cambridge University (UK), the Royal Marsden Hospital (UK), and Nijmegen University (Netherlands) [14].

Figure 17.5 shows a typical pre-treatment 1.5 T ^{31}P MR spectrum (with ^{1}H double irradiation) of an inguinal NHL tumor that was contained in a single $3 \times 3 \times 3\,cm^3$ voxel from an 8×8 matrix measured by chemical shift imaging (CSI). Three resonances originating from the three phosphate groups of nucleoside triphosphates appear at the high field (right hand) end of the spectrum. The β-phosphate is a triplet, and the α- and γ-phosphates are doublets. Also evident are resonances from phosphocreatine (PCr), phosphodiesters (PDE), inorganic phosphate (Pi), phosphocholine (Cho-P) and phosphoethanolamine (Etn-P). PCr probably originates from normal muscle contaminants in the voxel; the chemical shift of the Pi resonances measures the intracellular pH in the tumor.

In a preliminary analysis pre-treatment PME/NTP ratios from 41 NHL patients treated by a variety of different therapeutic protocols were grouped according to the International Prognostic Index (IPI)

according to tumor grade – low (L), low to high (LI), high to intermediate (HI), and high (H) (Figure 17.6). Eighteen of these patients went on to exhibit complete clinical response (CR) (i.e., total disappearance of their tumors) following treatment, whereas 23 did not achieve a CR (NR). A straight line was drawn between the means of the L and LI groups and extended over the HI and H groups. This line was used as the basis for predicting response over the entire group of patients. Note that positive predictive capacity of this test is a very poor 67%, but the negative predictive value is very high (96%). There is only one CR that falls above the line and one that falls on the line. Therefore, if a patient exhibits a pre-treatment PME/NTP ratio that falls above the line, there is 96% certainty that that patient will not exhibit a CR. In short, the test is identifying with a high degree of certainty patients who are likely to fail conventional treatment of NHL. If these data are confirmed over a much larger cohort of patients, then this pre-treatment test could identify the patients that should receive much more aggressive therapy from the inception of treatment with bone marrow transplantation to restore their immune system. This predictive capacity of ^{31}P MRS of tumors has now been observed in over 100 NHL patients treated with a variety of different

283

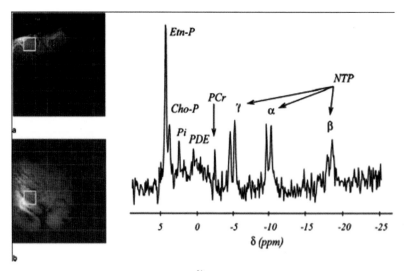

Figure 17.5. Example of an *in vivo* localized ^{31}P MR spectroscopy study in non-Hodgkin's lymphoma. Insets (a) and (b) show two orthogonal MR images (axial and coronal, respectively), illustrating tumor localization, in this case the right inguinal area. The images were overlaid with the [31]P 3D localization CSI grid, a cubic matrix with 8 steps per spatial dimension with a nominal cubic voxel of 30 mm³. The ^{31}P spectrum was sampled from the single tumor voxel projected on the images shown by a thick lined square. The assignments are phosphoethanolamine (Etn-P) and phosphocholine (Cho-P) in the phosphomonoester region; inorganic phosphate (Pi); phosphodiester region (PDE); phosphocreatine (PCr); and phosphates, γ, α, and β of nucleoside triphosphates (NTP). The chemical shift is expressed in parts per million (ppm) using the phosphoric acid as reference at 0 ppm (internal reference P of NTP at 10.01 ppm). The leftover glitch of PCr in the spectrum is minimal contamination from neighboring voxels caused by the CSI point spread function. The [Etn-P Cho-P]/NTP ratios reported throughout the article were obtained by summing the integrals of the Etn-P and Cho-P signals in the tumor spectra and dividing the result by the integral of the phosphate of NTP (assignments in bold). (Reproduced with permission from Arias-Mendoza *et al.*, *Acad Radiol* 2004; **11**: 368–76 [14].)

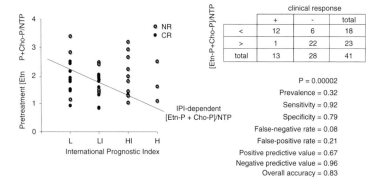

Figure 17.6. Analysis of pre-treatment PME/NTP as predictor of failure of NHL tumors to exhibit complete response. (F. Arias-Mendoza and T. R. Brown on behalf of Cooperative NMR group, unpublished data.)

	clinical response		
	+	–	total
<	12	6	18
>	1	22	23
total	13	28	41

$P = 0.00002$
Prevalence = 0.32
Sensitivity = 0.92
Specificity = 0.79
False-negative rate = 0.08
False-positive rate = 0.21
Positive predictive value = 0.67
Negative predictive value = 0.96
Overall accuracy = 0.83

methods and is even supported among small groups of patients with a particular type of NHL (diffuse large B-cell lymphoma, DLBCL) who have been treated with CHOP (cyclophosphamide, hydroxydoxorubicin, oncovin, prednisone) combination chemotherapy or CHOP plus rituximab (a monoclonal antibody against the CD20 antigen).

However, the ^{31}P MRS method for predicting therapeutic response has two major limitations: (1) because of its low sensitivity, it is limited to relatively large superficial tumors ($\geq 3 \times 3 \times 3\,cm^3 = 27\,cm^3$ at 1.5 T and ~ 10–$15\,cm^3$ at 3T), and (2) it is a negative

predictor, predicting response failure rather than success. To overcome these limitations, investigators at the University of Pennsylvania have been exploring the use of ^{1}H MRS and physiologically sensitive ^{1}H MRI methods that would be suitable for detecting much smaller deep-seated tumors. While these methods are generally not response-predictive, they are proving capable of detecting response at a very early stage of treatment. These studies have been performed on xenografts of the most common human NHL type, DLBCL. The tumor was implanted subcutaneously in the flanks of immunosuppressed mice. Drs. Mohammed and

Al-Katib at Wayne State University provided the DLCL2 cell line used in this study, which they established from cells obtained from a patient with a chemotherapy-resistant DLBCL tumor. These mice were treated with protocols that closely resembled treatments that are commonly administered to human NHL patients. The most common treatment of DLBCL NHL is combination chemotherapy with CHOP administered IV in six or more two-week cycles. Because of the more rapid growth rate of this tumor line in mice, the therapeutic cycle time was reduced to one week and the dose was slightly modified. The most significant recent advance in the treatment of NHL has been the introduction of the use of rituximab. This has improved survival dramatically, increasing the cure rate of DLBCL from about 33% to nearly 90%.

Figure 17.7 shows changes in volume of these tumors in a group of mice that were administered three cycles of CHOP, RCHOP (CHOP plus rituximab), R (rituximab only), or saline (sham-treated). CHOP and RCHOP cause a cessation of tumor growth that is evident within one cycle of treatment, whereas R alone only slightly diminishes the growth rate of the tumor. The figure also shows a dramatic decrease in tumor proliferation as indicated by the Ki67 monoclonal antibody assay, which is evident after two cycles of RCHOP or CHOP but not of R alone.

Figures 17.8 and 17.9 summarize the effects of treatment with these agents on levels of two metabolic markers that can be monitored by ^{1}H MRS of the tumors: steady-state lactate (Lac) and total choline (tCho), respectively. Lac exhibits a statistically significant decrease after one cycle of RCHOP or CHOP, but no significant change following treatment with R, whereas tCho decreased significantly after one cycle of RCHOP or R but not of CHOP. Therefore, Lac appears to be a very sensitive early indicator of response to combination chemotherapy with CHOP, whereas tCho is a very early sensitive indictor of response to R. RCHOP produces a decrease in both markers because it contains R and CHOP, which individually decrease Lac or tCho respectively. Recent studies show that rapamycin, a chemotherapeutic agent that inhibits proliferation of DLCL2 xenografts by selectively inhibiting phosphorylation of the signal-transduction protein mTOR, which controls tumor cell proliferation, also selectively lowers Lac but has no effect on tCho (S.-C. Lee, M. Marcek, M. A. Mariusz, and J. D. Glickson, unpublished). The reason for the selective

sensitivity of Lac to chemotherapy and tCho to immunotherapy is still unclear.

Preliminary measurements of tCho and Lac in humans are in progress. One study was performed on a DLCL2 patient who was examined by ^{1}H MRS on a Monday; treatment with RCHOP was initiated on Wednesday and a second ^{1}H MRS measurement was performed on Friday (within 48 hours of treatment). At the time of the second examination, the tumor had shrunk by 25%, Lac had decreased by 70%, and tCho had increased by 15%. These are very early results, but they look extremely promising, at least for Lac as a chemotherapeutic response marker.

Metabolic network analysis

In 1983, investigators at the University of Pennsylvania and University College London published a classic paper on ^{13}C MRS studies of isolated Langendorff perfused hearts of rats that were administered glucose and [2-^{13}C]acetate or [3-^{13}C]pyruvate in the perfusate [19]. The kinetics of ^{13}C-isotope exchange from acetate or pyruvate to specific carbons of glutamate and aspartate that were produced by the tricarboxylic acid (TCA) cycle were analyzed by ^{13}C MRS after the animals were sacrificed (three animals per time point), the hearts rapidly frozen, extracted with perchloric acid, lyophilized and dissolved in 33% D_2O/H_2O. Flux through the TCA cycle was analyzed by fitting the kinetic data on metabolism of acetate and pyruvate to the metabolic network model by solving a set of about 340 coupled differential equations. Using the computer program FACSIMILE, which at the time required a Cray supercomputer, a numerical solution to these differential equations was obtained. Even though the model generated a large number of equations, it still constituted a fully determined system since the equations were not independent, and the number of unknowns matched the number of observables. The model took into account two cellular compartments (cytosolic and mitochondrial) and dilution of the isotope over multiple turns of the TCA cycle. Today this same system of equations can be solved in less than three minutes on a conventional laptop computer. While others have developed simplified versions of this classic model [20–25], this remains the most sophisticated model for analysis of TCA cycle flux that has been published.

In 1995, Chatham et al. [26] refined and validated this model by incorporating glycolysis and the glycerol phosphate and malate–aspartate shuttles (Figure 17.10).

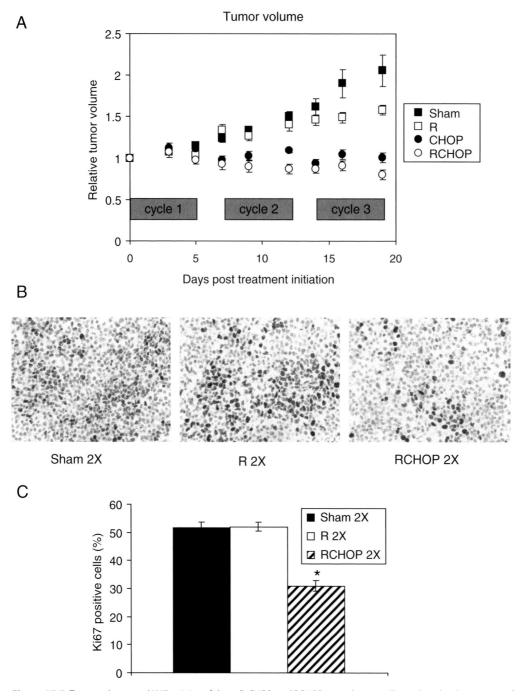

Figure 17.7. Tumor volumes and Ki67 staining of sham, R, CHOP, and RCHOP treated tumors. (Reproduced with permission from Lee *et al.*, *NMR Biomed* 2008; **21**: 723–33 [15].)

Isotopic labeling data were obtained by continuous measurement of ^{13}C MRS spectra of the Langendorff perfused rat heart contained in a 20 mm NMR tube rather than the laborious method used by Chance *et al.* [19], which required sacrifice of hundreds of animals (three for each time point) (Figure 17.11). These authors validated the model by comparison of predicted rates of oxygen consumption with

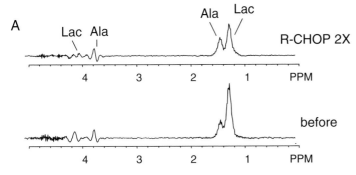

Figure 17.8. SelMQC spectra before and after RCHOP treatment, and comparison of Lac:H_2O ratios for sham, R, CHOP, and RCHOP treated tumors. (Reproduced with permission from Lee *et al., NMR Biomed* 2008; **21**: 723–33 [15].)

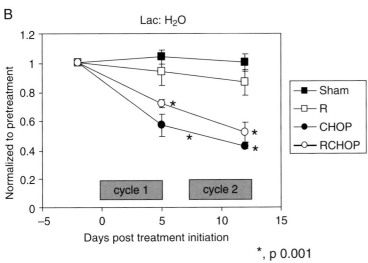

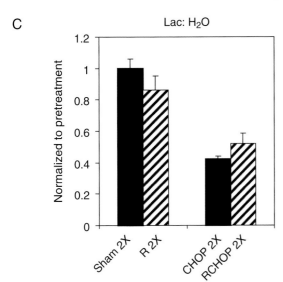

287

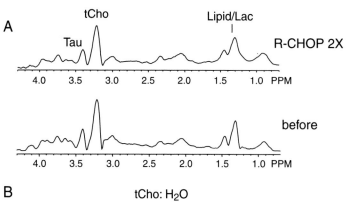

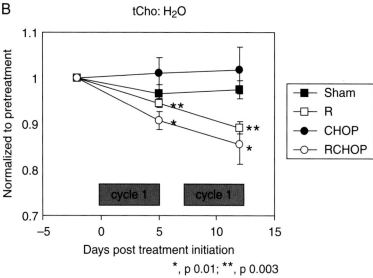

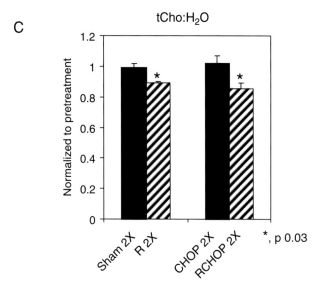

Figure 17.9. STEAM spectra before and after RCHOP treatment, and comparison of tCho:H_2O ratios for sham, R, CHOP, and RCHOP treated tumors. (Reproduced with permission from Lee *et al.*, *NMR Biomed* 2008; **21**: 723–33 [15].)

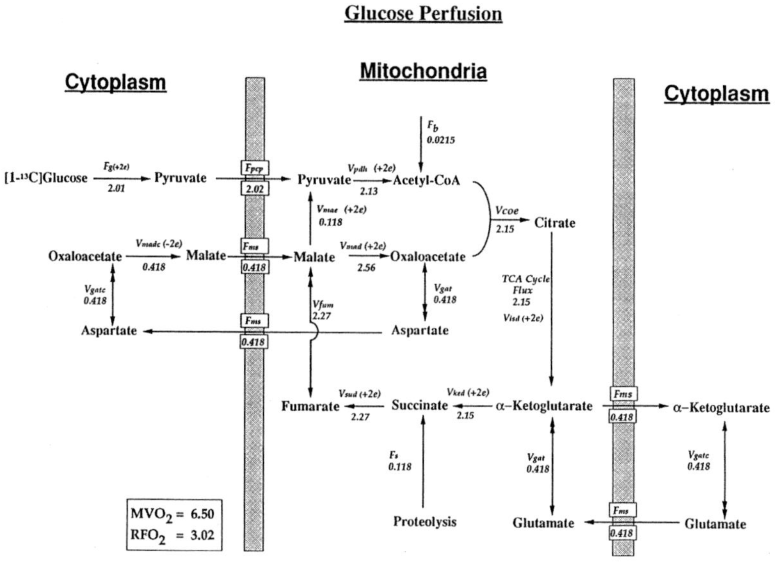

Glucose Perfusion

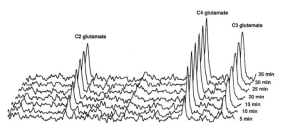

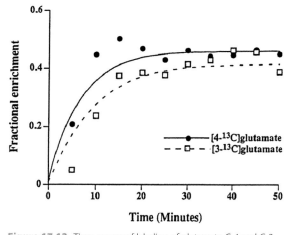

Figure 17.10. Reaction network used to analyze the kinetics of glutamate labeling for one of the experiments with [1-^{13}C] glucose as substrate and the calculated steady-state enzyme velocities (glucose experiment from Table II in reference [26]). The abbreviations of steady-state fluxes and flux relationships are as follows: Fg, total influx from glycolysis; Fpcp, pyruvate influx; Fms, malate–aspartate shuttle flux; Fs, proteolysis influx; Fb, flux from endogenous substrates; MVO$_2$, oxygen consumption; RFO$_2$, MVO$_2$/TCA cycle flux; +2e/−2e, two electron reduction/oxidation. Reactions with *double-headed arrows* indicate that the reaction is near equilibrium with a net flux in the direction of the *double-headed arrows*. Note that an additional redox shuttle was required to provide a hydrogen balance between the cytoplasm and the mitochondria; see results and discussion in reference [26] for more details. (Reproduced with permission from Chatham *et al.*, *J Biol Chem* 1995; **270**: 7999–8008 [26].)

Figure 17.11. Series of ^{13}C NMR spectra from isolated perfused rat heart with [4-^{13}C]β-hydroxybutyrate as substrate for 50 minutes. The spectra have been expanded to show the glutamate region only. Similar datasets were obtained for [1-^{13}C]glucose and [3-^{13}C]acetate. (Reproduced with permission from Chatham *et al.*, *J Biol Chem* 1995; **270**: 7999–8008 [26].)

Figure 17.12. Time course of labeling of glutamate C-4 and C-3 with [1-^{13}C]glucose as substrate from the data in Figure 17.11. (Reproduced with permission from Chatham *et al.*, *J Biol Chem* 1995; **270**: 7999–8008 [26].)

experimental values simultaneously measured polarographically (Figure 17.12). Inclusion of the malate–aspartate and glycerol phosphate shuttles was required for agreement with experimental oxygen consumption rates. The original model of Chance *et al.* [19] that lacked the shuttles consistently predicted low values of the oxygen consumption rate, whereas the refined model agreed with experimental measurements of this parameter (Figure 17.13).

Wehrle *et al.* have reported a study of metabolism of [1-^{13}C]glucose and [3-^{13}C]propionate by perfused EMT6/Ro breast cancer spheroids [27]. They have also performed a preliminary analysis of the ^{13}C kinetic data (E. M. Chance, J. Wehlre, C. Ng, and J. D. Glickson, unpublished). Data were analyzed utilizing the cardiac model validated by Chatham *et al.* [26] even though it

was recognized that this could lead to some small errors since a number of metabolic differences between glucose metabolism in the heart and tumors are known to exist: (1) lactate and alanine are present in the tumor model but are not observed in the non-ischemic heart; (2) the malic enzyme, which converts malate to pyruvate, occurs in the cytosol in the tumor (as indicated by labeling of lactate at C2 when [1-^{13}C] glucose and propionate are substrates) but is in the mitochondrial compartment in the heart; (3) glutamine is converted to glutamate in tumor mitochondria (i.e., glutaminolysis) but not in the

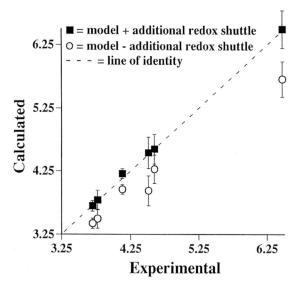

Figure 17.13. Comparison between the experimentally measured and the calculated oxygen consumption rates (MVO$_2$) with and without the glycerol phosphate and malate–aspartate shuttles. Both shuttles had the same effect on the model fit, so only the glycerol phosphate data are shown. Error bars represent 5% and 95% confidence limits of calculated values. (Reproduced with permission from Chatham *et al.*, *J Biol Chem* 1995; **270**: 7999–8008 [26].)

heart. Studies are now in progress to refine the cardiac model for application to tumors and to validate this model by comparison of experimental and predicted oxygen consumption rates. EMT6/Ro breast cancer spheroids were perfused in a 10 mm NMR tube with 5 mM [1-^{13}C]glucose. These tumor cells exhibit much higher levels of [3-^{13}C]lactate and lower levels of [4-^{13}C]glutamate than hearts, reflecting the higher levels of glycolytic metabolism and lower levels of oxidative metabolism in neoplastic tissues.

This model is being extended to include other critical pathways of tumor intermediary metabolism – the pentose shunt, fatty acid metabolism, and phospholipid metabolism. Translation of this approach to humans has already been demonstrated in the human brain [28]. These methods may prove suitable for identifying specific metabolic pathways that are modified by drugs targeting the signal transduction pathways. This can be conducted first on isolated perfused tumor cells, then in animal models, and finally in humans. The promise of molecular imaging lies in its ability to facilitate the development and implementation of strategies such as this in order to optimize the treatment of human diseases such as cancer, diabetes, Alzheimer's, and heart disease.

References

1. Tyagi S, Kramer FR. Molecular beacons: probes that fluoresce upon hybridization. *Nat Biotechnol*, 1996; **14**: 303–8.

2. Tung CH, Mahmood U, Bredow S, Weissleder R. In vivo imaging of proteolytic enzyme activity using a novel molecular reporter. *Cancer Res* 2000; **60**: 4953–8.

3. Stefflova K, Chen J, Li H, Zheng G. Targeted photodynamic therapy agent with a built-in apoptosis sensor for in vivo near-infrared imaging of tumor apoptosis triggered by its photosensitization in situ. *Mol Imaging* 2006; **5**: 520–32.

4. Tsien RY, Miyawaki A, Lev-Ram V, *et al.* Genetically encoded indicators of signal transduction and protein interaction. *FASEB J* 2000; **14**(8): 558.

5. Zhang L, Bhojani MS, Ross BD, Rehemtulla A. Molecular imaging of protein kinases. *Cell Cycle* 2008; **7**: 314–17.

6. Glickson JD, Lund-Katz S, Zhou R, *et al.* Lipoprotein nanoplatform for targeted delivery of diagnostic and therapeutic agents. *Mol Imaging* 2008; **7**: 101–10.

7. Shapiro EM, Sharer K, Skrtic S, Koretsky AP. In vivo detection of single cells by MRI. *Magn Reson Med* 2006; **55**: 242–9.

8. Goldstein JL, Brown MS. The LDL pathway in human fibroblasts: a receptor-mediated mechanism for regulation of cholesterol metabolism. *Curr Top Cell Regul* 1976; **11**: 147–81.

9. Li H, Zhang Z, Blessington D. Carbocyanine labeled LDL for optical imaging of tumors. *Acad Radiol* 2004; **11**: 669–77.

10. Corbin IR, Li H, Chen J, *et al.* Low-density lipoprotein nanoparticles as magnetic resonance imaging contrast agents. *Neoplasia* 2006; **8**: 488–98.

11. Zheng G, Chen J, Li H, Glickson JD. Rerouting lipoprotein nanoparticles to selected alternate receptors for the targeted delivery of cancer diagnostic and therapeutic agents. *Proc Natl Acad Sci USA* 2005; **102**: 17757–62.

12. Chen J, Corbin IR, Li H. *et al.* Ligand conjugated low-density lipoprotein nanoparticles for enhanced optical cancer imaging in vivo. *J Am Chem Soc* 2007; **129**: 5798–9.

13. Corbin IR, Chen J, Cao W, *et al.* Enhanced cancer-targeted delivery using engineered high-density lipoprotein-based nanocarriers. *J Biomed Nanotechnol* 2007; **3**: 367–76.

14. Arias-Mendoza F, Smith MR, Brown TR. Predicting treatment response in non-Hodgkin's lymphoma from the pretreatment tumor content of phosphoethanolamine plus phosphocholine. *Acad Radiol* 2004; **11**: 368–76.

15. Lee SC, Huang MQ, Nelson DS, *et al.* In vivo MRS markers of response to CHOP chemotherapy in the WSU-DLCL2 human diffuse large B-cell lymphoma xenograft. *NMR Biomed* 2008; **21**: 723–33.

16. Kurhanewicz J, Vigneron DB, Hricak H, *et al.* Prostate cancer: metabolic response to cryosurgery as detected with 3D H-1 MR spectroscopic imaging. *Radiology* 1996; **200**: 489–96.

17. Svoboda J, Andreadis C, Elstrom R, *et al.* Prognostic value of FDG-PET scan imaging in lymphoma patients undergoing autologous stem cell transplantation. *Bone Marrow Transplant* 2006; **38**: 211–16.

18. Evans SM, Kachur AV, Shiue CY, *et al.* Noninvasive detection of tumor hypoxia using the 2-nitroimidazole [F-18]EF1. *J Nucl Med* 2000; **41**: 327–36.

19. Chance EM, Seeholzer SH, Kobayashi K, Williamson JR. Mathematical analysis of isotope labeling in the citric acid cycle with applications to C-13 NMR studies in perfused rat hearts. *J Biol Chem* 1983; **258**: 3785–94.

20. Carvalho RA, Zhao P, Wiegers CB, *et al.* TCA cycle kinetics in the rat heart by analysis of ^{13}C isotopomers using indirect ^{1}H[^{13}C] detection. *Am J Physiol Heart Circ Physiol* 2001; **281**: H1413–21.

21. Hyder F, Chase JR, Behar KL, *et al.* Increased tricarboxylic acid cycle flux in rat brain during forepaw stimulation detected with H-1 [C-13] NMR. *Proc Natl Acad Sci USA* 1996; **93**: 7612–17.

22. Weiss RG, Gloth ST, Kalil-Filho R, *et al.* Indexing tricarboxylic acid cycle flux in intact hearts by C-13 nuclear magnetic resonance. *Circ Res* 1992; **70**: 392–408.

23. Portais JC, Schuster R, Merle M, Canioni P. Metabolic flux determination in C6 glioma cells using C-13 distribution upon [1-C-13]glucose incubation. *Eur J Biochem* 1993; **217**: 457–68.

24. Tran-Dinh S, Hoerter JA, Mateo P, Bouet F, Herve M. A simple mathematical model and practical approach for evaluating citric acid cycle fluxes in perfused rat hearts by C-13-NMR and H-1-NMR spectroscopy. *Eur J Biochem* 1997; **245**: 497–504.

25. Uffmann K, Gruetter R. Mathematical modeling of C-13 label incorporation of the TCA cycle: the concept of composite precursor function. *J Neurosci Res* 2007; **85**: 3304–17.

26. Chatham JC, Forder JR, Glickson JD, Chance EM. Calculation of absolute metabolic flux and the elucidation of the pathways of glutamate labeling in perfused rat heart by C-13 NMR spectroscopy and nonlinear least squares analysis. *J Biol Chem* 1995; **270**: 7999–8008.

27. Wehrle JP, Ng CE, McGovern KA, *et al.* Metabolism of alternative substrates and the bioenergetic status of EMT6 tumor cell spheroids. *NMR Biomed* 2000; **13**: 349–60.

28. Shulman RG, Rothman DL, Behar KL, Hyder F. Energetic basis of brain activity: implications for neuroimaging. *Trends Neurosci* 2004; **27**: 489–95.

Appendix 1: Linear systems

Paul A. Yushkevich

Objectives

- Overview the concepts of systems and signals
- Give examples of systems and signals in engineering, nature, and mathematics
- Define the properties of linearity and shift invariance
- Introduce the mathematical concepts of convolution and impulse function
- Analyze input/output relationship of systems via impulse response and transfer functions
- Describe discrete-time and multidimensional linear systems

Systems in engineering, biology, and mathematics

The term *system* has many meanings in the English language. In engineering and mathematics, we think of a system as a "black box" that accepts one or more inputs and generates some number of outputs. The external observer may not know what takes place inside the black box; but by observing the response of the system to certain test inputs, one may infer certain properties of the system. Some systems in nature behave in a very predictable manner. For example, once we have seen a magnifying glass applied to any printed image, or a megaphone applied to any person's voice, we can reliably predict how these devices would perform given any other image or voice. Other systems are more complex and less predictable. For example, if we use fMRI to measure the response of the language areas of the human cortex to hearing short sentences, the output in response to hearing "the sky is blue" is not enough to predict the response to "I love you" or to "*el cielo es azul*," since the brain responds quite differently to emotionally charged stimuli and unfamiliar languages. Most natural systems are stochastic, so that the same input presented at different times may lead to different outputs. Thus, even if we repeat the same phrase twice in an fMRI experiment, we are likely to measure slightly different fMRI responses each time. It turns out that many systems in engineering and biology, despite their complexity, can be approximated by simple deterministic systems with highly predictable behavior, called *linear shift-invariant systems*.

As we already see, the concept of system can be used to describe a variety of engineering devices and biological phenomena. A few more examples are: a compact disc player, which converts the grooves etched on the disc's surface into audible sound; photo cameras, which convert the distribution of photons hitting a sensor over a period of time into digital images; medical imaging devices, which convert the three-dimensional distribution of tissue in the human body into 3D digital images; neurons, which combine input from many synapses into the action potential in the axon; certain social and economic phenomena may also be represented as systems.

Some systems are purely mathematical. For instance, differential equations represent a type of a system. Consider the one-dimensional *diffusion equation*, which plays a very important role in image processing:

$$\frac{\partial u}{\partial t} - k\left(\frac{\partial^2 u}{\partial x^2}\right) = 0 \qquad x \in [x_0, x_1];\ t \in [0, \infty],$$

$$u(x, 0) = \phi(x) \qquad x \in [x_0, x_1]$$

$$u(x_0, t) = u(x_1, t) = 0 \qquad t \in [0, \infty] \qquad \text{(A1.1)}$$

The classical interpretation of this equation is to describe the distribution of heat u over time t in an infinitely thin

Introduction to the Science of Medical Imaging, ed. R. Nick Bryan. Published by Cambridge University Press. © Cambridge University Press 2010.

one-dimensional homogeneous rod.[1] At time zero, the heat distribution is given by the function $\phi(x)$. The temperature at the ends of the rod is always zero, perhaps because the rod is attached to a pair of heat sinks. We can treat this differential equation as a system, whose inputs are $\phi(x)$ and the constant k, which describes the heat conductivity of the rod. The output of the system is $u(x,t)$, the solution of the differential equation. Think of the algorithm used to solve this equation as a black box, such that as we pass in different inputs, we obtain different solutions. We can denote this by the relation:

$$u(x,t) = \mathcal{H}[k, \phi(x)]$$

It turns out that we can infer important properties of the system $\mathcal{H}$ without having to know the specific details of the underlying algorithm. Instead, by learning how $\mathcal{H}$ transforms *certain* inputs into outputs, we can predict its behavior for *any* input.

Signals

Inputs and outputs to systems are called *signals*. A signal is a generic term used to describe how a physical quantity varies over time and/or space. Sounds, images, recordings from biomedical devices, are all signals. A signal is described mathematically by a function:

$$f : \Omega \to \Psi \qquad (A1.2)$$

where Ω is the domain of the signal and Ψ is its range. The domain Ω is typically an interval of time, or a region of space, or a cross-product of the two. The range can be the set of all real numbers, the set of integers, or, for signals stored in the computer, the set {0,1}.

Consider the compact disc player. The input signal can be represented as a set of zeros and ones placed at equal intervals in time (as the player encounters these zeros and ones sequentially). Thus the domain is a set of time points and the range is the set {0,1}:

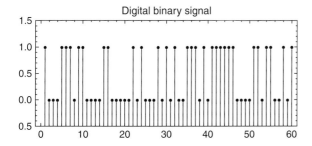

Signals like this, where the domain and the range are finite sets[2], are called *digital signals*. Digital signals can be stored and manipulated by computers, making them ubiquitous in modern communications and imaging systems. On the other hand, the output of each of the CD player's speakers is a sound wave form – a continuous function of time:

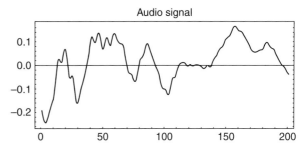

Signals that vary continuously over a continuous domain are called *analog signals*. Natural phenomena typically are associated with analog signals. In addition to analog and digital signals, we distinguish a third class: *discrete-time signals*. The domain of a discrete-time signal is a finite set, just as for digital signals, but the range is continuous, i.e., the signal may assume any real value. Such signals cannot be stored in a computer because computers have finite precision for storing data, but they can be approximated by digital signals. In the next few sections, we will focus our attention on systems that take as input and output one-dimensional analog signals. Later on, we will draw parallels to discrete-time systems.

Linearity and linear systems

Most systems in nature and engineering are very complex, and it is difficult to infer the inner workings of the system from the relationship between inputs and outputs. However, a special class of systems called *linear shift-invariant systems* open themselves to greater introspection. Luckily, it turns out that many real-world systems, including real imaging systems, can be accurately approximated by these simpler versions.

Let $\mathcal{H}$ be a system with one input and one output:

$$u(t) = \mathcal{H}[\phi(t)] \qquad (A1.3)$$

Let $\phi_1(t)$ and $\phi_2(t)$ be any two inputs to $\mathcal{H}$, and let $u_1(t)$ and $u_2(t)$ be the corresponding outputs. Then $\mathcal{H}$ is called a *linear system* if, and only if:

---

[1] See section *The diffusion equation in image analysis* below for the discussion of the equation's relevance to image processing.

[2] Technically, the domain of a digital signal may be a countable infinite set.

$$\mathcal{H}[\phi_1(t) + \phi_2(t)] = u_1(t) + u_2(t) \qquad (A1.4)$$

and, for any scalar a:

$$\mathcal{H}[a\phi_1(t)] = a\, u_1(t) \qquad (A1.5)$$

The first property, called *superposition*, states that the response of the system to the sum of two inputs is equal to the sum of the responses to the two inputs. The second property, *scaling*, states that scaling the input by a constant scales the response of the system by the same constant. The properties can be combined into a single relation that a system must satisfy in order to be linear:

$$\mathcal{H}[\phi_1(t) + a\phi_2(t)] = u_1(t) + au_2(t)$$

The reader may ask, what do these properties of linearity have to do with lines? Consider the simplest possible linear system, whose input and output are constants (or, more precisely, constant functions of time, $\phi(t) = const$). Let u_1 be the constant output corresponding to the input 1. Then, the output for the arbitrary input a can be expressed as:

$$\mathcal{H}[a] = a\mathcal{H}[1] = au_1 \qquad (A1.6)$$

So if we plot $\mathcal{H}[a]$ as a function of a, we would get a straight line passing through zero. Hence, linear systems exhibit behavior similar to lines, except that the inputs and outputs are more complex: general functions rather than constants:

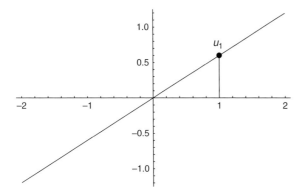

The diffusion equation (A1.1) is a linear system with respect to the input $\phi(t)$ – but not to the diffusion constant k. We leave it to the reader to verify this by letting $u_1(x,t) = \mathcal{H}[\phi_1(t), k]$ and $u_2(x,t) = \mathcal{H}[\phi_1(t), k]$ and

plugging $u^- = u_1 + au_2$ into Equation A1.1. It immediately comes out that $u^- = \mathcal{H}[\phi_1(t) + a\phi_1(t), k]$. The plots below show the response of the diffusion equation to a pair of input signals $\phi_1(t)$ and $\phi_2(t)$, as well as the response to their sum $\phi_1(t) + \phi_2(t)$. It can be clearly seen that the response to the sum of the inputs is the sum of the individual responses:

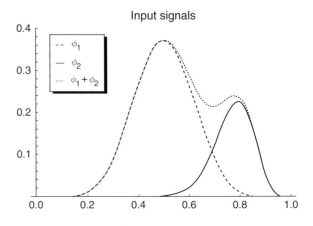

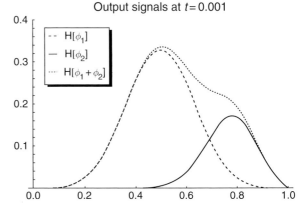

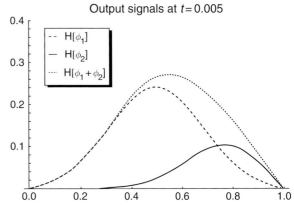

Whereas the diffusion equation (and many other differential equations) is an example of linear systems acting on analog inputs, matrix multiplication is an example of systems that act on discrete-time signals. An n-dimensional vector $\mathbf{x}$ is a discrete-time signal with n measurements $(x_1, x_2, \ldots, x_n)$. Multiplication of such vectors by an $n \times n$ matrix $\mathbf{A}$ is an operation that transforms input vectors into output vectors. Linear algebra tells us that $\mathbf{A}(\mathbf{x}_1 + a\mathbf{x}_2) = \mathbf{A}\mathbf{x}_1 + a\mathbf{A}\mathbf{x}_2$, so matrix multiplication satisfies the conditions of linear systems.

Strictly speaking, a compact disc player is not a linear system, since the input is a sequence of ones and zeros, and scaling it by a constant is meaningless. However, if we organize the series of bits into 32-bit "words," with each word representing an integer in the range $[-2^{31}, 2^{31}-1]$, the system becomes more linear. Scaling the words by a constant factor, as long as the factor is not so large as to cause overflow, will result in the amplitude of the output signal being scaled by the same constant, as long as the amplitude is within the power range of the speakers. Such is the case with many real-world systems: although they are not strictly linear, their behavior is nearly linear for signals within a certain "reasonable range."

Lastly, let us show that the superimposition property of linear systems can be generalized to infinite sums and integrals. The superimposition property of linear systems can be combined any number of times, i.e.,

$$\mathcal{H}[\phi_1(t) + \phi_2(t) + \phi_3(t)]$$
$$= \mathcal{H}[\phi_1(t)] + \mathcal{H}[\phi_2(t) + \phi_3(t)]$$
$$= \mathcal{H}[\phi_1(t)] + \mathcal{H}[\phi_2(t)] + \mathcal{H}[\phi_3(t)] \quad \text{(A1.7)}$$

Now let $u(t) = \mathcal{H}[\phi(t)]$ be a linear system, and suppose we have a family of functions $\phi_1(t)$, such that:

$$\phi_i(t) = \Phi(t, \tau_i) \quad \text{(A1.8)}$$

where $\tau_1, \tau_2, \ldots, \tau_N$ is a sequence of numbers such that $\tau_{i+1} = \tau_i + \Delta_\tau$. Then, naturally, the following holds:

$$\mathcal{H}\left[\sum_{i=0}^{N} \Phi(t, \tau_i)\Delta_\tau\right] = \sum_{i=0}^{N} \mathcal{H}[\Phi(t, \tau_i)]\Delta_\tau \quad \text{(A1.9)}$$

and, letting $N \to \infty$ and $\Delta_\tau \to 0$, we get the following integral relation:

$$\mathcal{H}\left[\int_a^b \Phi(t, \tau)d\tau\right] = \int_a^b \mathcal{H}[\Phi(t, \tau)]d\tau \quad \text{(A1.10)}$$

In other words, the response of a linear system to an integral is the integral of the responses. We will use this property below in the discussion of impulse response.

Shift-invariant systems

Another simplifying property of linear systems is *time invariance* or *shift invariance* (these terms have the same meaning, but time invariance refers to signals in the time domain, while shift invariance can be used to describe systems having multidimensional signal domains).

Formally, the system:

$$u(t) = \mathcal{H}[\phi(t)] \quad \text{(A1.11)}$$

is time-invariant if the following relation holds for all $\tau \in \mathbb{R}$:

$$u(t - \tau) = \mathcal{H}[\phi(t - \tau)] \quad \text{(A1.12)}$$

Inputs and outputs to time-invariant systems must be defined on the entire real line. If a signal is multidimensional, the shift-invariant property is likewise:

$$u(x_1 - \tau_1, x_2 - \tau_2, \ldots, x_n - \tau_n)$$
$$= \mathcal{H}[\phi(x_1 - \tau_1, x_2 - \tau_2, \ldots, x_n - \tau_n)] \quad \text{(A1.13)}$$

The diffusion equation (A1.1) for the finite length rod $[x_0, x_1]$ does not constitute a shift-invariant system because of the boundary conditions at the ends of the rod. However, if we extend the equation to the entire real line, making the rod infinitely long, as follows:

$$\frac{\partial u}{\partial t} - k\left(\frac{\partial^2 u}{\partial x^2}\right) = 0 \quad x \in (-\infty, \infty); \; t \in [0, \infty)$$

$$u(x, 0) = \phi(x) \quad x \in (-\infty, \infty) \quad \text{(A1.14)}$$

the system becomes a *linear shift-invariant system* (LSIS). Indeed, it is easy to verify that $u(x-\tau, t)$ is the solution of the equation with initial condition $\phi(x-\tau)$.

Informally, a system is time-invariant if it responds to a pattern in the signal the same way regardless of when in time the pattern occurs. For example, a compact disc player will transform a certain sequence of bits into the same sound whether the sequence occurs in the beginning of the disc or at the end. On the other hand, fMRI measurements are not time-invariant: due to drift in the BOLD response, the same stimulus presented at the beginning and the end of an fMRI session can generate a response that has a similar pattern but is scaled by a factor. The image below demonstrates fMRI response over a region of interest to a series of visual stimuli, with the drift over time clearly apparent:

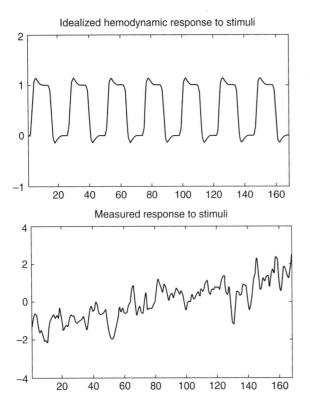

Idealized hemodynamic response to stimuli

Measured response to stimuli

Convolution

Convolution is a mathematical operation central to the study of linear systems. It is an operation that combines two functions into a single function by "blending them." Given functions $f: R \to R$ and $g: R \to R$, the convolution operation, denoted by the mathematical notation $f \circ g$, generates a new function $(f \circ g) : R \to \mathbf{R}$, given by the following expression:

$$(f \circ g)(t) = \int_{-\infty}^{\infty} f(\tau) \cdot g(t - \tau) d\tau$$

$$= \int_{-\infty}^{\infty} f(t - \tau) \cdot g(\tau) d\tau \qquad (A1.15)$$

Frequently, in engineering, the function f is some real-world signal, and the function g is a *filter* used to modify f, e.g., by removing high-frequency noise. For example, suppose f is a sound recording, and g is a "box-car" filter:

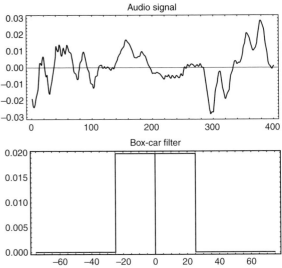

Audio signal

Box-car filter

The value of $f \circ g$ at a particular time point t_0 is computed by shifting the filter by t_0, multiplying f by the shifted filter, and integrating over time (i.e., taking the area under the curve), as this figure illustrates:

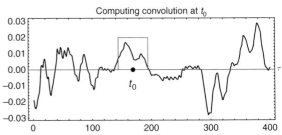

Computing convolution at t_0

When g is a box-car filter, this essentially averages the values of f over the interval $[t_1 0 - r, t_1 0 + r]$, where r is half the width of the box-car filter. Such averaging cancels out the effects of high-frequency unbiased noise on the signal, making the filtered signal smoother:

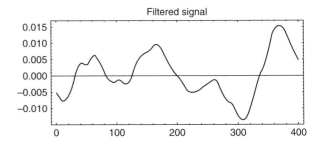

Filtered signal

Convolution itself constitutes a system, one that takes two inputs and generates a single output. In fact, convolution is a linear shift-invariant system, which the reader can easily verify. Moreover, as we will show shortly, every linear shift-invariant system is a convolution.

Convolution can be defined for functions of multiple variables. The definition simply becomes

$$h(x_1, \ldots, x_n) = f \circ g$$
$$= \int_{-\infty}^{\infty} \ldots \int_{-\infty}^{\infty} f(\tau_1, \ldots, \tau_n)$$
$$\cdot g(x_1 - \tau_1, \ldots, x_n - \tau_n) d\tau_1 \ldots d\tau_n$$

(A1.16)

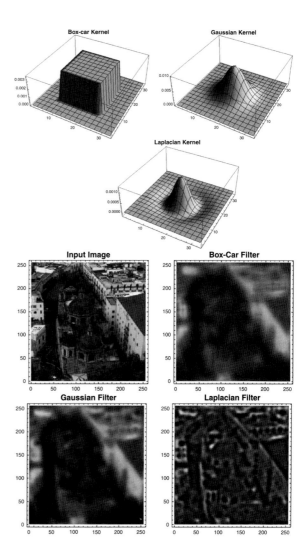

To the right are shown examples of convolution between a color image and three different kernels. Convolution is applied separately to the red, green, and blue channels of the image. The first kernel is the familiar box-car kernel, which replaces each pixel with the average of pixels in a $w \times w$ neighborhood. The second filter is the Gaussian, i.e., a normal probability function with two independent identically distributed variables. Both the box-car and the Gaussian filters smooth the image, although the box-car filter can increase the complexity of the image, while the Gaussian filter is considered an "ideal" smoothing filter because it always reduces complexity (expressed in terms of the edges in the image). The last filter is the Laplacian of the Gaussian. It highlights peak-like features in the image such as windows, statues, etc.

Impulse function and impulse response

The key property of shift-invariant linear systems is that their behavior is completely predictable. As long as we know the response of the system to one special input signal, $\delta(t)$, called the *unit impulse function*, we are able to infer the system's response to any other input signal. The unit impulse function, also known as the *Dirac delta function*, is a mathematical construct. Conceptually, it represents a function that is continuous, equal to zero everywhere, except at the origin, and integrates to one. One way to represent the delta function is as the limit of a family of the normal probability density functions (PDF) with zero mean and standard deviation tending towards zero. As the standard deviation σ decreases, the peak of the PDF gets higher and higher, the tails get flatter and flatter, but the area under the PDF graph remains equal to one. In the

limit, the PDF with shrinking σ approaches the delta function:

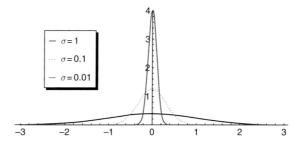

The delta function is not a function in the classical sense. Its rigorous treatment requires the theory of distributions, which is outside the scope of this

297

appendix. Nevertheless, it is possible to utilize it in the study of linear shift-invariant systems. One of the key properties of the delta function, called *sifting*, is that $f \circ \delta = f$, i.e., convolution with a delta function preserves the function. In other words:

$$f(t) = \int_{-\infty}^{\infty} f(\tau) \cdot \delta(t - \tau) \mathrm{d}\tau \qquad (A1.17)$$

The intuition behind this property is simple. Just as we previously thought of the delta function as the limit of a family of normal PDFs, we can think of it as the limit of a series of narrower and narrower box-car filters that integrate to 1. Recall that convolving f with a box-car function involves averaging f over an interval $[t - r, t + r]$. As the width of the box-car filter tends to zero, this average tends to $f(t)$.

Suppose now that we have some system $\mathcal{H}$, whose internal structure we wish to investigate. Suppose we know the output of the system when the input is the unit impulse function:

$$\xi(t) = \mathcal{H}[\delta(t)] \qquad (A1.18)$$

This output $\xi(t)$ is known as the *impulse response function* of the system $\mathcal{H}$. This function is very important in the study of systems. It turns out that if $\mathcal{H}$ is a linear shift-invariant system, the response of $\mathcal{H}$ for any input $\phi(t)$ can be predicted only by knowing the impulse response function. In other words, a linear shift-invariant system is fully characterized by the impulse response function.

Let us prove this important property. Suppose $u(t) = \mathcal{H}[\phi(t)]$ and $\mathcal{H}$ is linear shift-invariant. We can write:

$$\mathcal{H}[\phi(t)] = \mathcal{H}\left[\int_{-\infty}^{\infty} \phi(\tau) \cdot \delta(t - \tau) \mathrm{d}\tau\right] \qquad (A1.19)$$

Next, we recall from above that the response of a linear system to an integral is equal to the integral of the response:

$$\mathcal{H}\left[\int_{-\infty}^{\infty} \phi(\tau) \cdot \delta(t - \tau) \mathrm{d}\tau\right]$$
$$= \int_{-\infty}^{\infty} \mathcal{H}[\phi(\tau) \cdot \delta(t - \tau)] \mathrm{d}\tau \qquad (A1.20)$$

Now, inside the integral, $\phi(\tau)$ is a constant with respect to t, so multiplication by $\phi(\tau)$ can be carried outside the system as well:

$$\int_{-\infty}^{\infty} \mathcal{H}[\phi(\tau) \cdot \delta(t - \tau)] \mathrm{d}\tau$$
$$= \int_{-\infty}^{\infty} \phi(\tau) \cdot \mathcal{H}[\delta(t - \tau)] \mathrm{d}\tau \qquad (A1.21)$$

Finally, by the shift-invariance property, $\mathcal{H}[\delta(t - \tau)] = \xi(t - \tau)$, giving us:

$$\mathcal{H}[\phi(t)] = \int_{-\infty}^{\infty} \phi(\tau) \cdot \xi(t - \tau) \mathrm{d}\tau \qquad (A1.22)$$

So the response of $\mathcal{H}$ to $\phi(t)$ is simply the convolution of $\phi(t)$ with the impulse response function.

In differential equations, the impulse response function is known as Green's function. Let us revisit the example of the diffusion equation (A1.14) above. The impulse response function $\xi(x,t)$ is the solution of the following equation:

$$\frac{\delta \xi}{\partial t} - k\left(\frac{\partial^2 \xi}{\partial x^z}\right) = 0 \quad x \in (-\infty, \infty); t \in [0, \infty),$$
$$\xi(x, 0) = \delta(x) \qquad x \in (-\infty, \infty) \qquad (A1.23)$$

The physical analogy is an infinitely long homogeneous rod that at time zero is infinitely hot at the origin and completely cold everywhere else. The impulse response is a function describing the distribution of heat in the rod at time t. The solution turns out to be:

$$\xi(x, t) = \frac{1}{\sqrt{4\pi kt}} e^{\frac{-x^2}{4kt}} \qquad (A1.24)$$

which is the normal distribution with mean 0 and standard deviation $\sqrt{2kt}$. With the help of the impulse response function, we can solve the equation (A1.14) for any input ϕ, simply using convolution.

Eigenfunctions, Laplace transform, transfer functions

Eigenfunctions are a special kind of input to a system: the response to an eigenfunction is just the eigenfunction itself, scaled by a constant called the *eigenvalue*:

$$\mathcal{H}[\psi(t)] = \lambda \cdot \psi(t) \qquad (A1.25)$$

We can think of the eigenfunctions as inputs that are not "changed too much" by the system. Coming back to the diffusion equation (A1.3) on the infinite rod, we can see that $\sin(x)$ is an eigenfunction because the solution of the diffusion equation for every time t is the same sinusoid scaled by a constant:

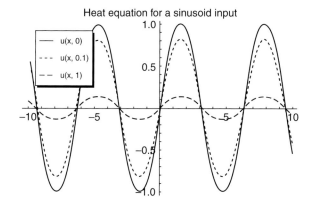

Heat equation for a sinusoid input

In fact, sinusoids are eigenfunctions of *all* linear shift-invariant linear systems. Recall that the general way to represent sinusoids is using the complex exponential notation:

$$e^{zt} = e^{(a+i-b)t} = a[\sin(bt) + i \cos(bt)] \qquad (A1.26)$$

where $z \in C$ is a complex number and $i = \sqrt{-1}$.

We can easily show that if $\mathcal{H}$ is a linear shift-invariant system, then for any complex number z, the function e^{zt} is an eigenfunction of $\mathcal{H}$ with corresponding eigenvalue $\lambda(z)$:

$$\mathcal{H}[e^{zt}] = \lambda(z) \cdot e^{zt} \qquad (A1.27)$$

Let $\xi(t)$ be the impulse response of $\mathcal{H}$. then:

$$\begin{aligned}
\mathcal{H}[e^{zt}] &= \int_{-\infty}^{\infty} e^{zt} \cdot \xi(t - \tau) \mathrm{d}\tau \\
&= \int_{-\infty}^{\infty} e^{z(t-\tau)} \cdot \xi(\tau) \mathrm{d}\tau \\
&= e^{zt} \cdot \int_{-\infty}^{\infty} e^{-zt} \cdot \xi(\tau) \mathrm{d}\tau \\
&= e^{zt} \cdot \lambda(z).
\end{aligned} \qquad (A1.28)$$

with the eigenvalues given by:

$$\lambda(z) = \int_{-\infty}^{\infty} e^{-zt} \cdot \xi(\tau) \mathrm{d}\tau \qquad (A1.29)$$

The function $\lambda(z)$ is known as the *transfer function* of the system $\mathcal{H}$. It describes how the system scales sinusoidal inputs into sinusoidal outputs. The transfer function is a powerful tool because it can be used to describe how the system responds to *any* input. For any input/output pair u,ϕ of a linear shift-invariant system:

$$\lambda(z) = \frac{\pounds[u(t)]}{\pounds[\phi(t)]} \qquad (A1.30)$$

where $\pounds$ denotes the bilateral *Laplace transform* of functions u and ϕ. The Laplace transform of a function of time is a function of frequency, given by the integral expression:

$$F(z) = \int_{-\infty}^{\infty} e^{-zt} \cdot f(t) \mathrm{d}t \qquad (A1.31)$$

Like the Fourier transform, the Laplace transform maps functions from time domain (or space domain) into the frequency domain. Thus, knowing the transfer function of a system, we can predict the response of the system to every output. The transfer function is itself the Laplace transform of the impulse response.

Why do we need to worry about eigenfunctions and the transfer function if the system's response to an arbitrary signal can be characterized by the impulse response? There are several compelling reasons. Firstly, the transfer function may be easier to estimate in a real-world application than the impulse response function. Whereas estimating the impulse response requires us to generate an infinitely high-contrast signal and to measure the system's response over all space/time, estimating the transfer function requires us to pass in an (infinite) series of sinusoidal inputs and to measure the constant ratio of the sinusoidal response to the sinusoidal input. The latter operation is more numerically stable. Furthermore, in most real-world systems, the transfer function is smooth and vanishes at infinity, making it possible to approximate it by measuring the response to just a few eigenfunctions. Lastly, the Laplace transform and multiplication by the transfer function, used to predict the response to an arbitrary signal in this approach, are less computationally expensive than the convolution operation, used in the impulse response method.

To demonstrate how the eigenfunction method can be useful, let us once more consider the diffusion equation (A1.23). We have shown that the system is linear and shift-invariant, so for any $\phi(x) = e^{zx}$, the solution must be of the form $u(x, t) = \lambda(z, t)e^{zx}$ – note that the transfer function λ is constant in x but varies over time. Substituting these sinusoidal input and output into the differential equation, we obtain (with some manipulation):

$$\left[\frac{\delta\lambda(z,t)}{\partial t} - kz^z\lambda(z,t)\right]e^{zx} = 0 \quad x \in (-\infty, \infty); t \in [0, \infty),$$

$$\lambda(z,0) \qquad = 1 \quad x \in (-\infty, \infty) \qquad \text{(A1.32)}$$

This is an ordinary first-order differential equation, whose solution is:

$$\lambda(z,t) = e^{ktz^2} \qquad \text{(A1.33)}$$

which is the transfer function for the diffusion equation. From this, the impulse response function can be derived by taking the inverse Laplace transform.

Discrete-time systems

Without going into detail, we note that the concepts of impulse response, convolution, and transfer function extend to discrete-time signals. Let us consider, without loss of generality, discrete-time signals that are sampled at intervals of 1, i.e., $t = -\infty, \ldots, -1, 0, 1, \ldots, \infty$.

For discrete-time linear shift-invariant systems, the equivalent of the impulse function is the Kronecker delta function, δ_i, equal to 1 when $i = 0$, and zero for all other i. The response of the linear shift-invariant system to the Kronecker delta is the impulse response, and convolution with the impulse response, defined for discrete-time functions as:

$$(f \circ \xi)_i = \sum_{j=-\infty}^{\infty} f_j \cdot \xi_{i-j} \qquad \text{(A1.34)}$$

gives the response to an arbitrary input signal.

Likewise, the eigenfunctions of discrete-time linear systems are complex exponentials of the form z^n, where $z = e^v, v \in C$. The equivalent of the Laplace transform is the z-transform:

$$Z[f] = \sum_{j=-\infty}^{\infty} f_j \cdot z^{-n} \qquad \text{(A1.35)}$$

The transfer function is the ratio $\frac{Z[u]}{Z[\phi]}$, given by the z-transform of the impulse response function.

The diffusion equation in image analysis

As was noted above, the diffusion equation plays an important role in image analysis. It is directly related to the process of *smoothing* images. Smoothing creates a smooth (i.e., continuous, with continuous derivatives) approximation of an image, in a way that preserves the important features of the images, while averaging out the

more noisy features. Here is an example of smoothing an image with different levels of approximation:

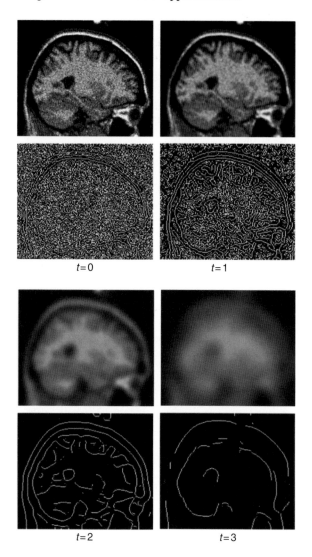

The top row shows an input MRI image (with some noise added to the image)[3] and the results of smoothing the image using the diffusion equation for different intervals of time. As smoothing proceeds, the image becomes more and more blurred. As the result, finer-scale features, including the noise, begin to disappear, while stronger, coarser-scale features remain. This is demonstrated in the bottom row by applying an *edge*

---

[3] Image from the *BrainWeb* simulated brain database: Collins DL, Zijdenbos AP, Kollokian V, *et al.* Design and construction of a realistic digital brain phantom. *IEEE Trans Med Imaging* 1998; **17**: 463–8. www.bic.mni.mcgill.ca/brainweb.

detector to each of the smoothed images. Edge detectors are a good way to extract salient features from an image. In this case, the edge detector finds all the pixels in the image where the magnitude of the image gradient exceeds a certain threshold. As we smooth the image, the number of salient features becomes smaller. Clearly, this is very relevant for image understanding.

There are many ways of smoothing an image (as demonstrated in the section on convolution), but smoothing based on the diffusion equation has unique and attractive properties. To understand them, we must first write down the diffusion equation in multiple dimensions, and then understand how the equation affects discrete images. In the case of two-dimensional images, the image intensity $u(x_1,x_2,t)$ is a function of two spatial directions x_1 and x_2 and of time t, and the diffusion equation takes the form:

$$\frac{\partial u}{\partial t} = k\left(\frac{\partial^2 u}{\partial x_1^2} + \frac{\partial^2 u}{\partial x_2^2}\right) \qquad \text{(A1.36)}$$

plus the appropriate boundary conditions, which we do not specify for the sake of brevity. In physics, this corresponds to heat diffusion on a plate with uniform heat density k. Thus the image intensity changes over time proportionally to the sum of the second derivatives in the cardinal directions. Let us discretize this equation on a sampling grid with inter-grid interval Δ_x. Using the Taylor series expression for the second derivative:

$$\frac{\partial^2 f}{\partial x^z} \cong \frac{f(x + \Delta_x) - 2f(x) + f(x - \Delta_x)}{\Delta_x^2} \qquad \text{(A1.37)}$$

we obtain the following discrete version of the equation:

$$\frac{\partial u}{\partial t} \cong k\,\frac{\begin{array}{c}u(x_1 + \Delta_x, x_2, t) + u(x_1, x_2 + \Delta_x, t)+\\ u(x_1, -\Delta_x, x_2, t) + u(x_1, x_2 - \Delta_x, t)-\\ 4u(x_1, x_2, t)\end{array}}{\Delta_x^2}$$

$$\text{(A1.38)}$$

The equation implies that as the diffusion progresses, the intensity of the image at the point (x_1,x_2) becomes a little closer to the average of the image intensities at the four neighboring grid points. In other words, the intensity from the four adjacent pixels slowly "bleeds into" the center pixel – at every pixel in the image. Over time, the intensity over the image becomes more and more uniform, eventually becoming constant.

As we have discussed before, smoothing via diffusion is equivalent to convolution with the Gaussian kernel. Thus in the literature this type of smoothing is called *Gaussian smoothing*. The property that makes Gaussian smoothing unique is the fact that *the information content (in the sense of Shannon's theory) of the image is guaranteed to reduce in the course of Gaussian smoothing*. Thus, for example, the output of the edge detector in the figure above becomes progressively simpler. This is not the case for other filters. For example, if we smooth the image by convolution with a box-car filter, we will create new small-scale features as we smooth:

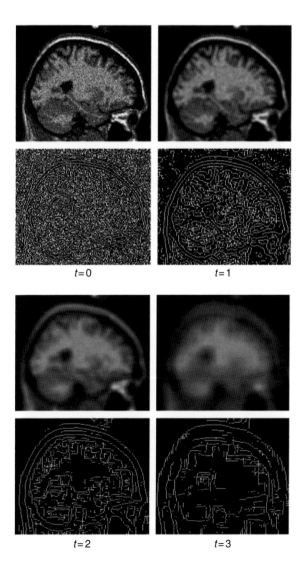

$t=0$ $t=1$

$t=2$ $t=3$

For this reason, as well as some other theoretical advantages, smoothing using the diffusion equation is used extensively in image processing and analysis.

Appendix 2: Fourier transform and *k*-space

Jeremy Magland

The Fourier transform in one dimension

In the context of medical imaging, we think of the Fourier transform as an operation on discrete vectors or discrete arrays of data. For example, the raw *k-space* data collected in MRI is usually a two- or three-dimensional array of complex numbers. The Fourier transform (actually the discrete Fourier transform, or DFT) is applied to reconstruct an image, which again is a discrete complex array. We will return to this DFT in a later section. In this section, however, we address the classical (continuous) Fourier transform (CFT) [1,2], which operates on functions, rather than vectors and arrays:

$$\hat{f}(k_x) := \int_{-\infty}^{\infty} f(x)e^{-2\pi i x k_x}\,\mathrm{d}x \qquad (A2.1)$$

According to this equation, the Fourier transform maps (or transforms) a continuous function $f(x)$ to a new continuous function $\hat{f}(x)$, and we write:

$$\mathrm{F}(f) = \hat{f} \qquad (A2.2)$$

or

$$f(x) \xrightarrow{\mathrm{F}} \hat{f}(k_x) \qquad (A2.3)$$

The criteria for convergence of the integral in Equation A2.1 is interesting in itself, but is beyond the present scope. One of the most famous examples, and of particular relevance to MRI, is the Fourier transform of a rectangular function (Figure A2.1a–b):

$$\chi_{[-1,1]}(x) \xrightarrow{\mathrm{F}} 2\,\mathrm{sinc}(2k_x) \qquad (A2.4)$$

where:

$$\chi_{[-1,1]}(x) = \begin{cases} 1 & \text{if } |x| < 1 \\ 0 & \text{otherwise} \end{cases} \qquad (A2.5)$$

is the characteristic function on the interval from −1 to 1, and:

$$\mathrm{sinc}(k_x) = \frac{\sin(\pi k_x)}{\pi k_x} \qquad (A2.6)$$

Perhaps the most important property of the Fourier transform is that it is essentially its own inverse. In other words, applying the Fourier transform twice essentially gives the original function back. The word *essentially* needs to be used here because of a technicality. The actual inverse Fourier transform varies slightly from the forward transform:

$$f(x) := \int_{-\infty}^{\infty} \hat{f}(k_x e^{2\pi i x k x}\,dk_x \qquad (A2.7)$$

Note the similarity between Equations A2.1 and A2.7. Equation A2.7 is known as the Fourier inversion formula. Along with the fast Fourier transform (FFT) algorithm, it is the basis for why the Fourier transform is so useful in medical imaging, and particularly MRI.

The one-dimensional Fourier transform has many other important properties and symmetries, some of which are depicted in Figure A2.1. In each pair, the function on the left is defined in the so-called spatial domain, or image space (*i*-space), whereas the function on the right (obtained via Fourier transform) is defined in the Fourier domain, or *k*-space. In MRI, raw data is collected directly from *k*-space, whereas the reconstructed image is in *i*-space.

Introduction to the Science of Medical Imaging, ed. R. Nick Bryan. Published by Cambridge University Press. © Cambridge University Press 2010.

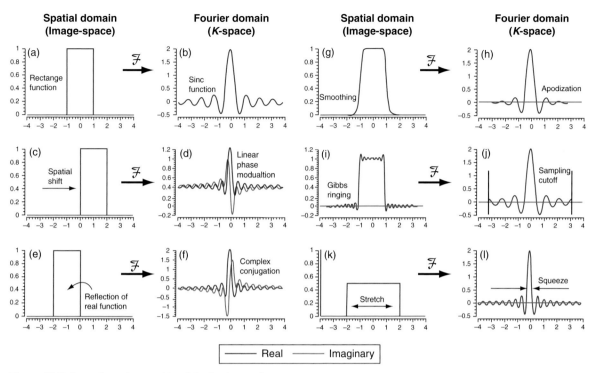

Figure A2.1. Properties and symmetries of the Fourier transform.

Figure A2.1c–d illustrates the *Fourier shift theorem*, which states that a spatial shift in *i*-space corresponds to a linear phase modulation in *k*-space. Mathematically this is written as:

$$\hat{f}_\tau(k_x) = e^{2\pi i \tau k_x} \hat{f}(k_x) \qquad (A2.8)$$

where f_τ is the same as f except shifted by τ units. Figure A2.1e–f shows that a reflection of a real function in *i*-space corresponds to complex conjugation in *k*-space. Both Figure A2.1g–h and Figure A2.1i–j show that suppression of high frequencies in *k*-space leads to a loss of resolution in *i*-space. In the case of a sharp cutoff (Figure A2.1i–j), transitions at sharp edges are lengthened, and a rippling artifact known as Gibbs ringing occurs. In the case of a smooth cutoff (Figure A2.1g–h), sharp edges are simply smoothed out, or blurred. Finally, if the function is stretched or dilated in *i*-space, then the corresponding *k*-space function is compressed (Figure A2.1k–l).

The Fourier transform in multiple dimensions

The Fourier transform in two dimensions is defined similarly to the one-dimensional transform:

$$\hat{f}(k_x, k_y) := \int_{-\infty}^{\infty} \int_{-\infty}^{\infty} f(x,y) e^{-2\pi i (xk_x + yk_y)} \, dx \, dy \qquad (A2.9)$$

More generally the *n*-dimensional Fourier transform is given by:

$$\hat{f}(k_{x_1}, \ldots, k_{x_n})$$
$$:= \int_{-\infty}^{\infty} \cdots \int_{-\infty}^{\infty} f(x_1, \ldots, x_n)$$
$$\times e^{-2\pi i (x_1 k_{x_1} + \ldots + x_n k_{x_n})} \, dx_1 \cdots dx_n. \qquad (A2.10)$$

Note that the integral in Equation A2.9 can be separated into two nested integrals:

$$\hat{f}(k_x, k_y) = \int_{-\infty}^{\infty} \int_{-\infty}^{\infty} f(x,y) e^{-2\pi i x k_x} dx \cdot e^{-2\pi i y k_y} dy. \qquad (A2.11)$$

with each integral being a Fourier transform in one dimension (a similar decomposition is possible for the *n*-dimensional transform). In this way, we can think of the multidimensional Fourier transform as simply a composition of one-dimensional Fourier transforms (each along a different dimension). Therefore all of the

303

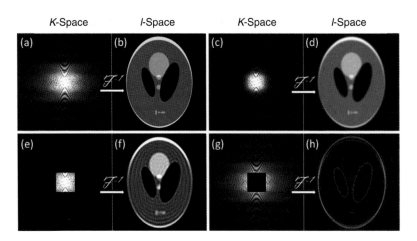

K-Space   I-Space   K-Space   I-Space

Figure A2.2. Contributions of low- and high-frequency portions of *k*-space to the reconstructed image.

properties mentioned in the previous section will apply to *n*-dimensional Fourier transforms.

Figure A2.2 shows the contributions of the low- and high-frequency portions of *k*-space to the reconstructed image. Figure A2.2a is the *k*-space data (or Fourier data) associated with the Shepp–Logan [3] phantom of Figure A2.1b. For practical reasons, we display only the magnitude (not the phase) of the complex Fourier data. Note that most of the signal intensity is concentrated toward the central portion of *k*-space, reflecting the strong tendency for the low-frequency components to be much larger in magnitude than the high-frequency components of the signal. Figure A2.2c–d shows the results of suppressing the high frequencies using a smooth Gaussian modulation in *k*-space. This results in an overall loss of resolution in *i*-space due to general blurring. Figure A2.2e–f shows the results of simply cutting out the high-frequency *k*-space data by setting them equal to zero. Note the Gibbs ringing artifact in Figure A2.2f. Similarly, Figure A2.2g–h shows the effect of setting the low-frequency data equal to zero.

The discrete Fourier transform (DFT)

In medical imaging we tend to deal with discrete sets of data, and not continuous functions. But it is useful to think of the underlying physical object being scanned as a continuous function, for example the spin-density function. As soon as we sample Fourier data in a finite collection of locations, we enter the realm of the *discrete* Fourier transform as opposed to the *continuous* Fourier transform.

The DFT can be thought of in either one of the following two ways:

(1) As an approximation of the CFT

(2) As a genuine CFT operating on the space of *periodic, band-limited* functions.

In this section we will take the first approach. By definition, the one-dimensional DFT operates on a vector $\bar{x} = (x_0, x_1, \ldots, x_{N-1})$ according to the formula:

$$X_m = \sum_{n=0}^{N-1} x_n e^{-2\pi imn/N}, \quad m = 0, 1, \ldots, N-1$$

(A2.12)

To see why this can be thought of as an approximation to the CFT, consider a continuous function $f(x)$ defined on the finite interval $-L/2 \leq x \leq L/2$ of length L. This is realistic, since in MRI we are dealing with a spin-density function which is defined over a finite region of space. Splitting this interval up into N equal pieces (assume N is even) of length $\Delta = L/N$, the Riemann approximation of the Fourier transform (Equation A2.1) is:

$$\hat{f}(k_x) = \int_{-L}^{L} f(x) e^{-2\pi ixk_x} dx \approx \Delta \sum_{n=-N/2}^{N/2-1} f(\Delta n) e^{-2\pi i\Delta nk_x}$$

(A2.13)

It is natural to sample the Fourier transform on a grid with spacing of $\Delta_k = 1/L$ in *k*-space (this is called Nyquist spacing). Plugging into Equation A2.13 we have:

$$\hat{f}(m\Delta_k) = \hat{f}(m/L) \approx \Delta \sum_{n=-N/2}^{N/2-1} f(\Delta n)e^{-2\pi i \Delta nm/L}$$

$$= \Delta \sum_{n=-N/2}^{N/2-1} f(\Delta n)e^{-2\pi i nm/N} \qquad (A2.14)$$

Finally, if we write $X_m = \Delta^{-1}\hat{f}(m\Delta_k)$ and $x_n = f(\Delta n)$, then we have:

$$X_m \approx \sum_{n=-N/2}^{N/2-1} x_n e^{-2\pi i mn/N} \qquad (A2.15)$$

which is *almost* the DFT. The trick is to consider the vectors $\bar{x}$ and $\bar{X}$ as periodic series with period N (Figure A2.3). This is natural, since the coefficients of Equation A2.15 are also N-periodic in both n and m. We can then simply rewrite the bounds in the summation of Equation A2.15 to obtain exactly the formula for the DFT in Equation A2.12. In this way the DFT can be thought of as a Riemann approximation to the CFT.

In MRI we do not actually deal with the *forward* DFT nearly as much as the *inverse discrete Fourier transform*, or IDFT. This is because the discrete sampling takes place in the Fourier domain, and we then reconstruct the image using the IDFT. As in the continuous case, the inversion formula resembles the forward transform:

$$x_n = \frac{1}{N}\sum_{m=0}^{N-1} X_m e^{2\pi i mn/N}, \quad n = 0, 1, \cdots, N-1$$

$$(A2.16)$$

Figure A2.4 illustrates the data acquisition process for MRI. We begin with a spin-density function, which is considered as a continuous function of space. Applying the CFT brings us to *k*-space where the samples are taken. Finally, the IDFT brings us back to *i*-space, where we have our (discrete) reconstructed image. Note that Figure A2.4(d) depicts some error in the reconstructed image (as compared to the original function). This error is caused by the finite sampling of Figure A2.4c. However, it should be noted that the finite sampling density is not the source of this error (the sampling density only needs to meet the Nyquist criterion). Rather the error comes from not sampling sufficiently far out in *k*-space. In other words, so long as the Nyquist criterion is met, if one samples far enough out in *k*-space, then (neglecting measurement noise) the reconstruction will be perfect (i.e., error-free).

The fast fourier transform

Efficient reconstruction in MRI depends almost exclusively on a fast implementation of the IDFT of

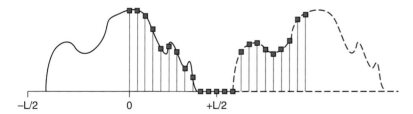

Figure A2.3. Sampling scheme for the DFT as an approximation to the CFT. The original continuous function is defined on the interval from −L/2 to L/2, but for sampling purposes we consider the function as periodic of period L.

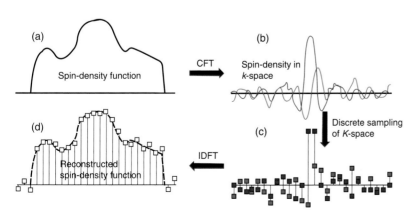

Figure A2.4. Decomposition of data acquisition in MRI.

(a) Spin-density function

(b) Spin-density in *k*-space

Discrete sampling of *K*-space

(c)

(d) Reconstructed spin-density function

CFT

IDFT

Equation A2.16. As written, this transform involves the addition of N^2 terms, or would take on the order of N^2 computer operations, i.e., $O(N)^2$ operations. For one-dimensional transforms, this is not a problem. However, typical reconstructions use two-dimensional $N \times N$ arrays, which involve $O(N)^4$ operations for inversion, or $O(N)^6$ operations for 3D reconstructions, becoming prohibitively time-consuming from a computational perspective. Fortunately, the fast Fourier transform (FFT), or in our case the inverse fast Fourier transform (IFFT), reduces the computation to $O(N)\log(N))$ operations for 1D, $O(N^2\log(N^2))$ operations for 2D, and $O(N^3\log(N^3))$ operations for 3D. Recall that log$N$ is usually much smaller than N. For example, $\log_2(512) = 9$. Therefore, the number of operations is almost linear in the number of array entries!

In this section, we describe the IFFT algorithm and demonstrate the claimed number of computational operations. For simplicity, we assume that N is always a power of 2, e.g. $N = 1, 2, 4, 8, 16, 32$, etc., or $N = 2^d$. We begin by handling the one-dimensional case (remember that higher-dimensional Fourier transforms can be decomposed into a series of one-dimensional transforms), and proceed by mathematical induction on the exponent d. First we take the base case of $d = 0$, or $N = 1$. In this case the IDFT of Equation A2.16 is trivial, taking a single operation to complete. Next, we assume that the fast Fourier transform has already been defined for $N/2 = 2^d$ and that it takes $O(N/2 \log(N/2))$ operations, and consider the transform of order $N = 2^d + 1$. The trick is to decompose the summation of Equation A2.16 into two pieces, each representing an IDFT of order $N/2$ (Figure A2.5).

Writing $w = e^{2\pi imn/N}$ we have:

$$
\begin{aligned}
x_n &= \frac{1}{N}\sum_{m=0}^{N-1} X_m e^{2\pi imn/N} \\
&= \frac{1}{N}\left(X_0 w^0 + X_1 w^1 + \ldots + X_{N-1}w^{N-1}\right) \\
&= \frac{1}{N}\left(X_0 w^0 + X_2 w^2 + X_4 w^4 + \ldots + X_{N-2}w^{N-2}\right) \\
&\quad + \frac{w}{N}\left(X_1 w^0 + X_3 w^2 + X_5 w^4 + \ldots + X_{N-1}w^{N-2}\right) \\
&= \frac{1}{N}\sum_{m=0}^{N/2-1} X_{2m} e^{2\pi imn/(N/2)} \\
&\quad + e^{2\pi imn/N}\frac{1}{N}\sum_{m=0}^{N/2-1} X_{2m+1} e^{2\pi imn/(N/2)} \quad (A2.17)
\end{aligned}
$$

which is the sum of two IDFTs of order $N/2$. By assumption, each of these takes $O(N/2 \log(N/2))$ operations, and then it takes $O(N)$ operations to do the sum, for a total of:

$$
\begin{aligned}
2O(N/2 &\log_2(N/2)) + O(N) \\
&= O(N(\log_2(N/2) + 1)) = O(N \log_2 N) \quad (A2.18)
\end{aligned}
$$

operations, as desired.

As mentioned above, the multidimensional CFT can be decomposed into a series of one-dimensional CFTs. Similarly, the multidimensional DFT (or IDFT) can be decomposed into a series of one-dimensional discrete transforms. For example, the 2D IDFT is given by:

$$
\begin{aligned}
x_{n_1,n_2} &= \frac{1}{N_1 N_2}\sum_{m_1=0}^{N_1-1}\sum_{m_2=0}^{N_2-1} X_{m_1 m_2} e^{2\pi i(m_1 n_1/N_1 + m_2 n_2/N_2)}, \\
&\quad m_j = 0, \cdots, N_j - 1 \quad (A2.19)
\end{aligned}
$$

and can be decomposed as:

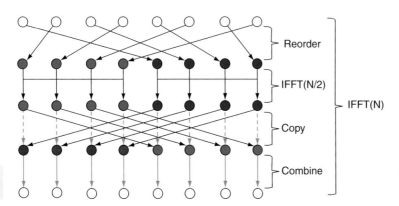

Figure A2.5. Graphical and recursive diagram of the fast Fourier transform algorithm.

Reorder

IFFT(N/2)

Copy

Combine

IFFT(N)

$$x_{n_1,n_2} = \frac{1}{N_1} \sum_{m_1=0}^{N_1-1} \left(\frac{1}{N_2} \sum_{m_2=0}^{N_2-1} X_{m_1 m_2} e^{2\pi i m_2 n_2/N_2} \right) e^{2\pi i m_1 n_1/N_1},$$

$$m_j = 0, \cdots, N_j - 1 \qquad (A2.20)$$

which can be seen as a series of N_1 IFFTs of order N_2 followed by N_2 IFFTs of order N_1. This yields a total of:

$$N_1 O(N_2 \log N_2) + N_2 O(N_1 \log N_1)$$
$$= O(N_1 N_2 (\log N_1 + \log N_2))$$
$$= O(N_1 N_2 \log(N_1 N_2)) \qquad (A2.21)$$

operations. Similar formulae hold for three- and higher-dimensional transforms.

References

1. Epstein CL. *Introduction to the Mathematics of Medical Imaging,* 2nd edn. Philadelphia, PA: Society for Industrial and Applied Mathematics, 2008.

2. Bracewell RN. *The Fourier Transform and Its Applications,* 3rd edn. Boston, MA: McGraw-Hill, 2000.

3. Shepp LA, Logan BF. The Fourier reconstruction of head sections. *IEEE Trans Nucl Sci* 1974: **NS-21**: 21–43.

Appendix 3: Probability, Bayesian statistics, and information theory

Edward H. Herskovits

If science represents humanity's endeavor to understand the universe, then probability theory is the language in which we encode this knowledge. In essence, probability theory formalizes the effect that evidence has on what we believe. Similarly, information theory quantitatively summarizes our knowledge. In this appendix, I briefly describe how probability theory and information theory developed, and how they serve to evaluate scientific hypotheses.

Probability theory
Basic concepts

This section briefly describes the central concepts required to understand the remainder of this appendix. For a more rigorous, detailed presentation of these concepts, please refer to [1,2].

Without loss of generality, we consider in this section only binary (i.e., two-valued) variables. Most of the concepts described in this section generalize to multi-state variables and continuous variables. The *marginal probability* that a statement S is true, written as $P(S)$, is the probability that statement S is true in the absence of any evidence. The *joint probability* of statements S_1 and S_2, written as $P(S_1, S_2)$, is the probability that both statements are true simultaneously, again in the absence of any evidence. *Mutually exclusive* statements cannot be true simultaneously; for example, the statements "the patient has squamous-cell carcinoma of the lung" and "the patient does not have squamous-cell carcinoma of the lung" are mutually exclusive. The *conditional probability* of a statement S given evidence E, written $P(S|E)$, is the probability that statement S is true, given evidence E. Conditional probability is defined as:

$$P(S|E) \equiv \frac{P(S, E)}{P(E)} \tag{A3.1}$$

This equation also tells us that $P(S|E)\, P(E) = P(E|S)\, P(S)$. Independent events have no probabilistic influence on each other; two events S_1 and S_2 are independent if $P(S_1, S_2) = P(S_1)\, P(S_2)$.

We can combine these definitions to construct useful propositions. For example, the *product rule* is often used to compute the conditional probability of a joint event:

$$\begin{aligned}
P(S_1, S_2|E) &= \frac{P(S_1, S_2, E)}{P(E)} \\
&= \frac{P(S_1|S_2, E)P(S_2, E)}{P(E)} \\
&= P(S_1|S_2, E)P(S_2|E)
\end{aligned} \tag{A3.2}$$

Similarly,

$$P(S_1, S_2|E) = P(S_2|S_1, E)P(S_1|E)$$

The *sum rule* is often used to compute the marginal probability of an event, by summing over all possible states of other variables in a joint-probability distribution. For example, in the case of two binary variables, S_1 and S_2, this rule can be expressed as:

$$\begin{aligned}
P(S_1 = T) &= P(S_1 = T, S_2 = T) + P(S_1 = T, S_2 = F) \\
&= P(S_1 = T|S_2 = T)P(S_2 = T) \\
&\quad + P(S_1 = T|S_2 = F)P(S_2 = F)
\end{aligned} \tag{A3.3}$$

where T and F represent true and false, respectively.

Introduction to the Science of Medical Imaging, ed. R. Nick Bryan. Published by Cambridge University Press. © Cambridge University Press 2010.

Examining the distribution of a continuous or discrete variable, we can compute summary statistics that are useful either descriptively or for hypothesis testing. A *probability density function* (PDF) represents a distribution over a continuous variable. There are a number of restrictions on PDFs; for example, a PDF must be integrable, must be non-negative throughout, and must integrate to 1. Examples of continuous PDFs include the uniform distribution, the exponential distribution, the chi-square distribution, and the Gaussian or normal distribution. The *cumulative distribution function* (CDF) is the probability that the variable will assume a value less than or equal to a specified value; the CDF is obtained by integrating the corresponding PDF over all values less than or equal to the specified value.

The *mean*, or *expected value*, of a distribution is defined as the sum (or integral, for a continuous distribution) of each possible value of a variable, weighted by its probability. For a variable X that can assume the states 1, 2, or 3, we compute the mean with the sum $(1 \times P(X = 1)) + (2 \times P(X = 2)) + (3 \times P(X = 3))$; if these probabilities were 0.1, 0.4, and 0.5, respectively, the mean value for X would be $(1 \times 0.1) + (2 \times 0.4) + (3 \times 0.5) = 2.4$. Similarly, if we accumulated a sample of 10 cases with 0 lesions, 25 cases with 1 lesion, and 15 cases with 2 lesions, the probabilities for 0, 1, and 2 lesions would be 0.2, 0.5, and 0.3, respectively, and the mean number of lesions per case would be $(0 \times 0.2) + (1 \times 0.5) + (2 \times 0.3) = 1.1$. The *median* of a distribution is the value below and above which half of the distribution lies; one advantage of working with the median, rather than the mean, in statistical inference, is the median's relative robustness to *outliers*, or very high or low values, even one of which in a sample can drastically change the value of the mean. The *mode* of a distribution is the most common value; for the distribution of the number of lesions described above, the mode would be 1. The mean, median, and mode are statistics that capture the central tendency of a distribution; the *variance* (or its square root, the *standard deviation*) of a distribution measures the spread of a distribution about its mean. For example, for a distribution with mean 100 and variance 1, we expect to see most values lie between 98 and 102, whereas for a distribution with mean 100 and variance 100, we expect to see most values lie between 80 and 120. Researchers use the mean and variance of a distribution to determine how likely it would be to observe the data at hand, and therefore estimate the plausibility of a hypothesis that could explain the observed data.

There are two principal schools of thought regarding the interpretation of probabilities. *Objectivists* define a probability as the ratio of successes in an experiment (e.g., the number of coin tosses that come up heads) divided by the total number of trials. Objectivists ground their viewpoint in data – that is, experimental results. *Subjectivists*, on the other hand, define a probability as a measure of belief; thus, a subjectivist might assign a prior probability of a coin toss resulting in heads to be 0.5, and then would update his or her belief in this probability distribution as the results of trials (i.e., coin tosses) are observed. Although these groups have debated the relative merits of their interpretations for decades [3–5], for our purposes the subjective viewpoint has the distinct advantage that it allows us to compute and interpret probabilities even in the case in which performing a series of experimental trials is difficult or impossible. For example, computing the probability that a radically new MR pulse sequence will be useful for angiography does not readily lend itself to an experiment in which we design many new MR pulse sequences, and determine the fraction that are useful for MR angiography. A subjectivist viewpoint to research allows us to incorporate evidence of any type when assessing the probability that a particular statement is true [6,7].

Theoretical underpinnings: why probability theory is the optimal way to quantify uncertainty

Starting with three simple statements regarding how a measure of certainty should behave, Cox [8] showed that probability theory is the unique quantitative system (to within a one-to-one mapping) that fulfills these criteria:

(1) The measure of belief in a statement, $Bel(S)$, can be expressed as a real number, and can be ordered: if $Bel(S_1)$ is greater than $Bel(S_2)$ and $Bel(S_2)$ is greater than $Bel(S_3)$, then $Bel(S_1)$ is greater than $Bel(S_3)$.

(2) $Bel(S)$ is related to belief in its negation, $Bel(\overline{S})$.

(3) Belief in a conjunctive statement $Bel(S_1, S_2)$ is a function of only $Bel(S_1|S_2)$, and $Bel(S_2)$.

The first of Cox's axioms states that we can use real numbers for measuring certainty; in practice, we use numbers in [0, 1], but these axioms do not require that we do so. The second axiom states that, once we know how likely a statement is to be true, we perforce know how likely its opposite is to be true. The third axiom states that we need know only how likely a statement is given another statement, and how likely the second statement is, to compute the likelihood of the joint statement. Although Halpern [9] and others have questioned the rigor of Cox's original work, there is general consensus that, with few modifications, these axioms form the basis for a rigorous proof. In any case, no one has derived a system for measuring uncertainty that can match probability theory with respect to two crucial properties:

(1) *Consistency*: results that could be computed by more than one approach always yield the same result.

(2) *Reasonableness*: results match common-sense expectations when the latter are available.

Bayes' rule

Although probability theory had been used for centuries in specific situations (e.g., to compute the probability of various outcomes in a game of chance), the first formal generalization of these models was put in writing by the Reverend Thomas Bayes and published posthumously [10]. In his presentation to the Royal Society of London, Bayes' friend, Richard Price, described how one should update one's belief in a hypothesis H, based on evidence E:

$$P(H|E) = \frac{P(E|H)P(H)}{P(E)} \qquad \text{(A3.4)}$$

This equation states that the probability of a particular outcome given the evidence at hand is equal to the probability that we would observe this evidence if this hypothesis were true, weighted by the probability that this hypothesis is indeed true, and divided by the probability that we would observe this evidence in *any* setting, not just in the context of the specified hypothesis. As a simple example, we could describe an experiment in which we are attempting to determine whether a coin is fair, i.e., heads and tails are equally likely. In this setting, H would represent the assertion, or hypothesis, that the coin is fair; E would represent the results of a number of coin tosses; $P(E|H)$ represents the likelihood that we would observe these results from a fair coin; $P(H)$ would represent our belief, prior to seeing any evidence, that this coin is fair; $P(E)$ would represent our belief, regardless of the coin used (fair or not), that we would observe these results; and $P(H|E)$ represents our belief that this coin is fair, given the results observed. Note that

the combination of a rarely observed series of coin tosses (i.e., $P(E)$ is relatively low), a high likelihood of seeing these results in the setting of a fair coin (i.e., $P(E|H)$ is relatively high), and a strong belief that this coin is fair (i.e., $P(H)$ is relatively high) would all contribute to a very high probability that the coin is fair, given the results observed. In other words, observing a series of coin tosses that is almost never seen except in the setting of a fair coin makes our belief in the fairness of this coin very strong.

Bayes' rule, in the context of the analysis of a scientific experiment, encodes the contribution of new information to our belief in a hypothesis. $P(H)$ encodes our prior belief in the hypothesis, $P(E|H)$ encodes our expectation of this experiment if H were in fact true, and $P(H|E)$ encodes our belief in H having observed the evidence E from the experiment.

Applications to the evaluation of (experimental) evidence

Bayesian evaluation of experimental evidence takes an approach different from that taken by hypothesis-based statistical tests. In the Bayesian approach, the researcher formulates a prior distribution over all hypotheses, collects data, computes the posterior probability distribution over hypotheses, and selects the hypothesis with maximum posterior probability, or perhaps considers an ensemble of hypotheses or models with high posterior probability [11].

Information theory
Basic concepts

As in previous sections, I provide here a brief introduction to basic concepts in information theory, to facilitate comprehension of the remainder of this appendix. For a more rigorous, detailed introduction to information theory, see [12].

A *bit* is the fundamental unit of information, analogous to a molecule of water flowing through a pipe. We often consider bits to be binary, that is, having exactly two states (e.g., on/off), although this requirement is not necessary for deriving any of information theory's theoretical results. A *channel* is an abstract term for a medium, analogous to a pipe, used to transmit information. The *bandwidth* of a channel indicates the maximum number of bits per unit time that can be transmitted through that channel. *Noise* indicates the frequency with which errors occur when receiving a transmission; a noiseless channel transmits each bit with perfect fidelity.

The logarithm of a number is approximately equal to the number of digits required to encode that number; in base 10, for example, the logarithm of 10 is 1, the logarithm of 100 is 2, the logarithm of 1000 is 3, and so on. This property makes the logarithm a very useful basis on which to quantify information: intuitively, the more complex something is, the more symbols we will require to represent it.

Entropy, often represented by H, quantifies the amount of information in a distribution, or alternatively, entropy quantifies our uncertainty about a statement. Consider a probability distribution over the possible values that a statement S can assume; let N_S be the number of possible values, and let p_i be the probability that S assumes value i, where i is in $[1, N_S]$. Then:

$$H \equiv - \sum_{i=1}^{N_S} p_i \log(p_i) \qquad \text{(A3.5)}$$

The entropy of a distribution is the sum (or integral) of terms, each of which can be thought of as the probability that S assumes value i multiplied by the number of bits required to represent that probability. In other words, H represents the expected number of bits required to represent, or transmit, one symbol. Note that, in the limit as a probability p decreases towards 0, $p \log(p)$ approaches 0; this allows us to compute the entropy of a distribution in which some probabilities will be 0. For example, for a trivial distribution in which S can assume only one of two states (e.g., $P(S = \text{True}) = 1$ and $P(S = \text{False}) = 0$), $H = 1 \log(1) + 0 \log(0) = 0$, which makes sense, in that there is no information in an event that is certain. In general, the entropy of a distribution is minimal (i.e., 0) when one probability is 1, and all remaining probabilities are 0; entropy is maximal (i.e., $\log(N_S)$) when the distribution is uniform, i.e., all probabilities are equal. As our uncertainty in the state of a variable increases, we require more bits, on average, to transmit the state of that variable.

The *conditional entropy* of two variables, X and Y, is derived from the definitions of conditional probability and entropy:

$$H(X|Y) = - \sum_{x,y} P(x,y) \log(P(x|y)) \qquad \text{(A3.6)}$$

where x and y are particular instantiations of X and Y, respectively. To the extent that Y increases our certainty about X, $H(X|Y)$ will be less than $H(X)$. Only when X and Y are marginally independent will $H(X|Y)$ be equal to $H(X)$.

The *mutual information* between two variables X and Y, $I(X; Y)$, is a measure of how well one distribution corresponds to another. Alternatively, from the description of conditional entropy above, we can see that mutual information quantifies the average decrease in uncertainty that we can expect upon observing Y. Mutual information is defined as:

$$I(X; Y) \equiv H(X) - H(X|Y). \qquad \text{(A3.7)}$$

Theoretical underpinnings: why information theory is the optimal way to quantify information

In the above discussion of the theoretical underpinnings of probability theory we presented Cox's three axioms, which together dictate that probability theory optimally represents a measure of belief. Similarly, in this section we present three statements put forth by Shannon regarding how a measure of information should behave. Shannon [13] has shown that entropy uniquely (to within a multiplicative constant) meets these criteria:

(1) Uncertainty must be a continuous measure.

(2) An event that has uniform probability has maximal uncertainty, and as the number of options increases uncertainty should increase; by implication, an event that is certain (i.e., $P(\text{event}) = 1$) has minimal uncertainty.

(3) If we decompose an event into two sub events, their overall measures of uncertainty should be equal.

The first criterion is similar to that for measuring belief: we require that a measure of uncertainty be a real number. The second criterion formalizes our intuition that, if we know something with certainty, our measure of uncertainty should be minimal, and if we have absolutely no information about something (i.e., all possible outcomes are equally likely), our measure of uncertainty should be maximal. The second criterion further states that, if we know nothing about two variables, the one with more states should have greater uncertainty; this statement is included because, even if we know nothing about which state a variable will assume, we have a greater chance of predicting its state if it has two possible states than if it has 20 possible states, and so our uncertainty about the latter is greater. The third criterion implies consistency: if we can compute the probability distribution for an event in two different ways, we should arrive at the same distribution, and therefore should necessarily have the same level of uncertainty regarding that event.

Applications to the evaluation of (experimental) evidence

If we consider science to be the gathering of data with the goal of synthesizing information, we can begin to understand how entropy can form the basis for analyzing data and evaluating hypotheses. Although there are many such entropy-based applications, we consider herein three of the most commonly applied approaches.

Minimum-description-length inference

The minimum-description-length (MDL) principle [14] prescribes selection of the model that minimizes an entropy-based metric with respect to the data at hand. The description-length metric consists of two parts: a description of the model, and the probability distribution of the data given the model. The former is a measure of how parsimonious the model is: complex models necessarily require more bits to describe them than do simple models. For example, if we have two models that explain our observation of 498 heads and 502 tails equally well, but one model is a fair coin and the other is the result of taking the mode of 17 simultaneously tossed fair coins, the former will be chosen by the entropy-based equivalent of Occam's razor. To the extent that a model explains the data observed, transmitting the data will require fewer bits; for example, if we have a fair coin as our model, but observe only heads for 1000 coin tosses, transmitting the data will require many more bits using this model than using the heads-only model. By summing the number of bits required to encode a model and to transmit the data given that model, we can compute an overall measure of how well that model explains the data. The MDL approach has additional complexity not described in this brief overview, primarily related to the precision with which parameters are encoded; see [14] for a more detailed description of this approach. Since MDL closely corresponds (by logarithmic transformation) to the Bayesian hypothesis evaluation described above, there are those who argue that MDL offers no advantage over the Bayesian approach [12].

Minimization of mutual information

If there are parameters that we can modify, which in turn affect two probability distributions, we can select as optimal those parameter settings that minimize mutual information between the distributions. In image processing, mutual information is commonly applied for registration [15]. In this approach, we select one image volume as the source, and the other as the target, for registration. We then select values for the affine-registration parameters, and apply that registration to the source image. Finally, we compute the mutual information between the signal-intensity distributions of the registered source image and the target image. We select as our final registration parameter settings the combination of parameter values that minimizes this mutual-information metric. One advantage of this approach relative to other registration techniques is that it can be applied to images acquired using different modalities or sequences; what matters is how well signal intensity in one image predicts signal intensity at the same voxel in the other image, not what those values actually mean.

Maximum-entropy evaluation of experimental evidence

Jaynes [1] has been the primary proponent of maximum-entropy inference. In essence, this principle uses the data to constrain the joint probability distribution over these variables. Any constraints that cannot be obtained from the data (e.g., probabilistic dependence) are not applied, leading to the fewest assumptions possible about this distribution, which will correspond to the distribution with highest entropy that still satisfies all of the constraints manifest in the data. For example, if we performed an experiment in which we tossed two coins simultaneously for many trials, we would assume that the results for each coin toss are marginally independent unless we had information to the contrary.

Example: segmentation

In this section we apply the concepts described in the previous sections to the problem of segmenting a magnetic resonance image of the brain into tissue classes, including lesions. Although the approach described is fairly simple, it illustrates the application of Bayesian and information-theoretic techniques to image processing.

Background

Given a collection of voxels or image data D, which are registered to a common standard A (e.g., an atlas), the goal is to produce the segmentation S that is most probable:

$$\operatorname*{argmax}_{S} P(S|D, A) \qquad \text{(A3.8)}$$

Let S_d be the classification of the dth voxel, and let N_S be the number of classes into which the image is being segmented. For convenience, we will assign each class an integer in $[1, N_S]$, and S_d is assigned a class index.

Our goal can be restated as:

$$\operatorname*{argmax}_{S} P(S|D, A) = \bigcup_{d} \operatorname*{argmax}_{S} P(S_d |d, A) \quad \text{(A3.9)}$$

This formulation allows us to utilize the information derived from registration, such as the atlas structure that corresponds to a particular location. For notational convenience, we will assume that conditioning on registration (i. e., on A) is implied in the remainder of this section.

Each datum, d, represents intensity and spatial vectors for a voxel:

$$P(S_d |d) \equiv P(S_d | I_d, L_d) \qquad \text{(A3.10)}$$

where I_d and L_d are the signal-intensity and spatial-location vectors for the dth voxel, respectively. We can restate the problem as maximization of $P(S_d, I_d, L_d)$:

$$\operatorname*{argmax}_{S} P(S|D) = \bigcup_{d} \operatorname*{argmax}_{S} P(S_d, I_d, L_d) \quad \text{(A3.11)}$$

By choosing classes that are spatially homogeneous in signal intensity on MR examination, even if they are not homogeneous microscopically, we can apply the notion of conditional independence to assert that each voxel's intensity and location are conditionally independent of each other, given their classification:

$$P(I_d, L_d | S_d) = P(I_d | S_d)P(L_d | S_d)$$

or equivalently:

$$P(I_d, L_d, S_d) = P(I_d | S_d)P(L_d | S_d)P(S_d) \qquad \text{(A3.13)}$$

In other words, by choosing classes that appear homogeneous in signal intensity, we ensure that if we know a voxel's classification (e.g., thalamus), knowing its intensity tells us nothing more about where the voxel is located, since the class is homogeneous in signal intensity. Similarly, knowing a voxel's location within a homogeneous structure tells us nothing more about its signal intensity than knowing that the voxel is *somewhere* within this structure. Clearly this assumption would not apply to a class such as *gyrus*, in which there is a heterogeneous distribution of signal intensities (gray matter surrounding white matter). This requirement is not restrictive, however, in that we can decompose structures of interest into relatively homogeneous substructures, such as cortex and subcortical white matter.

Combining Equations A3.11 and A3.13, our goal is to find:

$$P(I_d, L_d, S_d) = P(I_d|S_d)P(L_d|S_d)P(S_d) \qquad \text{(A3.14)}$$

We obtain $P(I_d|S_d)$, $P(L_d|S_d)$, and $P(S_d)$ empirically, from a training set. $P(I_d|S_d)$ could be modeled as a Gaussian distribution, or, if the distribution of voxel signal intensities for certain structures do not assume a Gaussian distribution, we could model $P(I_d|S_d)$ as a discrete distribution by using an integer-based $[0, 255]$ range. To compute the spatial distribution $P(L_d|S_d)$, for each image in the training set, we label all of the structures of interest, apply the registration algorithm, and, for each structure, compute the probability that a voxel in that structure will be in location S_d. We compute $P(S_d)$ by manually segmenting training images, and computing prior probabilities from the fractions of voxels that belong to each class.

If we have intensity, spatial, and prior distributions for each structure (class) of interest, we can apply Equation A3.14 to a voxel, and label that voxel as the structure that it is most likely to represent. Applying this algorithm to each voxel, we can obtain the most likely segmentation of the image, given our assumptions.

One way of defining a lesion is "unexpected signal intensity in a given location." The word "unexpected" indicates that entropy might be of use in quantifying this definition. Since the way we choose the most likely segmentation for each voxel involves computing a probability distribution, we can compute the entropy of that distribution. A voxel associated with high entropy is more likely to be within a lesion, since its signal intensity will be atypical for its spatial location. Conversely, a voxel that is classified with high probability will be associated with low entropy, and is relatively unlikely to represent a lesion.

In evaluating the certainty with which we have classified a new voxel V that was not in the training set, we must take into account how certain we are of

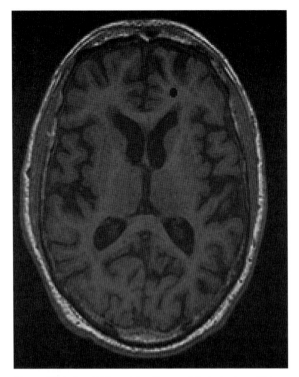

Figure A3.1. An axial T_1-weighted image of the brain, into which we placed a 22-voxel size lesion with CSF signal intensity, in left-frontal white matter.

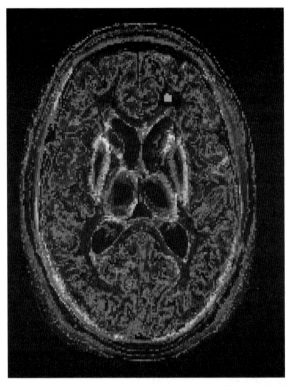

Figure A3.2. Entropy map after application of a simplified version of the segmentation algorithm.

classifying voxels in this location, overall. We therefore compare the entropy of V's posterior distribution to the average entropy value for that voxel location across all training images. We can compute the voxel-wise entropy values for each training image by classifying that image based on statistics from the remainder of the training set. For example, if a particular voxel were classified with high entropy (i.e., high uncertainty) in a region where voxels are usually classified with low entropy (i.e., high certainty), then this voxel probably represents a lesion rather than the normal (i.e., expected) tissue type at this site. Let us call the image of voxel-wise entropy difference an entropy-differential map (EDM). From this map, we can use Jaynes' entropy concentration theorem [16] to compute the probability of observing the entropy value for a voxel in the image to be segmented, given the corresponding values in the training set. Asymptotically in N, $2N\Delta H = \chi_k^2(1 - F)$, where N is the number of images in the training set, ΔH is the difference in entropy for a voxel between the image to be segmented and the average of the training set, N_S is the number of classes or structures, $k = (N_S - 1)$ is the degrees of freedom, and F is the p-value (e.g., 0.05). This formula yields the probability of observing the

entropy for a voxel, given the entropy values we have observed for the training set. This transformation yields a voxel-wise probability map of (ab)normality.

Application

To demonstrate how this algorithm might work, we applied it to $N = 13$ axial T_1-weighted gradient-echo MR images of the brain. Figure A3.1 shows the test image, which we used to illustrate use of this algorithm. We chose $N_S = 9$ classes: background, CSF, white matter, cortex, caudate, thalamus, putamen, skin, skull. Several of these classes, such as cortex, caudate, putamen, and thalamus, are not distinguishable by signal intensity alone. Each image was manually segmented, and underwent linear scaling and translation to maximize overlap of non-background voxels. One training image was arbitrarily chosen as the spatial standard. We obtained probability distributions for the signal intensity and spatial location of voxels in each structure over all subjects. We also computed entropy maps for each voxel in the training set, as described above. We then applied the same linear-registration algorithm to the test image, classified each voxel, and computed an entropy map

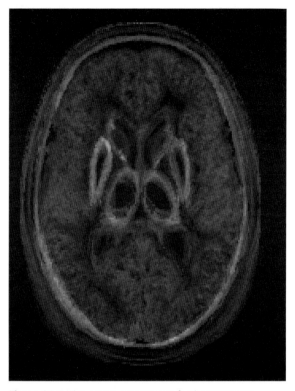

Figure A3.3. The average entropy map for the training set.

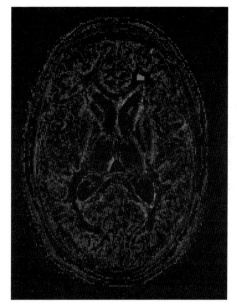

Figure A3.4. Subtraction of Figure A3.3 from Figure A3.2

for each voxel. To simulate a lesion, we placed a small CSF-signal intensity lesion in the white matter of the test image. The entropy map for the test image is shown in Figure A3.2; note that the shape and size of the head are slightly different, reflecting application of our very simple registration process.

Figure A3.3 is the average entropy map for the training images; as expected, uncertainty of classification is high at the boundaries of structures, and in regions of high spatial variability, such as gyri. Subtracting the average training entropy from segmentation entropy yields Figure A3.4. Although there is still high entropy along edges, the lesion demonstrates very high entropy relative to that expected for its location. Using Jaynes' concentration theorem, we find that the probability of having such high entropy for one of the lesion's voxels, given the entropy of the corresponding training-set voxels (all have approximately the same values) is approximately 10^{-6}.

References

1. Jaynes ET. *Probability Theory: the Logic of Science*, ed. GL Brethorst. Cambridge: Cambridge University Press, 2003.
2. Ross SM. *A First Course in Probability*, 2nd edn. New York, NY: Macmillan, 1984.
3. Bayarri MJ, Berger JO. The interplay of Bayesian and frequentist analysis. *Statist Sci* 2004; **19**: 58–80.
4. Efron B. Why isn't everyone a Bayesian? *Am Statistician* 1986; **40**: 1–5.
5. Good IJ. Kinds of probability. *Science* 1959; **129**: 443–7.
6. Jevning R, Anand R, Biedebach M. Certainty and uncertainty in science: the subjectivistic concept of probability in physiology and medicine. *Adv Physiol Educ* 1994; **267**: S113–19.
7. Poole C. Feelings and frequencies: two kinds of probability in public health research. *Am J Public Health* 1988; **78**: 1531–3.
8. Cox RT. Probability, frequency, and reasonable expectation. *Am J Phys*, 1946; **14**: 1–13.
9. Halpern JY. A counterexample to theorems of Cox and Fine. *J Artif Intell Res* 1999; **10**: 67–85.
10. Bayes T. An essay toward solving a problem in the doctrine of chances. *Philos Trans R Soc Lond*, 1763; **53**: 370–418.
11. Berger JO. *Statistical Decision Theory and Bayesian Analysis*. New York, NY: Springer-Verlag, 1985.
12. MacKay DJC. *Information Theory, Inference, and Learning Algorithms*. Cambridge: Cambridge University Press, 2003.
13. Shannon CE. A mathematical theory of communication. *Bell Syst Tech J*, 1948; **27**: 379–423.
14. Rissanen J. Hypothesis selection and testing by the MDL principle. *Comput J*, 1999; **42**: 260–9.
15. Jenkinson M, Smith SM. A global optimisation method for robust affine registration of brain images. *Med Image Anal*, 2001; **5**: 143–56.
16. Jaynes ET. On the rationale of maximum-entropy methods. *Proc IEEE* 1982; **70**: 939–52.

Index

Page numbers in *italics* refer to figures and tables

abdomen
    pre-/post-contrast CT *252*
    spatial heterogeneity *3*
acoustic impedance, ultrasound 149
active shape/appearance
        model-based delineation
        methods 220–223
Aequorea victoria 172, *173*
aequorin 172, *173*
aging, brain structural changes
        266–270, *268*
Akt kinase activity *179*
Akt protein 179
Allen Brain Atlas 238, *239*
aminocyclopentanecarboxylic acid
        (ACPC), carbon-11 labeling *204*
analog to digital (A/D) converter
        40, *40*
analysis of variance (ANOVA) 212
anaphylaxis, iodine-induced 184–185
anatomic correspondence *235*
anatomic localization *232*
anatomy, detailed from merged
        information *231*
Anger gamma camera/scanner 72–73,
        73, 123–124, *124*, 127
    single photon imaging *123*
angiogenesis 270
annexin V 180
ApoB100 *280*
apoptosis, optical imaging 180–181
area under the curve (AUC)
        102–104
arterial input function (AIF) 270, 271
arterial spin-labeled perfusion
        271–272
artificial intelligence 106
aspartate 285
astronomy 7–8, 36–37, 82
atlas building 230
    brain 231–232
        image registration 232–236
        diffusion tensor imaging *233*
        statistical atlases 240–249
atlas warping *232*
atoms 60–62, 117
    Bohr model *61*
    energy levels 122

attenuation 120–121
    Beer–Lambert law 148–149
    coefficients *184*
    CT 253
    PET 121, *121*
    SPECT 121, *121*
    ultrasound 148–149
    x-rays 136–137, 183, 253
Audubon, John James 2–3, *4*
automated computer feature
        extraction *109*
avalanche photodiodes 122–123

barium
    double contrast *184*
    x-ray contrast 183–185
Bayes' rule 310
    segmentation 312–315
Bayesian observers 88
Beer–Lambert law of attenuation
        148–149
beetles, spatial variation *17*
beta decay 117
bias 86
binding problem 95–96
binocular vision *94*
bioluminescence 172, *173*
bioluminescence imaging (BLI)
        172–173
    sensitivity 277–279
    tumor growth monitoring 174–175
Bloch equation *161*
block detector 124
blood flow
    arterial spin-labeled perfusion
        271–272
    assessment 270–271
    blood oxygen level determination
        272–273
blood oxygen level dependence (BOLD)
        272–273
blood–brain barrier
    contrast agents 185
    radiopharmaceuticals crossing 197
Bohr atomic model *61*
bone scan, ^{99m}Tc-MDP *199*
boundary-based methods of
        delineation 219–220

box-car filter 296, 297, 301
brain
    blood oxygen level dependence
        272–273
    evolutionary changes *238*
    function imaging *28*
    imaging *95*
    iodine contrast *186*
    MRI *11*
    structural changes with aging
        266–270, *268*
brain atlas construction 231–232
    anatomic variability 232
    average morphology 231–232
    challenges 231–232
    image registration 232–236
    volume registering 232
brain hemorrhage, MRI *260*
brain mapping 230–231
    Cartesian coordinate system 231
    MRI 230
    new technology 236–239
    RAVENS map 267–268, *268*
brain tumor growth *36*
breast, infrared thermography *56*
breast tumor
    contrast-enhanced MRI *263*
    see also mammography
bremsstrahlung 133–134
bright field microscopy *64*
brightness 263–264
Broad Street pump (cholera epidemic,
        London) *34*

cancer
    angiogenesis targeting 270
    apoptosis imaging 180–181
    hyperspectral imaging 175
    molecular beacon imaging
        179–180
    multispectral imaging 175
    optical imaging in research
        174–181
    post-translational modification
        monitoring 178–179
    protein–protein interaction
        monitoring 178–179
    stem cell imaging 175, *177*

transcriptional activity measurement 175–178
see also metastases; non-Hodgkin's lymphoma; thyroid cancer; tumor(s)
carbon-11 203, *204*
carbon-13 *289*
cardiac motion tracking *238*, 268–270
carfentanil *205*
carotid artery, Doppler ultrasonography *155*
Cartesian coordinate system 90–91, 111, *261*
  brain mapping 231
  morphological analysis 260
Cartesian geography *34*
Cartesian images *80*
cartography 5–6, *6*, 32–36
  measurement 41–42
  morphological analysis 260
certainty measures 311–310
change 252
characteristic radiation 134
charge capture device (CCD) camera 39–40
Chi-square statistic, classification tasks 102
cholera epidemic, London *34*
cholesterol esters 280
choline, carbon-11 labeling *204*
CHOP therapy 285
  tumor response to treatment *286*, *287*, *288*
classification tasks 100–104, *102*
coelenterazine 172
  bioluminescence imaging 172–173
cognition, visual search 96–98
Collider Detector (Fermilab) 39
collimators *128*
color detection *91*
color vision 89–90
communication
  biomedical system *85*
  imaging 82–83
  spatial information 114
  theoretical system *84*
Compton scattering 63, 120, *120*, *139*, 145
  x-rays 136–138
computed radiography (CR) systems 141–142, *142*
computed tomography (CT) 4, 143, 144–146, 185
  2D images *72*
  3D images 79–81
  acquisition *146*

brain evolutionary changes *238*
brain scan 37
  contrast agents 185
  data projection *5*
  direct/indirect image formation 77
  filtered back-projection 145
  heart *24*
  high-resolution *49*, *254*
  image reconstruction *146*
  images 145–146
  linear attenuation coefficient 253
  mouse skull/mandible 255–256
  multiple angular projections *80*
  phantom *92*
  pre-/post-contrast of abdomen *252*
  scanner for PET 121
  spatial information 79–81
  spatial resolution 254–255
  tumor progression *266*
computed tomography (CT) scanners 5, 143, *144*
computer-aided visualization and analysis (CAVA) 98–101, 215
computerized displays, image data manipulation 98–101
computers, observers 106–109
conduction band 122
constellations 82
  non-scientific imaging *83*
continuous systems 49
continuous/continuous systems 49
contrast agents
  blood–brain barrier 185
  CT 185
  kidney *185*
  MRA *188*
  MRI 185–194
  radiographic 183–185
  radiographic density *184*
  ultrasound 156–157, *156*, *157*, *158*
contrast-to-noise ratio (CNR) 87–88
  MRI 168
  x-rays 138–140
convolution, linear systems 296–297, 301
copper radionuclides, PET 204–206
correspondence mapping *237*
Crook's tubes 53
cumulative distribution function (CDF) 309

darkness 263–264
Darwin's finches *26*
decision making
  outcomes *210*, *211*
  terminology 211, *211*
delineation of images 218, 219

active shape/appearance model-based methods 220–223
  fuzzy region-based automatic 221–222
  fuzzy region-based human-assisted 223
  hard region-based automatic 221
  hard region-based human-assisted 222–223
  hybrid strategies 223
  approaches 219–223
  boundary-based methods 219–220
  fuzzy automatic 220
  hard human-assisted 220
  primary 219
delta function *50*, 297–298
depth
  fixed position monocular clues *94*
  perception *94*
dermatologic disease *8*
  image *8*
detectability index 213
detectors, signal 66–81
  arrangement 69
  field-of-view 69–73
  frequency modulation 73–76
  movement 72
  multiple 72–73
  non-projection spatial signal modulation 73–76
  performance 66–67
  sample size 70–73
  signal sampling 68–69
  signal source 67
  signal-to-noise ratio 67
  spatial resolution 70, 72
  x-rays 78
diagnostic imaging agents 196
diffusion equation 294–295
  image analysis 300–301
  one-dimensional 292–293
diffusion tensor images
  atlas building *233*
  manifolds 244
  scalar maps 241–242
digital images
  analysis 11
  data characteristics 214–215
  mammography *263*
  processing 214–229
digital radiography (DR) detectors 142–143, *142*
digital signals *40*, 293
digital subtraction angiography (DSA) *189*
Dirac delta function *50*, 297–298

discrete Fourier transform (DFT) 302,
304–305
inverse 306–307
sampling scheme *305*
discrete systems 49
discrete-time systems 300
discrimination measurement 210–213
ideal observer 213
receiver operating characteristic
211–213
terminology 211, *211*
discrimination tasks *210*
disease 251
prevalence *105*
disorder 84–85
distortion 86
distribution
entropy 311
mean 309
DNA
free radical damage 140–141
sample contamination *39*
Doppler shift 152–153
Doppler signal detection 154
Doppler ultrasonography 152–154,
154, 158
carotid artery *155*
d-prime 213
dsRed protein 173–174

echo planar imaging (EPI) 165–166
edge detectors *261*, 300–301
edge enhancement 98
visual processing *97*
eigenfunctions 298–299
electromagnetic energy 14–16
human visual system detection 30
waves 14
electromagnetic field, energy density/
flow 52–54
electromagnetic force 117
electromagnetic radiation *15*, 52–53,
117, *134*
MRI 59
NMR spectroscopy 68
signals 52
x-rays 133
electrons 60–62, 117
K-shell 134
L-shell 134
x-ray production 133–134
electro-stimulation 58
energy (E) 1–2, 8, 13, *14*, 17
external source 54–57
heating 58–59
ionizing radiation 59–62
imaging process 38

incident 65
ionizing radiation 59–62
measurement 38–42, *39*, 47, 49–51
metabolism pathways *284*
movement 52–57
potential 13–14
propagation 52–57
requirement for imaging 62
scientific image 22–25
sources *16*
spatial distribution 18–19
thermal 58–59
see also electromagnetic energy
enhancing filters 217
entropy 84–85, *86*, 311, *311*
conditional 311
edge detectors *261*
map *314*, *315*
voxels 313–315
error
elimination 42
image quality 50–51
measurement 42–45, 48, 49
estimation tasks 105–106
Euclidean geometry 33, 46–47
multidimensional measurements *47*
Euclidean space 46–47
eye
multimodality images *9*
see also retina; visual system

facial recognition *100*
false discovery rate (FDR)
comparisons 245
false positive fraction (FPF) 211, *213*
receiver operating characteristic 102
fast Fourier transform (FFT) 305–307
algorithm 302, *306*
inverse 306–307
see also discrete Fourier
transform (DFT)
ferromagnetic materials *191*
Ferumoxytol 192
fetal imaging *10*
ultrasound *25*
[18]F-fluorodeoxyglucose (FDG) 117,
119–120, 202
see also fluorodeoxyglucose PET
(FDG-PET)
field of view (FOV) *70*
detectors 69–73
MRI 163
SPECT scanners 128
filtered back-projection 145
firefly luciferase 172–173
transcriptional activity
measurement 176–178

Fischer discriminant analysis, kernel-
based (kFDA) 245
fluorescence energy transfer (FRET) 275
fluorescence imaging 173–174, *282*, *283*
schematic *174*
tumor growth monitoring 174–175
wavelength 67
fluorine-18 *118*, 202–203
DOPA labeling *203*
fluorodeoxyglucose PET (FDG-PET)
117, 119–120, 202–203, *203*
gastrointestinal tumor *204*
folate receptors 280–281
force 13–14
Fourier inversion formula 302
Fourier rebinning 127
Fourier transform 14, 126–127, *303*
continuous 302, 304, 305
discrete 302, 304–305
multiple dimensions 303–304
one dimension 302–303
rectangular function 302
wave properties *15*
see also discrete Fourier transform
(DFT); fast Fourier transform
(FFT)
Fourier zeugmatography 162–163
Fraunhofer zone 151
free induction decay (FID) 161, *161*
frequency
modulation 73–76
wave properties *15*
Fresnel zone 151
full width at half maximum
(FWHM) *51*
functional neuroimaging
brain mapping 230
MRI *110*
fuzzy boundary-based automatic
delineation methods 220
fuzzy region-based automatic
delineation methods 221–222
fuzzy region-based human-assisted
delineation methods 223

gadolinium
interaction with water molecules *187*
MRI contrast 186–189, *186*, *188*, *281*
MRI signal intensity 270–271
gadolinium-DTPA 186–189, *186*
adverse effects 189
Galileo 36–37, 82
moons of Jupiter *35*, 36, *84*
notebook *7*
gallium-67 199–200, *201*
gallium-68 199–200
gallstones, ultrasound *57*, *150*

gamma camera/scanner
  Anger 72–73, *73*, 123–124, *123, 124*, 127
  rectilinear 70–73, *71*
  thyroid cancer *57*
gamma radiation 117
Gaussian distribution *44*
  function 44–45, 313
Gaussian filter 297
Gaussian random variable 42
Gaussian smoothing 301
Gd-DTPA *see* gadolinium-DTPA
general kinetic model 270–271
geometric descriptors *257*
glutamate 285
  labeling *289*
glutaminolysis 289, 290
glycerophosphate shuttle 285–289
glycolysis 285–289, 290
gradient echo pulse sequences 165
gravity 13–14
green fluorescent protein (GFP) 172, *173, 174*
  fluorescence imaging 173–174
grids, radiographic 143
group average forming 245–246
Gulf Stream, seawater flow *20*

half-life 196–197
hard boundary-based human-assisted delineation methods 220
heart
  cardiac motion tracking 269
  CT *24*
  SPAMM *269*
heart beats 269
heart rate 269
HER-2 receptors 192–194, *194*
high-density lipoprotein (HDL) 281
high-dimensional data, statistical distribution 244–245
high-dimensional pattern classification 246–249
  dimensionality 248
  receiver operating curve 248–249
  spatial resolution 248
high-energy particle accelerator 39
holography 93
Hotelling's T-square statistic 245
Hounsfield units 37, 145–146
human observers 88–96, 207–213
hyperspectral imaging 175, *177*
hypothesis testing 11
  estimation tasks 105–106

image(s) 2–3, 22
  color 89–90

contrast *61*
decomposition 95–96
definition 13
hard copy 93
information
  content 63
  spatial representation 91–93
intensity 301
interpretation 8–10
media *32*
perception 31–32
presentation 93
processing algorithms 214
reconstruction process *126*
rectangular object *267*
remote *27*
scale *28*
similarity *235*
  measurement 234
soft copy 93
spatial components 90–91
two-dimensional *48*
volume registration 236–237
see also delineation of images; pre-processing of images; registration of images; scientific images
image analysis 8–10, 215–216, 228–229
  diffusion equation 300–301
  human 99
image data
  manipulation 98–100, *101*
  segmentation 313–314
image formation *71*
  direct/indirect 77–81
  nuclear medicine 125–126
  PET 125–126
  reconstruction algorithms 125–126
image operations
  analysis 215–216, 228–229
  classification 215
  manipulation 215–216, 228
  pre-processing 215–223
  visualization 215–216, 223–228
image operator performance metrics *51*
image quality 50–51, 100, 207
  expert opinion 209
  physical measurement 207–209
  spatial resolution 209
  subjective measures 209
  visibility measures 209
image-based surface rendering 225–226
image-based volume rendering 226
imaging 1
  2D projection 79–81
  communication 82–83

devices 8, *9*
energy requirement 62
forward problems 77
human involvement 10
inverse problems 77
measurements 47–48
process 38
response to therapy *180*
sample effect on signal 62–81
imaging system
  components 207
  discrimination measurement 210–213
  fundamental properties 207
  large-scale transfer characteristic 207–208
  model 49–51
  modulation transfer function 126–127, 208, 209
  real 51–62
  spatial resolution properties 208
  task-dependent performance 209–210
  see also noise; signal-to-noise ratio
impulse function 297–298
impulse response 297–298, 300
indium-111 198–199
  radiolabeled antibody *200*
individual patient analysis 246–249
information 83–85
  density 96
  merged *231*
  minimization of mutual 312
  spatial
    communication 114
    representation 91–93
  transfer 82–83
information theory 310–312
  concepts 310
  evidence evaluation 312
  quantification of information 311–312
  segmentation 312–315
infrared signals 54–57
infrared thermography, breast *56*
input–output transfer characteristic curve *208*
instrumentation 8
inverse discrete Fourier transform (IDFT) 306–307
inverse fast Fourier transform (IFFT) 306–307
inverse Radon transform *80*
iodinated compounds 201–206, *202*
iodine
  adverse effects 184–185
  SPECT contrast 200–206
  x-ray contrast 183–185, *185, 186*

iodine-123 54, 200–201, *201*
iodine-124 204, *205*
iodine-125 200
iodine-131 200–201
ionization detectors *67–68*
ionizing radiation 59–62
iron oxide contrast 189–194, *191, 192*
isosurfacing 219
isotopes
   nuclear medicine *119, 120*
   production for SPECT 119
iterative expansion technique 127

kernel-based Fischer discriminant
     analysis (kFDA) 245
kernel-based principal component
     analysis (kPCA) 245
kidney
   contrast agents *185*
   spatial heterogeneity *3*
   ultrasound *157–158*
kinetic energy 14
Kronecker delta function 300
k-space *77*, 161–165, *163*, 302–303, *304*
   coordinates *163*
   high-frequency *304*
   image reconstruction *164*
   low-frequency *304*

labeling grid, cardiac motion tracking
     269–270
Laplace transform 299–300
large-scale transfer characteristic 207–208
Larmor frequency 75, 160, *161*
   rotating frame of reference
     189–190, *190*
lateral geniculate nuclei (LGN) 95
Leeuwenhoek's microscope *27*
light
   microscopy signal 62–63
   properties 133
   signal 53–54
   visible *40*
linear attenuation coefficient 63, 253
linear shift-invariant systems 49–50,
     292, *293*, 295–296
   convolution 297
   eigenfunctions 299
linear superposition of filtered
     back-projection (LSFB) 126
linear systems 292–300
   convolution 296–297, 301
   discrete-time 300
   impulse function/response 297–298
   scaling 294, 295
   signals 293
   superimposition property 295

linearity 293–295
lines of response (LORs) 121
   oblique 125
   PET 129–131
lipoproteins, molecular imaging
     279–281
live-wire method *220, 221*
logarithms 311
low-density lipoprotein (LDL) 279–281
   structure *280*
low-density lipoprotein receptor
     (LDLR) 279–281
luciferase 172
   bioluminescence imaging 172–173
   p53-inducible reporter 176–178
   split molecule 277
D-luciferin 173
lungs
   anatomical variation 237–238
   display cutoffs of metastases *267*
   metastases *131, 267*
   motion *238*

machine learning 106
Macroscopic Prism and Reflectance
     Imaging Spectroscopy System
     (MACRO-PARISS) 175, *177*
magnetic resonance angiography
     (MRA) *108*, 188–189, *189*
   contrast-enhanced *188, 189*
   maximum intensity projection *224*
   pseudo-color display *225*
magnetic resonance imaging (MRI)
     160–171
   arterial spin-labeled perfusion *272*
   blood flow assessment 270–271
   blood oxygen level-dependent
     (BOLD) 272–273
   brain hemorrhage *260*
   brain mapping 230
   brain scan *11*
   cardiac motion tracking 268–270
   cerebrospinal fluid *222*
   contrast agents 185–194
     particle size 192–194
   contrast-enhanced 166–168, *263*
     dynamic 270–271, *271*
   contrast-to-noise ratio 168
   data sampling/reconstruction
     162–165
   decomposition of data
     acquisition *305*
   dephasing 189–190
   diffuse hyperintensities *259*
   diffusion tensor images 232
     manifolds 244
     scalar maps 241–242

dynamic contrast-enhanced
     270–271, *271*
echo planar imaging 165–166, *165, 166*
external magnetic field 74–75
field of view 163
frequency modulation 73–76
functional *110*
gadolinium contrast 186–189, *186,*
     188, 281
   signal intensity 270–271
gradient echo pulse sequences 165
gradient subsystem 168–169
hardware 168–169
image contrast *167*
image resolution 166–168
iron oxide contrast 189–194
k-space *77*, 161–165, *163*
   co-ordinates *163*
   image reconstruction *164*
live-wire method *220, 221*
longitudinal *268*
magnet 168–169
magnetic field strength 169–170
magnetization 160, *161*
molecular imaging 279
noise 169–170
Nyquist criterion 163
orbit *169*
phase angle 189–190
proton density-weighted *218*
protons 185–186
pulse sequence 188–189
radiofrequency pulse 166–167,
     185–186
radiofrequency transmit/receive
     assembly 168–169
relaxation 74–76, 187–188
rotating frame of reference 189–190
scan acquisition speed 165–166
segmentation 314–315
sensitivity 277–279
signal 160–161, 253
   characteristics 46
   intensity 247
   specificity for brain hematoma *262*
signal-to-noise ratio 167–168,
     169–170
spatial encoding 161–165
spatial frequency 162–163
spin echo sequence 89, 166–167, *170*
spin warp pulse sequence *163*
thermal energy 59
time (T_1 and T_2) constants 186,
     187–188, 190–192
tissue resistance 169–170
T-weighted images 166–167, *167*
T_1-weighted images 89, *168, 281, 314*

ventilation–perfusion ratio
mapping *237*
voxels 167–168
whole body scan *76*
magnetic resonance spectroscopy
(MRS) 279, *284*
clinical outcomes *114*
phospholipid metabolite detection
282–290
magnetite 190, *192*, *193*
magnetization 160, 161, *162*
ferromagnetic materials *191*
longitudinal *161*
magnocellular system 95, *99*
malate–aspartate shuttle 285–289
mammography 83
communication system *85*
digital images *263*
high-resolution digital monitors *96*
manifolds 243–244
statistical analysis 244, 246
manipulation of images 215–216, 228
mapping 41–42
correspondence *237*
maps *6*
thematic 35–36
margins, morphological analysis
260, *260*
marker genes 277
Mars, telescopic images *55*
mass (m) 1–2, 8, 13, *14*, 17
force 13–14
imaging process 38
measurement 38–42, 47, 49–51
scientific image 22–25
spatial distribution 18–19
mass spectrometry 58, *58*
maximum intensity projection (MIP)
98–101, 106–107, 225
magnetic resonance angiography *224*
maximum-entropy evaluation of
experimental evidence 312
m,E dimension 47–48
see also energy (E); mass (m)
m,E signal *52*
directionality 63–65
measurement 51–52
propagation 63–65
mean of distribution 309
measurement *41*
confounding signals 49
energy (E) 38–42, *39*, 47, 49–51
error 42–45, 48, 49
imaging 47–48
location 47
mapping 41–42
mass (m) 38–42, 47, 49–51

m,E dimension 47–48
m,E signal 51–52
multidimensional 45–47
noise 49
numerical 41
principles 38–42
spatial definition 48
spatial localization 52
time 47
types 41
variability 42–45, 48
variables 45–46
mechanical index (MI) 154–155
memory, visual search 96–98
metastases
lung *131*, 267
optical imaging 174–175
microbubbles, ultrasound contrast
156–157, *156*
microscopy *27*
bright field *64*
light signal 62–63
phase contrast *64*
minimization of mutual information 312
minimum description length
interference 312
modulation transfer function (MTF)
126–127, 208, 209
molecular beacon imaging 179–180, *180*
split luciferase molecule 277
molecular imaging 252–254, 275–290
coordinates *278*
lipoproteins 279–281
microbubbles *156*
MRI 279
nanoparticles 275, 279–281
prediction and early detection of
therapeutic response 282–290
signals 277–279
targets 275, *276*
tissues 279
Montreal Neurological Atlas 111
moons of Jupiter 35, *84*
morphological analysis 255–264
brightness 263–264
darkness 263–264
descriptors 256–257
margins 260, *260*
pattern matching 255
position 260
shape 259–261, *259*
signals 261–264
texture 264
volumetric 259
morphological imaging 251–264
spatial dimensions *254*
spatial resolution 254–255

morphological variability 111–112
morphology 251
average of brain 231–232
morphometric analysis *114*
morphometry, voxel-based *268*
mouse skull/mandible, CT *255–256*
multidimensional displays *92*
multimodality *46*
statistical analysis of data 243–245
multiparametric data, statistical
analysis 243–245
multi-reader multi-case (MRMC)
program 212
multispectral imaging, tumor
vasculature 175, *176*

nanoparticles 275, 279
lipoproteins 279–281
Napoleon's Russian Campaign,
Minard's graphic 91, *93*
nature *see* universe
near-infrared fluorophores 275
near-infrared imaging sensitivity
277–279
negative predictive values
(NPVs) 104
neuroreceptors/neurotransmitters,
PET 278–279
neutrons 60–61, 117
nitrogen-13 203–204
noise 49, 85–88, 208
images 87
signals 87
suppression 98
task performance 100
visualization *87*
see also contrast-to-noise ratio;
signal-to-noise ratio
non-Gaussian distribution *45*
non-Hodgkin's lymphoma
MRS *284*
treatment 284–285, *284*
non-projection spatial signal
modulation 73–76
nuclear factor-κB (NFκB) 178
nuclear force 117
nuclear imaging
biomedical 54–57
signal source 117–120
nuclear magnetic resonance
(NMR) *76*
k-space 161–162
signal 160
nuclear magnetic resonance (NMR)
spectroscopy
carbon-13 spectra *289*
irradiating RF signal 67–68

nuclear medicine *118*, 131
    attenuation 120–121
    Compton scattering 120, *120*
    gamma production by isotopes *120*
    image formation 125–126
    isotopes *119*
        gamma production *120*
    iterative expansion technique 127
    photoelectric effect 120, *120*
    physics 117
    scanner design 127–131
    series expansion technique 127
    signal detection 121–125
    signal/sample interaction 120
    transform algorithms 126–127
nuclear molecular labeling 196–206
    principles 196–197
nucleus 117
    decay 117–119
    forces 117
nuclides 61
Nyquist criterion 163, 252, 254
    discrete Fourier transform 305
Nyquist sampling theorem *29*
Nyquist spacing 304–305

object classification 98–100, *101*
    fuzzy connectedness *103*
    human observer feature
        extraction *106*
    ROC analysis *103*
    voxel thresholding *108*
object contrast 262–263
object edges *267*
object signal 262–263
object-based surface rendering 227, *227*
object-based volume rendering 227, *227*
observers 29–32, 88
    characteristics 88
    classification tasks 100–104
    computers 106–109
    human 88–96, 207–213
    ideal 213
    image presentation 93
    multidimensional data 91–93
    pattern extraction 100
    perception 88–90
    spatial components of images
        90–91
    task performance 100
    visual system 29–30, 88–90
optic chiasm 95
optical imaging 172–181
    bioluminescence imaging 172–173
    cancer research 174–181
    fluorescence imaging 173–174
    tumor growth monitoring 174–175

orbit, MRI *169*
order 84
ordered subset expectation
    maximization (OSEM)
    algorithm 127
oxidative metabolism 289
oxygen
    blood oxygen level determination
    272–273
    consumption rate measurement *290*
oxygen-15 204

p53-induced optical reporter
    176–178, *178*
pair production 63, 120
parallax 92–93
parallel image processing *98*
    human *99*
parallel imaging *73*
Parkinson's disease, fluorine-18 DOPA
    scan *203*
partial volume effect 71
parvocellular system 95, *99*
pattern analysis and recognition system
    246–248
pattern building *256*
pattern classification, high-dimensional
    246–249
    dimensionality 248
    receiver operating curve 248–249
    spatial resolution 248
pattern extraction 100
pattern learning *101*
    visual search 96–98
pattern matching *256*
    computerized 109
    facial recognition *100*
    morphological analysis 255
    radiology *101*
perception
    human 88–90
    images 31–32
phase contrast microscopy *64*
phosphatidylserine 180
phospholipid metabolites, MRS
    detection 282–290
photoacoustic imaging *68*
photocathode, quantum
    efficiency 122
photodynamic therapy 275–277
photoelectric absorption (PEA) *184*
photoelectric effect 63, 120, *139*, *145*
    absorption *120*
    x-rays 136–137
photomultiplier tubes 122–123
    Anger detector 123
    collimated 72–73

photons 14, 16
    emission from green fluorescent
        protein 173–174
    radionuclide decay *65*
    x-rays *184*
photopic vision 89–90, *89*
photoreceptors 30
photostimulable phosphor (PSP)
    plate 142
physiological imaging 251–252,
    265–274
    arterial spin-labeled perfusion
        271–272
    blood flow assessment 270–271
    blood oxygen level determination
        272–273
    brain structural changes with aging
        266–270
    cardiac motion tracking 268–270
    change detection in special
        dimensions over long time scale
        265–268
    dynamic contrast-enhanced MRI
        270–271
    tumor response assessment 265–266
piezoelectric crystals 57
    ultrasound 147, 149–150
pixels, artistic *25*
point response function (PRF) 50–51, *51*
point spread function (PSF) *51*,
    126–127
position analysis 260
positive predictive values (PPVs) 104
positron emission tomography
    (PET) 117
    attenuation 121, *121*
    camera *124*
    carbon-11 203
    carbon-11 labeled thymidine *205*
    clinical outcomes *114*
    coincidence measurement *129*
    copper radionuclides 204–206
    CT scanner 121
    data corrections *129*
    fluorine-18 202–203
    fluorodeoxyglucose 117, 119–120,
        202–203, *203*
        gastrointestinal tumor *204*
    image formation 125–126
    iodine-124 204, *205*
    isotope production 119
    lines of response 129–131
    lung metastases *131*
    neuroreceptors 278–279
    neurotransmitters 278–279
    nitrogen-13 203–204
    oxygen-15 204

radiolabeled tracers *119*, 197,
     202–206, *202*
radiometals 204–206
     rubidium chloride 206
     scanners 128–129, *129*
          time-of-flight 129–131, *130*
     scintillation detectors 124, 125, *125*
     sensitivity 277–279
     signal 253
post-translational modification
     monitoring 178–179
potential energy 13–14
predictive values, disease
     prevalence *105*
pre-processing of images *102*, 215–223
     delineation 218, 219
          approaches 219–223
          primary 219
     filtering 216–217
     interpolation 216
          image-based 216
          object-based 216
     recognition 218, 219
          human-assisted 219
     registration 217–218
     segmentation 218–219
principal component analysis,
     kernel-based (kPCA) 245
probability 43–45
     Bayes' rule 310
     conditional 308
     entropy of distribution 311
     interpretation 309
     uncertainty quantification 311–310
probability density function (PDF) *43*,
     297–298, 309
     parameters *43*
probability distribution 43–44, 46
probability theory 308–310
     concepts 308–309
product rule 308
projection imaging, visible light *75*
promoter activity 175–178
prostate, ultrasound imaging 157–158
protein–protein interaction
     monitoring 178–179
protons 60–61, 117
     magnetic perturbation 187
     MRI 185–186
Ptolemy 33
pulse repetition frequency 153
p-value maps 245

quantum efficiency (QE) 122

radiant energy 14, 16
radiocarbon dating, natural *56*

radiofrequency (RF) field 160–161
     MRI 185–186
radiofrequency (RF) pulse *161*, 166–167
     cardiac motion tracking 269
     signal modulation *75*
radiographic density, attenuation
     coefficients *184*
radiography, x-ray signal detection
     141–143
radioiodine *see* iodine
radiolabeled tracers *119*
     PET 202–206
     SPECT *119*, 197–206, *197*
radiology procedures, effective
     doses *141*
radiometals, PET 204–206
radionuclides
     half-life 196–197
     PET *119*, 197, *202*
     SPECT *119*, 197–206, *197*
radiopharmaceuticals 196
     blood–brain barrier crossing 197
     iodinated 201–206, *202*
     lipophilicity 197
     organic solubility 197
     specific activity 197
     technetium-99m labeled 200
     water solubility 197
RadLex lexicon 256, 259
     margins *260*
     morphological characteristic *257*
     shape *259*
     size modifiers *258*
Radon transform 145
     inverse *80*
randomness 84
RAVENS map *268*
     brain structural change assessment
          267–268
RCHOP therapy 285
     tumor response to treatment *286*,
          287, *288*
receiver operating characteristic (ROC)
     analog systems *105*
     bias *212*
     classification tasks 102–104, *104*
     computer-extracted feature *110*
     detectability *212*
     digital systems *105*
     discrimination measurement
          211–213
     high-dimensional pattern
          classification 248–249
     index of detectability 213
     localized quantitative analysis *107*
     manually extracted features *107*
     methodology 212–213

RECIST criteria 266, *266*
recognition of images 218, 219
     human-assisted 219
reconstruction algorithms, nuclear
     medicine images 125–126
dsRed protein 173–174
reflective imaging *74*
refraction, ultrasound beam 149
region of interest (ROI)
     analysis *113*
     scalar maps 242
registration of images 232–236, *233*
     anatomic labeling *113*
     elastic deformation 235–236
     image similarity measurement 234
     image volume 236–237
     information use 313
     minimization of mutual
          information 312
     multimodality study fusing *236*
     new technology 236–239
     ROI analysis *113*
     smoothness constraint 234
     solution estimation 234–235
     standard template *113*
     volume 236–237
Renilla luciferase 172–173
reproducible kernel Hilbert space
     (RKHS) 245
respiratory motion *238*
     cardiac motion tracking 269
retina 30, 89–90, *89*
     image decomposition 95
Roentgen, Conrad *4*
Rose–Burger phantom 209, *209*,
     210–212
rotating frame of reference (RFR)
     189–190
rubidium chloride 206

scalar maps
     diffusion tensor images
          241–242
     regions of interest 242
     statistical analysis 241–242
     statistical parametric mapping 242
scaling, linear systems 294, 295
scan acquisition speed, MRI
     165–166
scanner design, nuclear medicine
     127–131
scanners
     PET 128–129
          time-of-flight 129–131
     SPECT 127–129
scenes 17–22
     scientific images 25–29

science 1
scientific images 22
  analysis 4, 8–10
  content 22–29
  Darwin's finches *26*
  energy 22–25
  interpretation 8–10
  mass 22–25
  measurement 4
  observers 29–32
  scenes 25–29
  space 25–29
  spatial information 4–6
scintillation detectors 121–122
  performance *125*, 125
  PET 124, 125, *125*
  SPECT 125
scotopic vision 89–90, *89*
seawater flow *20*
segmentation 312–315
  algorithms 98–101, *101*, *314*
  application 314–315
self-preservation, visual tools 93–95
serial projection imaging *71*
series expansion technique 127
shape analysis *217*, 259–261, *259*, *260*, *261*
shape model-based boundary segmentation *221*
shape-based interpolation *217*
Shepp–Logan phantom 304
sifting 298
signal(s) 39–40
  confounding 49
  dependence on imaging modality *262*
  digital 293
  electromagnetic radiation 52
  external 54–57, 65
  image quality 50
  infrared 54–57
  intensity 65, 313–314
  intrinsic 65–66
  light 53–54
  linear systems 293
  magnetic resonance 160–161
  m,E 51–52
  modified 65–66
  molecular imaging 277–279
    sensitivity/specificity 252–253
  morphological analysis 261–264
  movement 63–65
  noise 87
  non-projection spatial modulation 73–76
  nuclear magnetic resonance 160
  object 262–263

propagation 63–65, *64*
  relating to function 265
  sample effect 62–81
  sampling detectors 68–69
  scattered 65
  source 53–54, *53*, 64–65
    detector design 67
    nuclear imaging 117–120
  ultrasound 147–148
    detection 149–151
    source 57, 147–148
    spatial encoding 150–151
  x-rays 133–136
    quantification 138
    source 133–136
signal detection 66–81, *66*, 121–125, *213*
  theory model 210–211, 213
  two-alternative forced choice 210–211
  ultrasound spatial encoding 150–151
  x-rays 141–143
  yes–no decision 210
signal/sample interaction 57–58, *58*, *66*
  nuclear medicine 120
  ultrasound 148–150
  x-rays 136–141
signal-to-noise ratio (SNR) 87, 207, 208–209
  detectors 67
  MRI 167–168, 169–170
  x-rays 138
single photon emission tomography (SPECT) 117
  Anger detector 123–124
  attenuation 121, *121*
  collimator arrangements 128
  field of view 128
  gallium-67/-68 199–200
  indium-111 198–199
  iodine 200–206
  isotope production 119
  principles 197
  radiolabeled tracers *119*, 197–206, *197*
  scanners 127–129
  scintillation detectors 125
  sensitivity 277–279
  technetium-99m 197–206
single photon imaging *123*
  collimators *128*
smoothing 300–301
  Gaussian 301
Snow, John 35–36
sonoelastography 158
space 4–6, 17–22
  scientific images 25–29

spatial analysis 109–112
  quantitative *113*
spatial attractors, human 97
spatial encoding, x-rays 143–144
spatial frequency 162–163
spatial heterogeneity 2, *61*
spatial homogeneity *61*
spatial independence, imaging modality *262*
spatial information
  communication 114
  representation 91–93
spatial labeling 109–112
spatial measurements 8
spatial modulation of magnetization (SPAMM) 269
spatial normalization 111–112
spatial patterns *18*
  non-random 85
spatial representation of information 91–93
spatial resolution
  bar pattern *209*
  CT 254–255
  detectors 70, 72
  full width at half maximum *51*
  image quality 209
  metric *90*
  morphological imaging 254–255
spatial variation *17*
speckle, ultrasound 151
statistical analysis
  high-dimensional data 244–245
  manifolds 244, 246
  multimodal data 243–245
  multiparametric data 243–245
  scalar maps 241–242
statistical atlases 240–249
  group analysis 241
  group average forming 245–246
  high-dimensional pattern classification 246–249
  individual patient analysis 246–249
  multiparametric statistics 241
  statistical analysis scalar maps 241–242
  uses 240
statistical decision theory 210, 211
statistical distribution, high-dimensional data 244–245
statistical parametric mapping (SPM) 107–109, 242
stereopsis 94
superimposition property of linear systems 295
superparamagnetic iron oxide (SPIO) 192–194, *194*

superparamagnetic magnetite 190
support vector machine (SVM)
    analysis 109
suppressing filters 216–217
Système International (SI) units *41*
systems 292–293
    mathematical 292–293
    natural 292
    transfer functions 299–300
    see also imaging system; linear
        systems

Talairach Brain Atlas 111, 231
    morphological analysis 260
Talairach Cartesian coordinate
        system *261*
task performance 100, 112–114
task-dependent performance 209–210
technetium-99m 117, *118*
    bone scan *199*
    chelating agents 198, *199*
    production 198
    radiopharmaceuticals *200*
    SPECT 197–206
technology assessment 112–115
temperature, continuous ratio
        measurement *42*
templates, deformation field *114*
temporal bone, high-resolution CT *254*
tensors 243–244
teratoma, ultrasound *148*
texture, morphological analysis 264
thermal energy 58–59
thermodynamics, laws of 84
thermography 54–57, *59*
thin-film transistor (TFT) array
        142–143
threshold analysis 106–107
thresholding 219
    voxels *108*
thymidine, carbon-11 labeling *205*
thyroid, ultrasound *152*
thyroid cancer
    gamma camera scan *57*
    iodine-123 diagnostic scan *201*
time
    images as function of 265
    long-scale change detection 265–268
    physiological imaging 252
    wave properties *15*
time-gain compensation, ultrasound 151
time-of-flight (TOF) scanners
        129–131, *130*
tissues
    ischemic and voxel classification *112*
    molecular imaging 279
    probabilistic classification *112*

tomography 143
    reconstructions *80*
    x-rays 144–146
    see also computed tomography (CT)
tracers 196
transcriptional activity measurement
        175–178
transfer functions of systems *208*,
        299–300
transferrin receptor 192–194
transform algorithms, nuclear
        medicine 126–127
tricarboxylic acid (TCA) cycle 285, 290
true positive fraction (TPF) 211, *213*
    observer performance *211*
    receiver operating characteristic 102
tumor(s)
    ATP production 289
    metabolic pathways 282–290
tumor assessment
    blood flow measurement 270
    physiological imaging 265–266
    size 265–266
tumor growth
    brain *36*
    monitoring 174–175
        optical imaging 174–175
    RECIST assessment 266, *266*
    WHO assessment 266
tumor response to treatment *286*,
        287, *288*
    assessment by physiological imaging
        265–266
tumor vasculature imaging 175
    multispectral 175, *176*
two-alternative forced choice 210–211

ultra-small paramagnetic iron oxide
        (USPIO) 192, *193*
ultra-small magnetic particles *193*
ultrasound 147–158
    acoustic impedance 149
    acoustic power 151, 154
    applications 157–*157*
    attenuation 148–149
    bicornuate uterus *153*
    biological effects 154–156
    cardiac motion tracking 268–270
    cavitation 154–155
    contrast agents 156–157, *156*,
        157, 158
    curvilinear array 149–150
    Doppler 152–154, *154*, 158
        carotid artery *155*
    dynamic range 151–152
    echo amplitude 149–150, *150*
    energy reflection 149

energy transmission 149
far field 151
fetal *25*
future developments 157–158
gallstones *57*, *150*
generation *148*
gray-scale images *31*, *90*, 150
high-frequency *157–158*
high-frequency, high-resolution
        scanners 157
hyper-/hypoechoic areas *150*
image contrast 151–152
kidney *157–158*
linear array 149–150
Mechanical Index 154–155
microbubbles 156–157
miniaturization of equipment 158
MRI-guided thermal ablation of
        uterine fibroid *60*
near field 151
pathologic areas 158
piezoelectric crystal 147, 149–150
prostate vascularity *157–158*
refraction 149
secondary mechanical effects
        154–155
signals 147–148
    detection 149–151
    source 57, 147–148
    spatial encoding 150–151
signal/sample interactions 148–150
spatial resolution of images 150–151
speckle 151
teratoma *148*
thermal effects 154
thermal energy 59
thyroid *152*
time-gain compensation 151
transducers 151–152, *154*
waves 148
unit impulse function 297–298
universe 1–3, 17–22, *21*, 82, 251
    discontinuous 20–22
    Newtonian 19–20
    spatial heterogeneity *2*
uterus
    bicornuate *153*
    ultrasound thermal ablation of
        fibroids *60*

valence band 122
variability 42–45
    measurement 48
variables, measurement 45–46
vector analysis 106
velocity 13
Visible Human Project *231*

visible light *40*
    projection imaging *75*
visual pathways, parvocellular/
    magnocellular *99*
visual processing, edge
    enhancement *97*
visual psychophysics, human
    93–96
visual system
    energy detection 30
    evolution 93–95
    human *30*, *89*, *98*
    observers 29–30, 88–90
    search 96–100
    self-preservation tools 93–95
    temporal resolution 30–31
visualization of images 215–216,
    223–228
    challenges 228
    image-based methods 223–226
    image-based surface rendering
        225–226
    image-based volume rendering 226
    maximum intensity projection 225
    modes *102*
    object-based methods 226–228
    object-based surface
        rendering 227
    object-based volume
        rendering 227
    slice mode 224
    volume mode 224–226
    voxel projection 226
VisualSonics Vevo 770 157
volumetric analysis 259
voxel-based morphometry *268*
voxel-based statistics 106

voxels
    classification *111*, 313–315
        ischemic tissue *112*
    entropy 313–315
    projection 226
    segmentation 313–314
    signal patterns 234
    spatial analysis 109
    thresholding *108*

water, free radical formation
    140–141
wavelength 14

x-ray(s) 133–146, 183
    2D projection views *79*
    adverse biological effects 141
    anodes 135
    atomic number of tissues 183
    attenuation 136–137, *138*, 183
    barium contrast agent 183–185
    bremsstrahlung 133–134
    characteristic radiation 134
    Compton scattering 136–138, *139*, *145*
    computed radiography systems
        141–142
    contrast agents 183–185
    contrast-to-noise ratio 138–140
    detection 78
    digital radiography detectors
        142–143
    effective doses *141*, 183
    electromagnetic radiation 133
    electron interactions 133–134
    electron–electron interactions
        140–141
    generation 53

    image production 77–79
    interactions with matter *139*
    iodine contrast agent 183–185
    ionization dose 183
    linear attenuation coefficient
        183, 253
    magnification 143–144
    mass attenuation coefficients *138*
    photoelectric effect 136–137,
        139, *145*
    photons *184*
    pixel values *140*
    production *136*
    projection *78*, 143–144
    projective geometry 143–144
    propagation *135*
    properties 133
    radiation dose 141
    radiographic grids 143
    Roentgen's wife's hand *4*
    sample effect on signal 136–140
    signal 133–136
        detection 141–143
        effect on sample 140–141
        quantification 138
        source 133–136
    signal/sample interaction
        136–141
    signal-to-noise ratio 138
    spatial encoding 143–144
    thoracic *145*
    tissue interaction 63
    tomography 143, 144–146
x-ray generators 136
x-ray tubes 133, 134–135, *137*
    components 134–135
    heat management 135